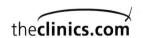

# EMERGENCY MEDICINE CLINICS OF NORTH AMERICA

Critical Care and
Emergency Medicine

GUEST EDITORS
Peter M. C. DeBlieux, MD
and Tiffany M. Osborn, MD

CONSULTING EDITOR
Amal Mattu, MD

August 2008 • Volume 26 • Number 3

**SAUNDERS**

An Imprint of Elsevier, Inc.
PHILADELPHIA   LONDON   TORONTO   MONTREAL   SYDNEY   TOKYO

**W.B. SAUNDERS COMPANY**

*A Division of Elsevier Inc.*

1600 John F. Kennedy Boulevard • Suite 1800 • Philadelphia, Pennsylvania 19103-2899

http://www.theclinics.com

| | |
|---|---|
| EMERGENCY MEDICINE CLINICS | Volume 26, Number 3 |
| OF NORTH AMERICA | ISSN 0733-8627 |
| August 2008 | ISBN-13: 978-1-4160-6289-9 |
| Editor: Patrick Manley | ISBN-10: 1-4160-6289-0 |

*Emergency Medicine Clinics of North America* (ISSN 0733-8627) is published quarterly by Elsevier Inc., 360 Park Avenue South, New York, NY, 10010-1710. Months of issue are February, May, August, and November. Business and Editorial Offices: 1600 John F. Kennedy Boulevard, Suite 1800, Philadelphia, PA 19103-2899. Customer Service Office: 6277 Sea Harbor Drive, Orlando, FL 32887-4800. Periodicals postage paid at New York, NY, and additional mailing offices. Subscription prices are $109.00 per year (US students), $212.00 per year (US individuals), $339.00 per year (US institutions), $145.00 per year (international students), $285.00 per year (international individuals), $400.00 per year (international institutions), $145.00 per year (Canadian students), $261.00 per year (Canadian individuals), and $400.00 per year (Canadian institutions). International air speed delivery is included in all *Clinics'* subscription prices. All prices are subject to change without notice. POSTMASTER: Send address changes to *Emergency Medicine Clinics of North America*, Elsevier Periodicals Customer Service, 6277 Sea Harbor Drive, Orlando, FL 32887-4800. Customer Service: 1-800-654-2452 (US). From outside the United States, call 1-407-563-6020. Fax: 1-407-363-9661. E-mail: JournalsCustomerService-usa@elsevier.com.

*Reprints.* For copies of 100 or more of articles in this publication, please contact the Commercial Reprints Department, Elsevier Inc., 360 Park Avenue South, New York, NY 10010-1710. Tel.: 212-633-3812; Fax: 212-462-1935; E-mail: reprints@elsevier.com.

*Emergency Medicine Clinics of North America* is covered in *MEDLINE/PubMed (Index Medicus), Current Contents/Clinical Medicine, EMBASE/Excerpta Medica, BIOSIS, SciSearch, CINAHL, ISI/BIOMED,* and *Research Alert.*

Printed in the United States of America.

# CONSULTING EDITOR

**AMAL MATTU, MD,** Program Director, Emergency Medicine Residency; and Associate Professor, Department of Emergency Medicine, University of Maryland School of Medicine, Baltimore, Maryland

# GUEST EDITORS

**PETER M. C. DEBLIEUX, MD,** Pulmonary/Critical Care, Section of Emergency Medicine, Charity Hospital, New Orleans, Los Angeles

**TIFFANY M. OSBORN, MD,** Department of Emergency Medicine, University of Virginia Health System, Charlottesville, Virginia

# CONTRIBUTORS

**LAURA K. BECHTEL, PhD,** Research Associate, Division of Medical Toxicology, Department of Emergency Medicine, University of Virginia School of Medicine, Charlottesville, Virginia

**HUGO BONATTI, MD,** Clinical Fellow in Surgical Critical Care, University of Virginia School of Medicine, Charlottesville, Virginia

**TRISHA N. BRANAN, PharmD,** Critical Care Pharmacy Resident, Department of Pharmacy Services, University of Virginia Health System, Charlottesville, Virginia

**JAMES FORREST CALLAND, MD,** Assistant Professor of Surgery, Department of Surgery, University of Virginia School of Medicine, Charlottesville, Virginia

**MICHAEL H. CATENACCI, MD,** Assistant Professor, Department of Emergency Medicine and Critical Care Transport, University of Alabama at Birmingham School of Medicine, Birmingham, Alabama

**BRIAN DANIEL, RRT,** Clinical Specialist, Respiratory Care Service, University of California, San Francisco, San Francisco, California

**STEPHEN G. DOBMEIER, BSN,** Director, Blue Ridge Poison Center, University of Virginia Health System, Charlottesville, Virginia

**TIMOTHY J. ELLENDER, MD,** Assistant Professor of Clinical Emergency Medicine, Department of Emergency Medicine, Indiana University Hospital, Emergency Medical Group, Inc.; Multidisciplinary Critical Care Fellowship, Methodist Hospital/Clarian Health, Indianapolis, Indiana

**J. MATTHEW FIELDS, MD,** Chief Resident in Emergency Medicine, Department of Emergency Medicine, University of Pennsylvania School of Medicine, Philadelphia, Pennsylvania

**J. CHRISTIAN FOX, MD, RDMS,** Director, Division of Emergency Ultrasound; and Associate Clinical Professor of Emergency Medicine, Department of Emergency Medicine, University of California Irvine Medical Center, Orange, California

**CHRIS A. GHAEMMAGHAMI, MD,** Associate Professor of Emergency Medicine, Department of Emergency Medicine, University of Virginia School of Medicine; Director, Fellowship in Cardiovascular Emergencies, Chest Pain Center, University of Virginia Health System, Charlottesville, Virginia

**MUNISH GOYAL, MD, FACEP,** Assistant Professor of Emergency Medicine, Department of Emergency Medicine, University of Pennsylvania School of Medicine, Philadelphia, Pennsylvania

**JAMES W. HARRIS, MD,** Resident, Department of Emergency Medicine, University of Virginia Health System, University of Virginia School of Medicine, Charlottesville, Virginia

**CHRISTOPHER P. HOLSTEGE, MD,** Director, Division of Medical Toxicology; and Associate Professor, Department of Emergency Medicine; and Associate Professor, Department of Pediatrics; University of Virginia School of Medicine; Blue Ridge Poison Center, University of Virginia Health System, Charlottesville, Virginia

**ZARETH IRWIN, MD, MS,** Fellow, Division of Emergency Ultrasound, Department of Emergency Medicine, University of California Irvine Medical Center, Orange, California

**KAIRA KING, MD,** Attending Physician, Trinity Medical Center, Birmingham, Alabama

**MARIAN P. LAMONTE, MD, MSN,** Chief, Neurological Services; and Director, Stroke Center, St. Agnes Hospital, Baltimore, Maryland

**MICHAEL T. MCCURDY, MD,** Department of Emergency Medicine; and Chief Resident, Combined Emergency Medicine/Internal Medicine/Critical Care Program, University of Maryland School of Medicine, Baltimore, Maryland

**ROBIN M. NAPLES, MD,** Fellow, Cardiovascular Emergencies, Department of Emergency Medicine, University of Virginia School of Medicine, Charlottesville, Virginia

**JAIRO I. SANTANILLA, MD,** Fellow, Division of Critical Care Medicine, University of California, San Francisco, San Francisco; Emergency Medicine Faculty, Alameda County Medical Center, Highland Hospital, Oakland, California

**JOSEPH C. SKINNER, MD,** Volunteer Clinical Lecturer, Department of Emergency Medicine, Indiana University Hospital, Emergency Medical Group, Inc.; Multidisciplinary Critical Care Fellowship, Methodist Hospital/Clarian Health, Indianapolis, Indiana

**DAVID F. VOLLES, PharmD,** Clinical Pharmacy Specialist, Department of Pharmacy Services, University of Virginia Health System, Charlottesville, Virginia

**MICHAEL E. WINTERS, MD, FAAEM, FACEP,** Assistant Professor, Department
of Emergency Medicine, and Assistant Professor, Department of Medicine; and
Director, Combined Emergency Medicine/Internal Medicine Program;
and Co-Director, Combined Emergency Medicine/Internal Medicine/Critical Care
Program, University of Maryland School of Medicine, Baltimore, Maryland

**MEI-EAN YEOW, MD,** Fellow, Division of Critical Care Medicine, University of California,
San Francisco, San Francisco, California

**JEFF ZILBERSTEIN, MD,** Department of Emergency Medicine; and Chief Resident,
Combined Emergency Medicine/Internal Medicine/Critical Care Program, University
of Maryland School of Medicine, Baltimore, Maryland

# CONTENTS

> With an increasing incidence of sepsis, increasing use of the
> emergency department by populations at risk, and an increase in
> time spent in the emergency department awaiting hospital
> admission, emergency medicine practitioners are offered a valuable
> opportunity to make a significant difference in the fight against
> sepsis. By administering appropriate antibiotics in a timely fashion,
> removing possible sources of infection, practicing early goal-
> directed hemodynamic optimization, using lung-protective ven-
> tilation strategies, and judiciously using corticosteroids and
> intensive insulin therapy, the goal of reducing mortality from
> sepsis can be achieved.

> In terms of cost and years of potential lives lost, injury arguably
> remains the most important public health problem facing the
> United States. Care of traumatically injured patients depends on
> early surgical intervention and avoiding delays in the diagnosis of
> injuries that threaten life and limb. In the critical care phase,
> successful outcomes after injury depend almost solely on diligence,
> attention to detail, and surveillance for iatrogenic infections and
> complications.

management of the critically poisoned patient. Specific clinical characteristics are identified that may clue the clinician into a specific toxin class as a diagnosis. Appropriate testing in the poisoned patient is reviewed. Complications of poisoning that may bring a rapid demise of the critically ill poisoned patient are highlighted and the management of those complications is discussed.

Many critically ill patients are remaining in the emergency department for extended periods of time, and delays in diagnosis and/or therapy may increase patient morbidity and mortality. All emergency physicians use monitoring modalities in critically ill patients to detect early cardiovascular compromise and impaired oxygen delivery before disastrous collapse occurs. The authors hope the discussion in this article regarding the monitoring of oxygenation, ventilation, arterial perfusion pressure, intravascular volume, markers of tissue hypoxia, and cardiac output will help the EP provide optimal care for this complicated patient population.

Shock is a final common pathway associated with regularly encountered emergencies including myocardial infarction, microbial sepsis, pulmonary embolism, significant trauma, and anaphylaxis. Shock results in impaired tissue perfusion, cellular hypoxia, and metabolic derangements that cause cellular injury. The clinical manifestations and prognosis of shock are largely dependent on the etiology and duration of insult. It is important that emergency physicians, familiar with the broad differential diagnosis of shock, be prepared to rapidly recognize, resuscitate, and target appropriate therapies aimed at correcting the underlying process. This article focuses on the basic pathophysiology of shock states and reviews the rationale regarding vasoactive drug therapy for cardiovascular support of shock within an emergency environment.

Care for patients who have time-sensitive disease processes in the emergency department and critical care settings is optimized with rapid diagnosis and intervention. Recent advances in medical imaging have increased portability, decreased image acquisition time, improved data resolution, and increased use of noninvasive studies. This article discusses the use of portable imaging techniques such as bedside ultrasound and radiography as well as CT and CT angiography in the diagnosis and care of critically ill patients.

Antibiotic resistance is increasing faster than the drug industry can develop and market new antibiotics. Medical personnel commonly must deal with the resistant gram-positive pathogens including MRSA and VRE, in addition to the problem gram-negative bacteria, Pseudomonas, Acinetobacter, and ESBL producing strains of Klebsiella and E. coli. Clinicians should be familiar with treatment strategies for these resistant pathogens. Because of the lack of novel agents to treat resistant infections, clinicians must use antibiotics judiciously and appropriately to limit further development of resistance. Early, appropriate cultures of the blood, urine, sputum and suspected source, ideally obtained before antibiotic initiation, allow for future de-escalation of antibiotics, or the decision to discontinue antibiotics.

Noninvasive positive pressure ventilation (NPPV) is becoming more commonplace, both in the ICU and also in the Emergency Department. This article addresses the rationale and mechanism of action for NPPV. A review of the indications for using NPPV and a discussion detailing the initiation of NPPV follows. NPPV has been shown to decrease length of hospital stay and the need for intubation in patients who have chronic obstructive pulmonary disease and acute cardiogenic pulmonary edema. NPPV should be considered for most patients who have respiratory distress who are being considered for intubation. After NPPV is initiated, very close monitoring and follow-up must be employed to identify those patients who are at risk for treatment failure.

Over the past several years, there has been an introduction of numerous modes of mechanical ventilation, each with their own advantages and limitations. This article reviews the common modes of mechanical ventilation, new technologies, and specific ventilator strategies that have been shown to be beneficial. In addition, it reviews the steps that should be taken when troubleshooting a ventilator.

# FORTHCOMING ISSUES

# RECENT ISSUES

**The Clinics are now available online!**

Access your subscription at
**www.theclinics.com**

## GOAL STATEMENT
The goal of *Emergency Medicine Clinics of North America* is to keep practicing physicians up to date with current clinical practice in emergency medicine by providing timely articles reviewing the state of the art in patient care.

## ACCREDITATION
The *Emergency Medical Clinics of North America* is planned and implemented in accordance with the Essential Areas and Policies of the Accreditation Council for Continuing Medical Education (ACCME) through the joint sponsorship of the University of Virginia School of Medicine and Elsevier. The University of Virginia School of Medicine is accredited by the ACCME to provide continuing medical education for physicians.

The University of Virginia School of Medicine designates this educational activity for a maximum of *15 AMA PRA Category 1 Credits™*. Physicians should only claim credit commensurate with the extent of their participation in the activity.

The Emergency Medicine Clinics of North America CME program is approved by the American College of Emergency Physicians for 60 hours of ACEP Category I Credit per year.

The American Medical Association has determined that physicians not licensed in the US who participate in this CME activity are eligible for *15 AMA PRA Category 1 Credits™*.

Credit can be earned by reading the text material, taking the CME examination online at: http://www.theclinics.com/home/cme, and completing the evaluation. After taking the test, you will be required to review any and all incorrect answers. Following completion of the test and evaluation, your credit will be awarded and you may print your certificate.

## FACULTY DISCLOSURE/CONFLICT OF INTEREST
The University of Virginia School of Medicine, as an ACCME accredited provider, endorses and strives to comply with the Accreditation Council for Continuing Medical Education (ACCME) Standards of Commercial Support, Commonwealth of Virginia statutes, University of Virginia policies and procedures, and associated federal and private regulations and guidelines on the need for disclosure and monitoring of proprietary and financial interests that may affect the scientific integrity and balance of content delivered in continuing medical education activities under our auspices.

The University of Virginia School of Medicine requires that all CME activities accredited through this institution be developed independently and be scientifically rigorous, balanced and objective in the presentation/discussion of its content, theories and practices.

All authors/editors participating in an accredited CME activity are expected to disclose to the readers relevant financial relationships with commercial entities occurring within the past 12 months (such as grants or research support, employee, consultant, stock holder, member of speakers bureau, etc.). The University of Virginia School of Medicine will employ appropriate mechanisms to resolve potential conflicts of interest to maintain the standards of fair and balanced education to the reader. Questions about specific strategies can be directed to the Office of Continuing Medical Education, University of Virginia School of Medicine, Charlottesville, Virginia.

**The authors/editors listed below have identified no professional or financial affiliations for themselves or their spouse/partner:**
Laura K. Bechtel, PhD; Hugo Bonatti, MD; Trisha N. Branan, Pharm.D.; James Forrest Calland, MD; Michael H. Catenacci, MD; Brian M. Daniel, RCP, RRT; Stephen G. Dobmeier, BSN; Timothy J. Ellender, MD; Jason Matthew Fields, MD; Chris A. Ghaemmaghami, MD; Munish Goyal, MD, FACEP; James W. Harris, MD; Christopher P. Holstege, MD; Zareth Irwin, MD, MS; Kaira K. King, MD; Marian P. LaMonte, MD, MSN; Patrick Manley (Acquisitions Editor); Amal Mattu, MD (Consulting Editor); Michael T. McCurdy, MD; Robin M. Naples, MD; Tiffany Osborn, MD (Guest Editor); Jairo Ignacio Santanilla, MD; Joseph C. Skinner, MD; Michael E. Winters, MD, FAAEM, FACEP; Bill Woods (Test Author); Mei-Ean Yeow, MD; and Jeff Zilberstein, MD.

**The authors/editors listed below have identified the following professional or financial affiliations for themselves of their spouse/partner:**
**Peter M.C. DeBlieux, MD (Guest Editor)** is a consultant, serves on the Speakers Bureau, and serves on the Advisory Committee for MERCK and Ortho McNeil, and serves on the Advisory Committee for Covidien.
**John Christian Fox, MD, RDMS** has loaned equipment from Sonosite, Inc.
**David F. Volles, Pharm.D.,** BCPS serves on the Speakers Bureau for Wyeth Pharmaceuticals and Cubist Pharmaceuticals.

*Disclosure of Discussion of non-FDA approved uses for pharmaceutical products and/or medical devices:*
**The University of Virginia School of Medicine, as an ACCME provider, requires that all faculty presenters identify and disclose any "off label" uses for pharmaceutical and medical device products. The University of Virginia School of Medicine recommends that each physician fully review all the available data on new products or procedures prior to instituting them with patients.**

## TO ENROLL
To enroll in the Emergency Medicine Clinics of North America Continuing Medical Education program, call customer service at 1-800-654-2452 or visit us online at: www.theclinics.com/home/cme. The CME program is available to subscribers for an additional fee of $195.00.

ELSEVIER
SAUNDERS

Emerg Med Clin N Am
26 (2008) xiii–xiv

EMERGENCY
MEDICINE
CLINICS OF
NORTH AMERICA

# Foreword

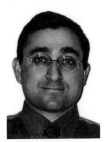

Amal Mattu, MD
*Consulting Editor*

Critical care medicine has always been a significant part of the specialty of emergency medicine (EM). The diagnosis and resuscitation of critically ill patients is at the heart of EM's core curriculum. The physicians that make the initial management decisions of the most critically ill patients are emergency physicians. Intubation and initiation of mechanical ventilation often begins in the emergency department (ED). Placement of chest tubes and central lines for fluid resuscitation and initiation of vasopressors occurs in the ED, and the "golden hour" of trauma care (the period of time during which many of these patients' fate is determined) usually occurs in the ED.

Despite this longstanding presence of critical care medicine in EM, emergency health care providers are under more pressure than ever before to increase their knowledge of critical care medicine and to practice critical care medicine in the ED. The simultaneous occurrence of hospital overcrowding, an aging population, and increasing nursing home referrals to EDs has resulted in an substantial increase in critically ill patients in the ED. Emergency physicians are routinely required to manage patients for prolonged periods on ventilators, to initiate and sustain sepsis protocols, and to perform advanced techniques in hemodynamic monitoring.

Educators in EM are working to meet these new demands of the specialty in several ways. Residency directors have added increased ICU rotations to emergency medicine training. Continuing medical education conference organizers have added numerous critical care-related topics to their conferences. Directors of medical simulation have increased training in resuscitation.

0733-8627/08/$ - see front matter © 2008 Elsevier Inc. All rights reserved.
doi:10.1016/j.emc.2008.06.002

Finally, textbook and journal editors have promoted increased publications focused on the care of the critically ill patient in the ED.

In this issue of *Emergency Medicine Clinics of North America*, critical care experts Dr. Peter DeBlieux and Dr. Tiffany Osborn have provided yet another invaluable resource for emergency physicians to improve their skills in caring for the critically ill patient. The enclosed articles cover general topics (such as the use of vasopressors, antibiotic choices, mechanical ventilation, and imaging) and specific conditions (such as acute coronary syndrome, trauma, sepsis, and stroke). The authors, all of whom are experienced and accomplished educators in emergency medicine, intentionally focus their attention on the issues that are most relevant to critically ill patients, and they address challenges, myths, and pitfalls in common ED practice.

This issue of *Emergency Medicine Clincs of North America* represents a valuable addition to EM education. This issue should be considered a must-read, not only for practicing emergency physicians, but also for EM trainees and any other health care providers responsible for caring for critically ill patients. Knowledge and practice of the concepts that are discussed in the following pages will certainly save lives. The guest editors and authors are commended for providing this outstanding resource for our specialty.

Amal Mattu, MD
*Program Director*
*Emergency Medicine Residency*
*Associate Professor*
*Department of Emergency Medicine*
*University of Maryland School of Medicine*
*110 S. Paca Street, 6th Floor, Suite 100*
*Baltimore, MD 21201, USA*

*E-mail address:* amattu@smail.umaryland.edu

ELSEVIER
SAUNDERS

Emerg Med Clin N Am
26 (2008) xv–xvi

EMERGENCY
MEDICINE
CLINICS OF
NORTH AMERICA

# Preface

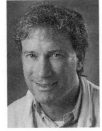 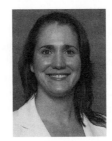

Peter M. C. DeBlieux, MD     Tiffany M. Osborn, MD
*Guest Editors*

Many concepts and practice requirements of critical care medicine and emergency medicine are indistinguishable. Thanks to collaborative giants and leaders in the fields of critical care and emergency medicine, these specialties are being championed as the keys to improving patient outcomes in the "golden hours of critical care." The collegiality and cross training of intensivists, surgeons, and emergency medicine clinicians have yielded multispecialty clinical breakthroughs that directly and positively impact patient survival. These survival benefits are most pronounced when critical care concepts are implemented early, with specific goals set for physiologic and laboratory measures. These pathways and interventions begin with emergency medicine clinicians identifying critically ill patients early, promptly initiating appropriate antibiotics when indicated, aggressively resuscitating patients using defined parameters, and involving consultants emergently for definitive care. As a specialty, emergency medicine is poised to become an equal partner in the management of critically ill patients. This issue of *Emergency Medicine Clinics of North America* is a testament to how far the specialty of emergency medicine has traveled in its young existence to claim an important seat at the critical care table. Our patients deserve our critical care expertise, and our training reflects a knowledge base that is growing closer to a critical care curriculum.

This issue of *Emergency Medicine Clinics of North America* focuses on a broad clinical spectrum of critical care medicine, from sepsis and trauma to acute coronary syndromes and neurologic events. Articles on the topics of toxicology and venothromboembolism complete the clinical offerings, before an updated review of critical care monitoring, vasopressor therapy, critical care imaging, antibiotic therapy and mechanical ventilation is provided. It is impossible to include all topics germane to critical care, but we feel that these selected areas will offer emergency medicine clinicians an update in common areas that are vital to improving patient outcomes. We trust that you will enjoy these topics as much as we have enjoyed editing them.

We thank Patrick Manley and the Elsevier crew for their patience and persistence in making this publication a reality. We acknowledge our talented authors, who worked diligently to bring you quality works that advance our critical care efforts in emergency medicine. Lastly, we thank our families for their unending love, support, and understanding, which enabled us to bring this effort to press.

Peter M. C. DeBlieux, MD
*Pulmonary/Critical Care*
*Section of Emergency Medicine*
*Charity Hospital*
*1532 Tulane Avenue, Room 1351*
*New Orleans, LA 70112, USA*

*E-mail address:* pdebli@lsuhsc.edu

Tiffany M. Osborn, MD
*Department of Emergency Medicine*
*University of Virginia Health System*
*MSB-1172, Suite 2266*
*PO Box 800699*
*Charlottesville, VA 22908, USA*

*E-mail address:* tmosbornmd@msn.com

ELSEVIER
SAUNDERS

Emerg Med Clin N Am
26 (2008) 603–623

EMERGENCY
MEDICINE
CLINICS OF
NORTH AMERICA

# Severe Sepsis and Septic Shock: Improving Outcomes in the Emergency Department

## Michael H. Catenacci, MD[a],*, Kaira King, MD[b]

[a]Department of Emergency Medicine and Critical Care Transport,
University of Alabama at Birmingham School of Medicine, JTN 266,
619 19th Street South, Birmingham, AL 35249, USA
[b]Trinity Medical Center, Birmingham, AL, USA

The incidence of severe sepsis is increasing [1–3]. There are an estimated 750,000 cases of sepsis per year in the United States and a projected annual increase of 1.5% [4]. The reasons for the increasing incidence include a rise in the United States' elderly population, increasing antimicrobial resistance, and more prevalent immunocompromised states due to an increase in solid organ transplants, more effective chemotherapy, and prolonged survival of HIV/AIDS patients [3,4]. Because of the greater incidence of severe sepsis, the overall mortality associated with sepsis has also risen. This has not been a proportionate rise, as the case–fatality rate appears to be decreasing [1–3]. Estimates for mortality have ranged from 20%–50%, depending on the stage of the disease studied [5–7]. Costs are staggering and an estimated $16.7 billion is spent annually [4].

Over the past two decades, emergency department (ED) use has also increased, especially use by populations at risk for sepsis. Increasing ED volumes have been principally driven by patients who are age 45 and older, with the highest overall rates of use in the elderly [8]. These patients are at a far greater risk for developing sepsis than younger populations. Angus and colleagues [4] reported a 100-fold increased incidence in the elderly as compared with children (0.2/1000 in children versus 26.2 per 1000 in those older than 85 years). Increasing volume has also been associated with an increase in illness severity; Lambe and colleagues [9] reported a 59% increase in

* Corresponding author. Department of Emergency Medicine and Critical Care Transport, University of Alabama at Birmingham School of Medicine, JTN 266, 619 19th Street South, Birmingham, AL 35249.

*E-mail address:* mcaten@uab.edu (M.H. Catenacci).

critically ill patients presenting to the ED between 1990 and 1999. National estimates report an increase in cases of potential shock (ie, a presentation requiring emergent resuscitation within 15 minutes) with an estimated 1.1 million Americans presenting to EDs nationally with potential shock. This marks an estimated increase in emergent resuscitation requirements from 17% (1998) to 22% (2002) [8].

In addition to the higher patient volumes and acuity levels, the ED physician is challenged by overcrowding from boarding patients awaiting admission [10]. This was reflected in a recently published study analyzing data from the National Hospital Ambulatory Medical Care Survey. Between 2001 and 2004, ED visits for suspected severe sepsis totaled over 500,000 patients annually, with a mean ED length of stay of 4.7 hours and with 20.4% staying in the ED greater than 6 hours [11].

With the increased incidence of severe sepsis, increased ED use by high-risk populations, and the protracted time spent in the ED awaiting admission, emergency medicine practitioners are offered a valuable opportunity to make a significant contribution in the fight against sepsis. This article reviews therapies that may improve outcomes in patients with sepsis.

## Improving outcomes in sepsis

### Refining definitions

The word "sepsis" is derived from the Greek word sēpein meaning to putrify or to make rotten [12]. Before the 1990s, clinical usage of the terms sepsis, septicemia, and septic shock varied, which made diagnoses, research endeavors, and communications between practitioners challenging. A consensus statement published in 1992 by the American College of Chest Physicians and Society of Critical Care Medicine provided some clarity [13]. This statement defined the systemic inflammatory response syndrome (SIRS) as the physiologic response of the human body to a variety of clinical insults. SIRS is reflected in the physiologic variables listed in Box 1, and can develop as a response to multiple stressors: infectious, toxicologic, traumatic, ischemic, or immunologic. Sepsis was then defined as SIRS resulting from a documented or presumed Infection. Infection, in turn, was defined as a pathologic process caused by the invasion of normally sterile tissues by pathogenic microorganisms (eg, bacteria, viruses, or fungi).

Although the 1992 consensus statement helped clarify definitions, a survey of European Intensivists in 2000 indicated that only 17% of clinicians agreed on a common definition of sepsis, and 83% said it was likely that sepsis was frequently missed [14]. Collaborators at the 2001 International Sepsis Definitions Conference refined the previous definitions, and created a list of potential signs of systemic inflammation in response to infection [15]. Ultimately, the collaborators were seeking to make the definitions more clinically applicable via objectifying those physical examination and

---

**Box 1. Summary of definitions**

*SIRS*
SIRS, manifested by:
- Temp >38.3° or <36°
- HR >90
- RR >20 or PaCO2 <32
- WBC >12,000 or <4000 or >10% bands

*Infection*
A pathologic process caused by the invasion of normally sterile tissue by pathogenic microorganisms

*Sepsis*
SIRS and a presumed or documented focus of infection

*Severe sepsis*
Sepsis complicated by organ dysfunction, hypotension before fluid challenge, or lactate ≥4 mmol/L

*Septic shock*
Sepsis with persistent hypotension

---

lab findings that result in the experienced clinician's gestalt that a patient "looks septic". These diagnostic criteria are listed in Box 2.

Severe sepsis is defined as sepsis complicated by either hypotension before fluid challenge, organ dysfunction, or lactate ≥4 mmol/L. Examples of organ dysfunction commonly seen with sepsis include respiratory failure, acute renal failure, acute liver failure, coagulopathy, and thrombocytopenia. Sepsis with persistent hypotension is described as septic shock. Persistent hypotension is defined as systolic blood pressure <90 mm Hg or <40 mm Hg from baseline, or mean arterial pressure <70 mm Hg, despite adequate fluid resuscitation (20–40 cc/kg of crystalloid). The above definitions are listed in summary form in Box 1.

*Increasing awareness*

Increasing provider awareness and promoting early recognition of the disease process is essential in improving outcomes in patients with sepsis. The Surviving Sepsis Campaign (SSC) is an ongoing international effort to increase awareness and improve outcomes in patients with sepsis. The campaign was formed under the administration of the Society of Critical Care Medicine, the European Society of Intensive Care Medicine, and the International Sepsis Forum. Since its inception, eight additional organizations have joined the effort, including the American College of Emergency Physicians (ACEP) [16].

**Box 2. Diagnostic criteria for sepsis**

*Sepsis: suggested by a documented or suspected infection plus some of the following:*
General variables
- Fever (core temperature >38.3°C)
- Hypothermia (core temperature <36°C)
- Heart rate >90 min or >2SD above the normal value for age
- Tachypnea
- Hyperglycemia >120 mg/dL with no history of diabetes
- Altered mental status
- Significant edema or positive fluid balance (>20 mL/kg over 24 h)

Inflammatory variables
- Leukocytosis (WBC count >12,000 µL)
- Leukopenia (WBC count <4000 µL)
- Normal WBC count with >10% immature forms
- Plasma C-reactive protein level >2SD above the normal value
- Plasma procalcitonin >2SD above the normal value

Hemodynamic variables
- Arterial hypotension (SBP <90 mm Hg, MAP <70, or an SBP decrease >40 mm Hg in adults or <2SD below normal for age)
- $ScvO_2$ >70%
- Cardiac index >3.5 L/min/m$^2$

Organ dysfunction variables
- Arterial hypoxemia ($Pao_2/Fio_2$ <300)
- Acute ologuria (UOP <0.5 mL/kg/h for at least 2 hours)
- Creatinine increase (>0.5 mg/dL)
- Coagulation abnormalities (INR >1.5 or aPTT >60 sec)
- Ileus
- Thrombocytopenia (<100,000 µL)
- Hyperbilirubinemia (plasma total bilirubin >4 mg/dL)

Tissue perfusion variables
- Elevated lactate (>2 mmol/L)
- Decreased capillary refill (>2 sec or mottling)

---

*Abbreviations:* $Fio_2$, fractional inspired concentration of oxygen; MAP, mean arterial pressure; $PaO_2$, arterial partial pressure of oxygen; SBP, systolic blood pressure; $ScvO_2$, central venous oxygen saturation; SD, standard deviation; UOP, urine output.

*Data from* Levy MM, Fink MP, Marshall JC, et al. 2001 SCCM/ESICM/ACCP/ATS/SIS International Sepsis Definitions Conference. Crit Care Med 2003;31: 1250–6.

Phase I of the SSC was initiated in October of 2002 with the Barcelona Declaration at the 15th Annual Congress of the European Society for Intensive Care Medicine. The Barcelona Declaration called for increased public and provider awareness and an improvement in the diagnosis and treatment of sepsis, with the goal of decreasing mortality by 25% within 5 years [17]. The SSC issued an initial set of guidelines in 2001 based on the preceding 10 years of data that were coordinated by the International Sepsis Forum. Phase II of the SSC brought together critical care and infectious disease experts representing 11 international organizations to develop practical guidelines for the bedside clinician. A new set of guidelines was formulated in 2004, which incorporated the latest information through the end of 2003. The 2004 guidelines were supported by unrestricted educational grants from industry. The most recent set of guidelines was published in 2008, which included information through 2007. These guidelines were coordinated by the Society of Critical Care Medicine and the European Society of Intensive Care Medicine, with no industry funding supporting guideline committee activities. To provide the most advanced information on guideline development for the 2008 revisions, the SSC enlisted the Grades of Recommendation, Assessment, Development, and Evaluation (GRADE) system [18,19].

Phase III of the SSC is almost complete. The aim was to create a focused plan to assist clinicians with guideline application at the bedside. Web site based tools were provided to assist with identification and implementation. Additionally, a data tracker was provided so institutions could follow improvements in guideline application and mortality. A separate study group was established with over 100 sites internationally to examine the process impact on outcomes. This data is currently being processed.

*Early, appropriate antibiotics*

The early administration of appropriate antibiotics makes practical physiologic sense. If targeted antibiotics are given earlier, offending organisms will be destroyed faster, toxin production may be limited, and the detrimental effects of a robust cytokine and inflammatory response may be held in check.

Several studies have looked at the timing of antibiotics with regard to clinical outcomes. There are no randomized prospective trials on delayed or inappropriate antibiotics given to patients with sepsis for obvious ethical reasons. However, there is strong evidence to suggest improvement in outcome with faster antibiotic delivery in septic shock. In a retrospective study of 2731 septic shock patients admitted to 14 ICUs in the United States and Canada, researchers found a significant correlation between the rapidity with which antibiotics were administered and the outcome [20]. Administration of antibiotics within the first hour of onset of hypotension resulted in an overall survival rate of 79.9%. For each hour that antibiotics were delayed, there was an average increase in mortality of 7.6%. In multivariate analysis, time to initiation of effective antibiotic therapy was the single strongest predictor of outcome. Similar results have been shown in a study investigating mortality in patients with cancer and septic shock. A delay in receiving antibiotics greater than two hours after admission resulted in a 7-fold increase in mortality [21]. Similarly, in patients presenting to a Canadian hospital with community-acquired meningitis, greater than 6 hour delays in receiving antibiotics resulted in an 8.4-fold increase in mortality [22].

Antibiotics should be given without delay in the critically ill patient. Additionally, empiric antibiotics need to be selected appropriately, anticipating the most likely causative organism. In a large cohort of patients with microbiologically confirmed severe sepsis, inappropriate initial antibiotic therapy was associated with excess mortality (odds ratio 1.8) [23]. In this study, inappropriate antibiotics were defined as antibiotics given within 24 hours of the diagnosis of sepsis, which did not match the in-vitro susceptibility of a pathogen eventually isolated. In another retrospective study of 2158 bacteremic patients, appropriate empiric antibiotic treatment resulted in a decrease in mortality from 34% to 20%. The odds ratio for fatality with inappropriate antibiotics and septic shock was 1.6 [24]. In a prospective study of 492 patients with bacteremia admitted to the ICU, mortality rates for patients treated with inappropriate antibiotics was 61.9%, while appropriately treated patients was 28.4% [25].

The goal in selecting antibiotics for patients with sepsis is to treat the most likely affecting organisms, often attempting to do so with a limited amount of data. The factors that are important in this process include: an assessment of the most likely site of infection, host predispositions to infection, and local antibiotic resistance patterns. Secondary factors include drug cost, potency, pharmacodynamics, and drug–drug interactions.

Bacteria are the most common microorganisms causing sepsis, with a transition over the past 20 years from a gram-negative to a gram-positive predominance. In one study examining data collected at hospital discharge, Martin and colleagues [3] showed that in the year 2000, gram-positive bacteria accounted for 52.1% of cases while gram-negative bacteria accounted for 37.6% of cases. Infections were polymicrobic in 4.7% of cases, anaerobic in 1.0% of cases, and fungal in 4.6% of cases. In another study examining only community-acquired sepsis, Valles and colleagues [26] showed a preponderance of gram-positive organisms at 43.6%, with two-thirds due to *Streptococcus pneumonia* or *Staphylococcus aureus*.

In general, an ascertainment of the most likely site of infection helps narrow the list of bacteria involved considerably. Studies have consistently shown that the most common sites of initial infection in sepsis, in descending order, are: the respiratory tract, the abdomen, and the genitourinary tract [20,26]. Rapid history and physical examination, targeted imaging, and focused laboratory testing can help confirm the most likely source of infection.

Host factors are also important to consider when selecting empiric antibiotics. Chemotherapy-induced neutropenia is a risk for serious infection, and it is commonly encountered in the ED. The most common opportunistic organisms causing infections in neutropenic patients are bacteria and fungi. The most common bacteria involved are three aerobic gram-negative rods (*Escherichia coli, Klebsiella pneumoniae*, and *Pseudomonas aeruginosa*) and four gram-positive cocci (*Staphylococcus aureus, Staphylococcus epidermidis, Streptococcus viridians,* and *Enterococcal* species) [27]. There appears to be a shift in the bacteriology of these infections over the past three decades from predominantly gram-negative to gram-positive infections. Reasons for this shift may include: increasing use of in-dwelling intravascular devices, the use of fluoroquinolones as prophylaxis in neutropenia, and an increased prevalence of high-dose chemotherapy-induced mucositis [28]. Besides neutropenia, other common predisposing conditions for sepsis include HIV/AIDS and organ transplantation with immunosuppresion. These patients are at risk for infections with common organisms (eg, *Pneumococcus*), as well as opportunistic and unusual pathogens (eg, *Pneumocystis jiroveci*).

Finally, resistance patterns are important to keep in mind when selecting antibiotics. Two important bacteria with increasing rates of resistance include drug-resistant *Streptococcus pneumonia* (DRSP) and methicillin-resistant *Staphylococcus aureus* (MRSA). DRSP's penicillin resistance has increased over the last decade, and correlates with its resistance to other antibiotics (eg, other beta-lactams, macrolides, and TMP-SMX) [29,30]. In two recent studies, rates of high-level resistance to penicillin (MIC $>2ug/mL$) were 8%–26%, with marked geographic variability in 20,000 samples [30,31]. Resistance to broad spectrum antibiotics such as third generation cephalosporins was 6.4–8.1% during the years 1998–2001 [32], while resistance to fluroquinolones has remained low at 0.5%–1.0% [29,30].

Community-acquired MRSA (CA-MRSA) infections have increased dramatically over the past decade in the United States [33]. In many areas, CA-MRSA infections are now the leading cause of skin and soft tissue infections [34,35]. A 2004 study of 11 academic EDs showed that 59% of the isolates from community-acquired skin and soft-tissue infections were MRSA [34]. CA-MRSA is also being increasingly isolated from more invasive infections. A recent study using data from nine centers in the United States estimated that there were 94,360 cases of invasive disease in 2005, with 29% of cases due to the USA-300 Pulse Field Type, the most common type of CA-MRSA [36]. In addition, CA-MRSA has been reported to cause a rapidly progressive post-influenza pneumonia and sepsis in previously healthy, young adults [37].

Due to the rapid progression of sepsis and multi-organ failure, initiating appropriate antibiotics promptly will save lives. If severe sepsis is being considered, administration of broad spectrum antibiotics should be completed expeditiously. Appropriate cultures should be obtained before antibiotic administration if feasible.

*Source control*

Besides timely and appropriate antibiotics, the identification and removal of infectious foci will eliminate continued exposure to pathogenic micro-organisms. Identification through history, physical, and rapid diagnostic imaging is important. For example, physical examination may reveal cellulitis, induration, and fluctuance in the vicinity of an in-dwelling intra-vascular device. Plain films of the chest may reveal a parapneumonic effusion or empyema requiring drainage. Abdominal ultrasound is a nonin-vasive, rapid, and accurate way to delineate biliary pathology that may require decompression. Abdominal CT scanning can help identify intrabdo-minal, intrapelvic, or genitourinary foci that may require surgical or endo-scopic debridement.

Removal of infected prosthetic devices may be required in the ED. Research has shown that bacteria resist destruction by antimicrobials through adherence to medical devices in protective biofilms [38]. Types of devices that can be removed in the ED may include in-dwelling urinary cath-eters, vascular access devices (central venous catheters, peripherally inserted central venous catheters, and hemodialysis catheters), peritoneal dialysis catheters, and intrauterine devices. More invasive removal may be required for ureteral stents, prosthetic joints, indwelling vascular devices, vascular grafts, and prosthetic heart valves.

The lung is the most commonly identified source of sepsis in both trauma and nontrauma patient populations [7,20,26]. Drainage of a parapneumonic effusion or empyema may be essential. Thoracentesis of a parapneumonic effusion should be attempted if pleural fluid thickness is greater than 10 mm on a lateral decubitus chest xray [39]. Thoracostomy tube placement is generally indicated for gross purulence aspirated on thoracentesis, fluid pH <7.2, pleural fluid glucose <40 mg/dL, positive gram stain or culture of fluid, and loculated fluid aspirated on thoracentesis [40].

Superficial skin infections are rarely the source of sepsis. Simple incision and drainage of skin abscesses and debridement of decubiti may be warranted. Immediate surgical consultation for operative exploration and management is indicated if there is a suspicion of a necrotizing skin infec-tion. Examples of these infections include necrotizing fasciitis, invasive *Streptococcal* and *Staphylococcal* cellultis, *Clostridial* myonecrosis, and Fournier's gangrene. These necrotizing skin infections may be monomicro-bial, but are more often polymicrobic. The most common bacteria isolated in necrotizing infections are Group A Beta-hemolytic *Streptococcal* species, *Staphylococcal* species, non-Group A *Streptococcal* species, *Enterobacteria-ceae*, and anaerobes such as *Clostridial* and *Bacteroides* species [41]. These infections are suggested by the combination of a skin infection with signs of sepsis, pain out of proportion to examination, rapid progression, bullae formation, subcutaneous crepitus, and visible gas on imaging studies. One retrospective study showed a low sensitivity (85%) in detecting these infections when crepitance, blistering, or gas detected on imaging studies were used [42]. This highlights the importance of confirmatory testing such as CT or MRI when a high clinical suspicion exists.

Intra-abdominal sources of infection may be approached via open or percutaneous drainage. Percutaneous drainage is an attractive option given the high operative risk of these seriously ill patients. There is an expanding body of literature on this topic and recommendations continue to evolve. CT-guided drainage of intra-abdominal abscesses has been shown to be effective in a recent European study [43]. In this study of 75 patients, 83% of patients who underwent CT-guided drainage had complete resolution with no operative management required. There were higher success rates in patients with APACHE (Acute Physiology and Chronic Health Evaluation) III scores <30 and in patients with smaller, more accessible abscesses. In contrast, one randomized trial of 123 patients with acute cholecystitis and APACHE III scores ≥12 demonstrated no difference in mortality between non-operative therapy and percutaneous cholecystostomy tube placement [44].

*Early goal directed therapy*

In 2001, a landmark study by Rivers and colleagues [45] investigated early goal-directed therapy (EGDT) in severe sepsis and septic shock. Goal directed therapy previously had been used in the ICU to match systemic oxygen delivery with demand through manipulating cardiac preload, afterload, and contractility. Rivers and colleagues studied patients before ICU admission, on arrival to a busy urban ED. Patients were randomized to EGDT or usual care and were followed for 72 hours to investigate mortality, end points of resuscitation, and APACHE-II scores.

The EGDT protocol is shown in Fig. 1. The protocol identifies septic patients in the ED and attempts to match oxygen supply with demand within the first 6 hours of presentation. Patients first were oxygenated with either endotracheal intubation or supplemental oxygen. Central venous and arterial pressure monitoring were then instituted. If central venous pressure (CVP) was <8, patients were given fluid boluses in 500 cc aliquots every 30 minutes until CVP was >8. An assessment of mean arterial pressure (MAP) was then performed. If MAP was <65 with CVP >8, patients were given vasopressors to keep MAP >65. An assessment of central venous oxygen saturation (ScvO$_2$) was then made. If ScvO$_2$ was <70% despite CVP 8-12 and MAP >65, patients were transfused with packed red blood cells until the hematocrit was >30%. If ScvO$_2$ remained <70% after transfusion, inotropic agents (dobutamine) were given. All patients were admitted to the ICU.

Results of the study showed that in the patients who received EGDT, absolute mortality was decreased by 16% (30.5% versus 46.5%), APACHE-II scores were lower (6.3 versus 13.0), and end-points of resuscitation were

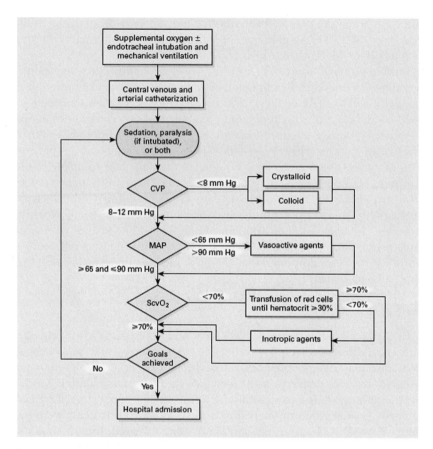

Fig. 1. Protocol for early goal-directed therapy. (*From* Rivers E, Nguyen B, Havstad S, et al. Early goal-directed therapy in the treatment of severe sepsis and septic shock. N Engl J Med 2001;345:1368–77; with permission. Copyright © 2001, Massachusetts Medical Society.)

improved (lower serum lactate levels, higher serum pH values, and higher central venous oxygen saturation) as compared with the control group.

After the initial EGDT study was published, questions of external validity as well as the practicality of instituting the protocol in other centers were raised. One recent review identified 11 peer-reviewed publications and 28 abstracts from academic, community, and international settings that have investigated the use of the EGDT protocol since the initial study [46]. These studies have provided both external validation and generalizability of the protocol, showing decreases in morbidity, mortality, and health care resource consumption.

*Lung-protective ventilation strategies*

The pulmonary parynchyma is the most common site of initial infection in sepsis. In addition, sepsis-induced pulmonary dysfunction is a common source of morbidity and mortality in these patients. Acute respiratory distress syndrome (ARDS) is a syndrome of diffuse pulmonary parenchymal injury associated with noncardiogenic pulmonary edema. ARDS occurs with high frequency in patients with sepsis and results in varying degrees of hypoxemic respiratory failure. The diagnosis of ARDS is made clinically, according to the criteria set forth by the American-European Consensus Conference (Box 3).

Initial studies in the early 1990s showed that mechanical ventilation using lower tidal volumes reduced mortality in ARDS [47,48]. The term "lung protective ventilation" (LPV) was coined. It was shown that patients who have ARDS do not have a homogenous distribution of infiltration within the pulmonary parenchyma; overdistension of the remaining normal alveoli was thought to lead to injury [49].

Injury to the pulmonary parenchyma due to mechanical ventilation is termed "ventilator-induced lung injury" (VILI). VILI is thought to occur secondary to both volutrauma and barotrauma. Volutrauma is damage to the lung caused by excessive ventilator volumes; it is due to end-inspiratory alveolar overdistension and stretch [50,51]. Volutrauma leads to pulmonary edema, increased inflammatory cells and cytokines in the lungs, and results in diffuse alveolar damage. Barotrauma is damage to the lung caused by excessive ventilation pressures. Excessive intra-alveolar pressures focused at the closely opposed alveolar-bronchovascular sheath can result in air entrance into the insterstitial tissues [52,53]. This may result in various forms of air leaks commonly seen as a pneumothorax, pneumomediastinum, pneumoperitoneum, pneumopericardium, and subcutaneous emphysema. Additionally, elevated pressures and volume may cause diminished venous return, decreased in cardiac output, and worsening hypotension.

The ARDSNET study was the most successful and largest trial to investigate the use of LPV in patients with ARDS [54]. ARDSNET enrolled

---

**Box 3. Criteria for the diagnosis of acute respiratory distress syndrome**

- Acute onset
- $PaO_2/FiO_2$ <200 regardless of PEEP
- Bilateral infiltrates
- PCWP <18 mm Hg

---

*Abbreviations:* $FiO_2$, fractional inspired concentration of oxygen; $PaO_2$, arterial partial pressure of oxygen; PCWP, pulmonary capillary wedge pressure; PEEP, positive end-expiratory pressure.

*Data from* Bernard GR, Artigas A, Brigham KL, et al. The American-European Consensus Conference on ARDS: definitions, mechanisms, relevant outcomes, and clinical trial coordination. Am J Respir Crit Care Med 1994;149:818–24.

greater than 800 patients in a prospective multicenter design. ARDSNET compared ventilation with tidal volumes of 6 cc/kg and 12 cc/kg using predicted body weight. A degree of hypoventilation and mild respiratory acidosis (pH 7.30–7.45) termed "permissive hypercapnea" was tolerated in the reduced tidal volume group. Results of the study showed that lower tidal volume ventilation was associated with a 9% absolute reduction in mortality when the plateau pressure was kept below 30 cm $H_2O$.

There are strong recommendations to use reduced tidal volumes for patients with sepsis and evidence of early ARDS. Practically, when using lower tidal volumes (6 cc/kg of ideal body weight), one must tolerate a degree of hypercapnea using PEEP to improve oxygenation, while maintaining plateau pressures less than 30 cm $H_2O$.

## Corticosteroids

Sepsis demands high levels of counter-regulatory hormones, such as cortisol, glucagon, and growth hormone. Primary adrenal insufficiency may be life threatening and occurs with destruction of the adrenal gland (autoimmune adrenalitis, adrenal hemorrhage, adrenal thrombosis) [55]. Secondary adrenal insufficiency occurs with dysfunction of the pituitary or hypothalamus (postpartum pituitary necrosis, sarcoidosis, pituitary malignancy). Relative adrenal insufficiency is said to exist when adrenal response is not sufficient to meet increased metabolic demands (sepsis, trauma, burns).

The therapeutic use of steroids in sepsis spans several decades of research. The first prospective randomized trial of intravenous hydrocortisone versus placebo in septic patients was published in 1963 [56]. Most early clinical trials investigated supraphysiologic doses of steroids. The consensus showed no benefit or possible increased harm [57–60]. Next, low doses of steroids were suggested ("physiologic doses") based on the results of cosyntropin stimulation testing. In this test, cosyntropin (a synthetic adrenocorticotropic hormone analog) is given and cortisol levels are measured at zero, thirty, and sixty minutes. If the cortisol level increases by less than 9ug/L, the patient is said to be a nonresponder. If, on the other hand, cortisol levels increase by greater than 9ug/L, the patients is said to be a responder.

In 2002, Annane and collegues examined outcomes in steroid replacement therapy in a placebo-controlled, randomized, double-blinded study in 19 French ICUs [61]. Septic patients with vasopressor-resistant shock (hypotension despite fluid administration and vasopressors) were all given a cosyntropin stimulation test. Patients were then randomly assigned to receive either hydrocortisone 50 mg intravenously every 6 hours and fludrocortisone 50-mcg by mouth every day, or placebo for 7 days. The results of the trial showed that cosyntropin nonresponders given steroid replacement had decreased mortality compared with nonresponders given placebo (53% versus 63%, $P = .02$) and a decrease in total length of time on vasopressors.

Cosyntropin responders had no significant differences whether they received steroids or not. Overall, there were no differences in adverse events such as superinfection, bleeding, and psychiatric disorders.

A more recent trial has challenged the use of low-dose steroids in sepsis. The recently published CORTICUS study was conducted with nearly 500 patients as a multicenter (52 ICUs in nine countries), blinded, and placebo-controlled trial [62]. Septic patients with evidence of shock that persisted for one hour up to 72 hours prior to enrollment, were given a cosyntropin stimulation test. The patients were then randomized to receive hydrocortisone 50 mg intravenously every 6 hours for 5 days or placebo. There were several important differences between the study by Annane and colleagues and the CORTICUS trial. CORTICUS patients were enrolled if their blood pressure was less than 90 systolic for 1 hour, regardless of response to vasopressor therapy, whereas Annane's patient's were vasopressor-dependent. This may have resulted in a less severely ill patient population enrolled in CORTICUS, as reflected by lower mortality rates and lower simplified acute physiology II scores in the placebo group as compared with the Annane trial. Secondly, the Annane study enrolled septic shock patients within the first 8 hours of shock onset, whereas CORTICUS allowed enrollment for up to 3 days after onset of shock. Finally, Annane excluded patients that received etomidate within 6 hours of randomization, while CORTICUS did not. Results showed that there was no difference in 28-day mortality between the hydrocortisone and placebo group in nonresponders (39.2% versus 36.1% respectively, $P = .69$) or in responders. In addition, there were more episodes of superinfection, including new sepsis and septic shock, in the patients who received hydrocortisone.

Further studies with larger numbers of patients are required to refine the guidelines for steroid administration in patients with sepsis [63]. For now, the 2008 SSC guidelines emphasize the use of intravenous hydrocortisone to adult septic shock patients only if their blood pressure is poorly responsive to fluid resuscitation and vasopressor therapy as in the patient population enrolled by Annane and colleagues [18]. The guidelines recommend: against using the cosyntropin stimulation test to identify the subset of patients who should receive hydrocortisone; against the use of dexamethasone as a substitute for hydrocortisone (due to immediate and prolonged suppression of the hypothalamic-pituitary axis); and against the routine use of steroids in septic patients without shock, unless warranted by the patient's endocrine or corticosteroid use history.

*Etomidate use and sepsis*

Etomidate is a carboxylated imidazole derivative with sedative and hypnotic effects that appear to be mediated through the γ-aminobutyric acid (GABA)-adrenergic system [64]. Etomidate may be the most common choice of sedative used by United States emergency physicians for rapid sequence induction (RSI), used in over 80% of cases in one recent observational study of 610 intubations at one academic center [65]. Advantages of etomidate include a rapid onset, short duration of action, and favorable hemodynamic response even in patients with cardiovascular instability [65–67]. Etomidate also appears to have cerebroprotective effects. One study of patients with intracranial space-occupying lesions undergoing induction with etomidate demonstrated reductions in intracranial pressure with maintenance of cerebral perfusion pressure [68].

One well-known disadvantage of etomidate is that it inhibits adrenal steroid production by reversibly inhibiting 11-β hydroxylase and cholesterol side chain cleavage enzyme [69]. In 1984, a retrospective study by Watts and colleagues [70] of 428 trauma patients admitted to a surgical ICU found increased mortality in patients who underwent continuous sedation with morphine and etomidate versus morphine and benzodiazepines (77% versus 28%, $P = <0.0005$). In the same year, Wagner and colleagues [69] showed that in surgical patients receiving prolonged etomidate infusions, low plasma cortisol levels were associated with decreased responsiveness to ACTH testing even days after discontinuation of infusions. Because of these early studies, the use of continuous sedation with etomidate in the ICU has been abandoned.

The ability of a single dose of etomidate to inhibit adrenal function, and what clinical effect this may have, is the center of great current debate [71–73]. In the CORTICUS trial, the odds ratio from the crude analysis for death in the 244 patients who received etomidate compared with those who did not receive etomidate was 1.53 (95% confidence interval, 1.06–2.26). However, the association between etomidate exposure and outcome was lost in multivariate analysis that included a confidence interval of 1 [62]. One review of multiple small studies revealed transient (2–24 hr) adrenal suppression after a single bolus of etomidate [74]. However, there is a considerable paucity of outcomes data linking this transient laboratory effect to clinical outcomes. In one small, randomized study by Absalom and colleagues [75] (n = 35), subjects were randomized to receive thiopentone or etomidate for induction. Results showed that there was a trend toward decreased responsiveness to ACTH stimulation in patients who received etomidate, but no measurable difference in outcome. A retrospective study by Ray and colleagues [76] investigating induction agents used in septic shock patients showed no relation between choice of induction agent and vasopressor requirements, steroid administration, or clinical outcome. Furthermore, supplemental corticosteroid therapy for patients who received etomidate did not affect outcome. Dmello and colleagues [72] showed similar results in their retrospective study of 224 patients who had septic shock.

What is the practicing ED physician to do when faced with an unstable septic shock patient that is in need of safe induction for endotracheal intubation? Currently, there is no clear evidence against the use of etomidate in septic shock patients. ED physicians should weigh the known immediate beneficial effects of etomidate on maintaining hemodynamic stability and tissue perfusion with the possibility of future harmful effects on adrenal steroidogenesis. Alternative agents such as ketamine, a short-acting agent with a favorable hemodynamic profile, appear to be a reasonable alternative. The automatic dosing of corticosteroids if etomidate is employed is of unproven benefit and is not currently recommended [73,76]. Regardless, if etomidate is chosen, communication of this to inpatient providers seems prudent to help direct future diagnostic and therapeutics.

## Recombinant human-activated protein C

In sepsis, there is a complex host response to infection that involves significant interplay between inflammatory cytokines and coagulation mediators. In severe sepsis, the end result of these interactions may be diffuse endothelial injury, inappropriate coagulation in the microcirculation, multiple organ dysfunction, and death [77].

There are three main defense mechanisms employed by the body to inhibit coagulation: the tissue factor pathway inhibitor, antithrombin, and the protein C system [78]. Activated protein C (APC) is an endogenous mediator in the coagulation cascade that inhibits thrombosis, inflammation, and apoptosis [79]. Reduced levels of APC are found in most patients with sepsis and are associated with an increased risk of death [80,81].

The efficacy of recombinant human APC (rhAPC) was studied in severe sepsis and septic shock in the Recombinant Human Protein C Worldwide Evaluation in Severe Sepsis (PROWESS) study [77]. This was an international, multicenter, randomized, placebo-controlled study of 1690 patients. Efficacy was demonstrated and the trial was stopped early after the second interim analysis. Results showed that the 28-day mortality was reduced from 30.8% in the placebo group to 24.7% in the treatment group (relative reduction in mortality of 19.8%). Major bleeding (defined as life-threatening, or requiring transfusion of 3 units of packed cells per day for 2 consecutive days) was 3.5% in the rhAPC group and 2.0% in the placebo group ($P = .06$). Increased survival was associated with higher severities of illness, as reflected in higher APACHE-II scores and greater number of sepsis-induced organ dysfunctions.

Since the PROWESS study, other studies investigating rhAPC have been conducted. The administration of Drotrecogin alfa (activated) in Early Stage Severe Sepsis Trial showed that rhAPC in less severely ill patients (APACHE-II <25 or single organ dysfunction) confers no benefit [82]. The Extended Evaluation of Recombinant Human Activated Protein C (ENHANCE) study was a global, nonblinded, single-arm trial, designed to provide supplementary safety efficacy data to PROWESS [83]. ENHANCE enrolled 2375 patients and showed a similar mortality benefit to PROWESS (mortality 25.3% at 28 days), but increased rates of bleeding (6.5% at 28 days). ENHANCE also showed greater benefit if rhAPC was started within 24 hours from the first sepsis-induced organ dysfunction (22.9% mortality if started between 0–24 hours versus 27.4% mortality if started greater than 24 hours).

Indications for rhAPC use in the ED are limited. As demonstrated by ENHANCE, there is data to suggest that earlier therapy may confer decreased mortality. There are studies showing that ED use is feasible when used as one component in a sepsis pathway [84]. However, based on risks of bleeding and cost, it seems that rhAPC should be considered only after hemodynamic optimization has been achieved, appropriate antibiotics have been given, and if there is significant delay in admission to the ICU. Practically, rhAPC is recommended for adult patients with sepsis-induced organ dysfunction associated with a high risk of death (most patients with APACHE II scores $\geq 25$ and multiple organ failures) [18]. Recombinant human APC is given as an infusion of 24mcg/kg/h for 96 hours. Absolute contraindications are listed in Box 4.

*Intensive glycemic control*

Hyperglycemia is common in critically ill patients, regardless of whether they have a history of diabetes. Previously it was thought this "stress glycemic response" was adaptive. In 2001, Van den Berghe and colleagues [85] studied intensive control of blood glucose in a population of critically ill patients. The authors conducted a prospective, randomized, controlled trial of 1548 mechanically ventilated patients admitted to a single surgical intensive care unit (SICU). Patients were randomized to intensive glycemic control (serum blood glucose maintained between 80–110 mg/dL) through the use of an insulin infusion protocol, versus conventional care. Results

---

**Box 4. Absolute contraindications to the use of rhAPC**

- Active internal bleeding
- Hemorrhagic cerebrovascular accident within 3 months
- Intracranial surgery, spinal surgery, or severe head trauma within 2 months
- Trauma with an increased risk of life-threatening bleeding
- Presence of an epidural catheter
- Central nervous system neoplasm, mass lesion, or cerebral herniation
- Known allergy to rhAPC

---

*Abbreviation:* rhAPC, recombinant human activated protein C.

showed a reduction in overall ICU mortality in the group randomized to intensive glycemic control (4.6% versus 8%, $P<.04$). The greatest reduction in mortality was seen in patients who stayed in the SICU for greater than 5 days (10.6% versus 20.2%), and in patients with a proven septic focus and multiple organ failures. Other beneficial outcomes seen with intensive glycemic control were decreases in overall hospital mortality by 34%, bloodstream infections by 46%, acute renal failure by 41%, total number of red blood cell transfusions, the incidence of critical illness polyneuropathy, the duration of mechanical ventilation, and intensive care length of stay.

In 2005, the same authors repeated the study in a population of medical intensive care unit (MICU) patients [86]. This was a prospective, randomized, controlled study of 1200 mechanically-ventilated patients admitted to a single center's MICU. Results showed that intensive glycemic control did not reduce overall mortality (37.3% in tightly controlled group versus 40% in conventional group, $P = .33$) and resulted in more cases of hypoglycemia. However, intensive glycemic control did reduce morbidity by preventing newly acquired kidney injury, accelerating weaning from mechanical ventilation, and hastening discharge from both the ICU and hospital. Additionally, although length of stay in the ICU could not be predicted at admission, patients who stayed in the ICU for greater than 3 days who underwent intensive insulin therapy had decreased mortality (43% versus 52.5%, $P = .009$).

Why septic patients seem to benefit more from intensive glycemic control with prolonged ICU stays is not clear at this time. Additional large multicenter studies are needed to elucidate the best strategy for glycemic control in sepsis. The 2008 SSC Guidelines stress the reduction in morbidity and mortality of intensive glycemic control with longer ICU stays and recommend that adult patients with severe sepsis and hyperglycemia receive IV insulin therapy to a targeted glucose level of <150 mg/dL [18]. In addition, it is recommended that all patients on IV insulin therapy receive a glucose calorie source, have glucose levels monitored every 1–2 hours until stable, and have point-of care glucose determinations interpreted cautiously, as these values may overestimate arterial or plasma values.

## Summary

The last two decades have seen tremendous advancements in sepsis research. Definitions have been clarified, and awareness has increased. There remain many questions to be answered and complexities to be unraveled. However, one fact remains: morbidity and mortality can be decreased with timely intervention. With the increasing incidence of sepsis, increasing use of the ED by populations at risk, and an increase in time spent in the ED awaiting hospital admission, emergency medicine practitioners are offered a valuable opportunity to make a significant difference in the fight against sepsis. By administering appropriate antibiotics in a timely fashion, removing possible sources of infection, practicing early goal-directed hemodynamic optimization, using lung-protective ventilation strategies, and judiciously using corticosteroids and intensive insulin therapy, this goal of reducing mortality in sepsis can be achieved.

## References

[1] Dombrovskiy VY, Martin M, Sunderrram J, et al. Rapid Increase in hospitalization and mortality rates for severe sepsis in the United States: A trend analysis from 1993 to 2003. Crit Care Med 2007;35:1244–50.

[2] The EPISEPSIS Study Group. EPISEPSIS: a reappraisal of the epidemiology and outcome of severe sepsis in French intensive care units. Intensive Care Med 2004;30:580–8.

[3] Martin GS, Mannino DM, Eaton S, et al. The epidemiology of sepsis in the United States from 1979 through 2000. N Engl J Med 2003;348(16):1546–54.

[4] Angus D, Linde-Zwirble WT, Lidicker MA, et al. Epidemiology of severe sepsis in the United States: analysis of incidence, outcome, and associated costs of care. Crit Care Med 2001;29:1303–10.

[5] Rangel-Frausto MS, Pittet D, Costigan M, et al. The natural history of the systemic inflammatory response syndrome (SIRS). A prospective study. JAMA 1995;273:117–23.

[6] Dellinger RP. Cardiovascular management of septic shock. Crit Care Med 2003;31:946–55.

[7] Osborn TM, Tracy JK, Dunne JR, et al. Epidemiology of sepsis in patients with traumatic injury. Crit Care Med 2004;32:2234–40.

[8] McCaig LF, Burt CW. National Hospital Ambulatory Medical Care Survey: 2002 emergency department summary. Adv Data 2004;340:1–34.

[9] Lambe S, Washington DL, Fink A, et al. Trends in the use and capacity of California's emergency departments, 1990–1999. Ann Emerg Med 2002;39:389.

[10] Steele R, Kiss A. EMDOC (emergency department overcrowding) internet-based safety net research. J Emerg Med 2007. DOI 10.1016/j.jemermed.2007.03.022.

[11] Wang H, Shapiro N, Angus D, et al. National estimates of severe sepsis in United States emergency departments. Crit Care Med 2007;35:1928–36.

[12] Merriam-Webster's Collegiate Dictionary. 11th edition. Merriam-Webster Incorporated; 2003.

[13] Anonymous. American College of Chest Physicians/Society of Critical Care Medicine Consensus Conference. Definitions for sepsis and organ failure and guidelines for the use of innovative therapies in sepsis. Crit Care Med 1992;20:864–74.

[14] Poze MRG, Ramsay G, Gerlach H, et al. An international sepsis survey: a study of doctors' knowledge and perception about sepsis. Crit Care 2004;8:R409–13.

[15] Levy MM, Fink MP, Marshall JC, et al. 2001 SCCM/ESICM/ACCP/ATS/SIS International sepsis definitions conference. Crit Care Med 2003;31:1250–6.

[16] Osborn TM, Nguyen HB, Rivers EP. Emergency medicine and the surviving sepsis campaign: an international approach to managing severe sepsis and septic shock. Ann Emerg Med 2005;46:228–31.

[17] The Surviving Sepsis Campaign. Available at: http://www.survivingsepsis.org/background/barcelona_declaration. Accessed April 1, 2008.

[18] Dellinger RP, Levy MM, Carlet JM, et al. Surviving Sepsis Campaign: international guidelines for management of severe sepsis and septic shock: 2008. Crit Care Med 2008;36:296–327.

[19] Dellinger RP, Carlet JM, Masur H, et al. Surviving Sepsis Campaign guidelines for management of severe sepsis and septic shock. Crit Care Med 2004;32:858–73.

[20] Kumar A, Roberts D, Wood KE, et al. Duration of hypotension before initiation of effective antimicrobial therapy is the critical determinant of survival in human septic shock. Crit Care Med 2006;34:1589–96.

[21] Larche J, Azoulay E, Fieux F, et al. Improved survival of critically ill cancer patients with septic shock. Intensive Care Med 2003;29:1688–95.

[22] Proulx N, Frechette D, Toye B, et al. Delays in the administration of antibiotics are associated with mortality from adult acute bacterial meningitis. QJM 2005;98:291–8.

[23] Harbarth S, Garbino J, Pugin J, et al. Inappropriate initial antimicrobial therapy and its effect on survival in a clinical trial of immunomodulating therapy for severe sepsis. Am J Med 2003;115(7):529–35.

[24] Leibovici L, Shraga I, et al. The benefit of appropriate empirical antibiotic treatment in patients with bloodstream infection. J Intern Med 1998;244:379–86.

[25] Ibrahim EH, Sherman G, Ward S, et al. The influence of inadequate antimicrobial treatment of bloodstream infections on patient outcomes in the ICU setting. Chest 2000;118(1): 146–55.

[26] Valles J, Rello J, Ochagavia A, et al. Community-acquired bloodstream infection in critically ill adult patients: impact of shock and inappropriate antibiotic therapy on survival. Chest 2003;123:1615–24.

[27] Kanamaru A, Tasumi Y. Microbiological data for patients with febrile neutropenia. Clin Infect Dis 2004;39:S7–10.

[28] Zinner SH. Changing epidemiology of infections in patients with neutropenia and cancer: emphasis on gram-positive and resistant bacteria. Clin Infect Dis 1999;29(3):490–4.

[29] Doern GV, Pfaller M, Kugler K, et al. Prevalence of antimicrobial resistance among respiratory tract isolates of streptococcus pneumonia in north america: 1997 results from the SENTRY antimicrobial surveillance program. Clin Infect Dis 1998;27:764–70.

[30] Thornsberry C, Sahm DF, Kelly LJ, et al. Regional trends in antimicrobial resistance among clinical isolates of *Streptococcus pneumonia, Haemophilus influenza*, and *Moraxella catarrhalis* in the United States: results from the TRUST Surveillance Program, 1999–2000. Clin Infect Dis 2002;34:S4–16.

[31] Doern GV, Brown SD. Antimicrobial susceptibility among community-acquired respiratory tract pathogens in the USA: data from PROTEKT US 2000–01. J Infect 2004;48:56–65.

[32] Centers for Disease Control and Prevention. Effect of new susceptibility breakpoints on reporting of resistance in *Streptococcus pneumonia*: United States, 2003. MMWR Morb Mortal Wkly Rep 2004;53(7):152–4.

[33] Crum NF, Lee RU, Thornton S, et al. Fifteen-year study of the changing epidemiology of methicillin-resistant Staphylococcus aureus. Am J Med 2006;119(11):943–51.

[34] Moran GJ, Krishnadasan A, Gorwitz RJ, et al. Methicillin-resistant S. aureus infections among patients in the emergency department. N Engl J Med 2006;355:666–74.

[35] Frazee BW, Lynn JL, Charlebois ED, et al. High prevalence of methicillin-resistant staphylococcus aureus in emergency department skin and soft tissue infections. Ann Emerg Med 2005;45(3):311–20.

[36] Klevens MK, Morrison MA, Nadle J, et al. Invasive methicillin-resistant Staphylococcus aureus infections in the United States. JAMA 2007;298(15):1763–71.

[37] Centers for Disease Control and Prevention. Severe methicillin-resistant Staphylococcus aureus community-acquired pneumonia associated with influenza–Louisiana and Georgia, December 2006–January 2007. MMWR Morb Mortal Wkly Rep 2007;56(14):325–9.

[38] Costerton JW, Stewart PS, Greenberg EP. Bacterial biofilms: a common cause of persistent infections. Science 1999;284:1318–21.

[39] Sahn SA, Light RW. The sun should never set on a parapneumonic effusion. Chest 1989; 95(5):945–7.

[40] Light RW. A new classification of parapneumonic effusions and empyema. Chest 1995; 108(2):299–301.

[41] Elliott DC, Kufera JA, Myers RA, et al. The microbiology of necrotizing soft tissue infections. Am J Surg 2000;179:361–6.

[42] Elliott DC, Kufera JA, Myers RA. Necrotizing soft tissue infections: risk factors for mortality and strategies for management. Ann Surg 1996;224:672–83.

[43] Betsch A, Wiskirchen J, Trubenbach J, et al. CT guided percutaneous drainage of intra-abdominalabscesses: APACHE III score stratification of 1-year results. Eur Radiol 2002; 12:2883–9.

[44] Hatzidakis AA, Prassopoulos P, Petinarakis I, et al. Acute cholecystitis in high-risk patients: percutaneous cholecystomy vs conservative treatment. Eur Radiol 2002;12:1778–84.

[45] Rivers E, Nguyen B, Havstad S, et al. Early goal-directed therapy in the treatment of severe sepsis and septic shock. N Engl J Med 2001;345:1368–77.

[46] Rivers E, Coba V, Whitmill M. Early goal-directed therapy in severe sepsis and septic shock: a contemporary review of the literature. Curr Opin Anaesthesiol 2008;21:128–40.

[47] Hickling KG, Henderson SJ, Jackson R. Low mortality associated with low volume pressure limited ventilation with permissive hypercapnea in severe adult respiratory distress syndrome. Intensive Care Med 1990;16:372–7.

[48] Hickling KG, Walsh J, Henderson S, et al. Low mortality rate in adult respiratory distress syndrome using low-volume, pressure-limited ventilation with permissive hypercapnea: a prospective study. Crit Care Med 1994;22:1568–78.

[49] Rouby J-J, Puybasset L, Nieszkowska A, et al. Acute respiratory distress syndrome: lessons from computed tomorgraphy of the whole lung. Crit Care Med 2003;31(Suppl):S285–95.

[50] Dreyfuss D, Soler P, Basset G, et al. High inflation pressure pulmonary edema: respective effects of high airway pressure, high tidal volume, and positive end-expiratory pressure. Am Rev Respir Dis 1988;137:1159–64.

[51] Ricard JD, Dreyfuss D, Saumon G. Production of inflammatory cytokines in ventilator-induced lung injury: a reappraisal. Am J Respir Crit Care Med 2001;163:1176–80.

[52] Rouby JJ, Lherm T, Martin De Lassale E, et al. Histologic aspects of pulmonary barotraumas in critically ill patients with acute respiratory failure. Intensive Care Med 1993;19:383–9.

[53] Petersen GW, Baier H. Incidence of pulmonary barotraumas in a medical ICU. Crit Care Med 1983;11:67–9.

[54] The Acute Respiratory Distress Syndrome Network. Ventilation with lower tidal volumes as copmpared with traditional tidal volumes for acute lung injury and the acute respiratory distress syndrome. N Engl J Med 2000;342:1301–8.

[55] Oelkers W. Adrenal insufficiency. N Engl J Med 1996;335:1206–12.

[56] Bennett IL, Finland M, Hamburger M, et al. The effectiveness of hydrocortisone in the management of severe infections. JAMA 1963;183:462–5.

[57] The Veterans Administration Systemic Sepsis Cooperative Study Group: Effect of high-dose glucocorticoid therapy on mortality in patients with clinical signs of sepsis. N Engl J Med 1987;317:659–65.

[58] Sprung CL, Caralis PV, Marcial EH, et al. The effect of high-dose corticosteroids in patients with septic shock. N Engl J Med 1984;311:1137–43.

[59] Bone RC, Fisher CJ, Clemmer TP, et al. A controlled clinical trial of high-dose methylprednisolone in the treatment of severe sepsis and septic shock. N Engl J Med 1987;317:653–8.

[60] Lefering R, Neugebauer E. Steroid controversy in sepsis and septic shock: a metanalysis. Crit Care Med 1995;23:1294–303.

[61] Annane D, Sebille V, Charpentier C, et al. Effect of treatment with low doses of hydrocortisone and fludrocortisone on mortality in patients with septic shock. JAMA 2002;288: 862–71.

[62] Sprung CL, Annane D, Keh D, et al. Hydrocortisone therapy for patients with septic shock. N Engl J Med 2008;358:111–24.

[63] Finfer S. Cotricosteroids in septic shock. N Engl J Med 2008;358:188–9.

[64] Evans RH, Hill RG. The GABA-mimetic action of etomidate [proceedings]. Br J Pharmacol 1977;61:484P.

[65] Sakles JC, et al. Airway management in the emergency department: A one-year study of 610 tracheal intubations. Ann Emerg Med 1998;31:325–32.

[66] Weiss-Bloom LJ, Reich DL. Haemodynamic responses to tracheal intubation following etomidate and fentanyl for anaesthetic induction. Can J Anaesth 1992;39(8):780–5.

[67] Gooding JM, Weng JT, Smith RA, et al. Cardiovascular and pulmonary responses following etomidate induction of anesthesia in patients with demonstrated cardiac disease. Anesth Analg 1979;58:4–10.

[68] Modica PA, Tempelhoff R. Intracranial pressure during induction of anaesthesia and tracheal intubation with etomidate-induced EEG burst suppression. Can J Anaesth 1992; 39:236–41.

[69] Wagner RL, White PF, Kan PB, et al. Inhibition of adrenal steroidogenesis by the anesthetic etomidate. N Engl J Med 1984;310:1415–21.

[70] Watt I, Ledingham IM. Mortality amongst multiple trauma patients admitted to an intensive therapy unit. Anaesthesia 1984;39:973–81.

[71] Annane D. ICU physicians should abandon the use of etomidate! Intensive Care Med 2005; 31:325–6.

[72] Dmello D, Taylor S, O'Brien J, et al. ICU physicians should not abandon the use of etomidate! Crit Care Med 2006;34:A110.

[73] Jackson WL Jr. Should we use etomidate as an induction agent for endotracheal intubation in patients with septic shock? A critical appraisal. Chest 2005;127:1031–8.

[74] Lundy JB, Slane ML, Frizzi JD. Acute adrenal insufficiency after a single dose of etomidate. J Intensive Care Med 2007;22:111–7.

[75] Absalom A, Pledger D, Kong A. Adrenocortical function in critically ill patients 24 h after a single dose of etomidate. Anaesthesia 1999;54:861–7.

[76] Ray DC, McKeown DW. Effect of induction agent on vasopressor and steroid use, and outcome in patients with septic shock. Crit Care 2007;11:R56. Available at: http://ccforum.com/content/11/3/R56.

[77] Bernard GR, Vincent JL, Laterre PF, et al. Efficacy and safety of recombinant human activated protein C for severe sepsis. N Engl J Med 2001;344:699–709.

[78] Fourrier F. Recombinant human activated protein C in the treatment of severe sepsis: an evidence based review. Crit Care Med 2004;32(S):S534–41.

[79] Joyce DE. Recombinant human activated protein C attenuates the inflammatory response in endothelium and monocytes by modulating nuclear factor-kappaB. Crit Care Med 2002; 30(5 Suppl):S288–93.

[80] Fisher CJ, Yan SB. Protein C levels as a prognostic indicator of outcome in sepsis and related diseases. Crit Care Med 2000;28(S):S49–56.

[81] Yan SB, Helterbrand JD, Hartman DL, et al. Low levels of protein C are associated with poor outcome in severe sepsis. Chest 2001;120:915–22.

[82] Abraham E, Laterre PF, Garg R, et al. Drotrecogin alfa (activated) for adults with severe sepsis and a low risk of death. N Engl J Med 2005;353:1332–41.

[83] Vincent JL, Bernard GR, Beale R, et al. Drotrecogin alfa(activated) treatment in severe sepsis from the global open-label trial ENHANCE: further evidence for survival and safety and implications for early treatment. Crit Care Med 2005;33:2266–77.

[84] Nguuyen HB, Corbett SW, Menes K, et al. Early goal-directed therapy, corticosteroid, and recombinant human activated protein C for the treatment of severe sepsis and septic shock in the emergency department. Acad Emerg Med 2006;13:109–13.

[85] Van den Berghe G, Wouters P, Weekers F, et al. Intensive insulin therapy in critically ill patients. N Engl J Med 2001;345:1359–67.

[86] van den Berghe G, Wilmer A, Hermans G, et al. Intensive insulin therapy in the medical ICU. N Engl J Med 2006;354:449–61.

ELSEVIER
SAUNDERS

Emerg Med Clin N Am
26 (2008) 625–648

EMERGENCY
MEDICINE
CLINICS OF
NORTH AMERICA

# Trauma

## Hugo Bonatti, MD, James Forrest Calland, MD*

*University of Virginia School of Medicine, 1215 Lee Street,
Charlottesville, VA 22908, USA*

Trauma accounts for approximately one third of all intensive care admissions in the United States and poses a major burden on the health care system [1]. With more than 50 million individuals seeking medical care for injury annually, trauma has become the leading cause of death for Americans under the age of 45 [2,3].

Severity of traumatic injury depends on the inflicted force, rate of deceleration, protective factors (eg, restraining devices or helmets), and constitution of the individual. Individual response to traumatic injury is critically important and is impacted by many factors, including age, comorbidities, and genetics. A considerable upcoming challenge facing our trauma systems is the combination of aging and obesity [4]. Exciting new developments are emerging in the acute management of traumatic injury. The late Dr. Peter Safar [5] noted that acute resuscitation initiates at presentation in the field and extends to acute resuscitation in the emergency department, culminating in intensive care management. Further developments in all phases of acute injury management contribute to improved outcomes [6]. Data from Montreal and Upper New York State from the late 1990s independently found that rapid transportation of severely injured patients to level 1 trauma centers was associated with a reduction in mortality and morbidity [7,8]. According to MacKenzie and colleagues [6], the case-mix adjusted 1-year mortality of injured patients cared for at designated trauma centers patients is significantly lower than at nondesignated centers (10.4% versus 13.8%; relative risk, 0.75; 95% confidence interval, 0.60–0.95). Many critical and practical considerations regarding damage control techniques, including our understanding of the importance of their application, have matured during the second Iraq war [9,10].

---

* Corresponding author.

*E-mail address:* jfc3t@hscmail.mcc.virginia.edu (J.F. Calland).

doi:10.1016/j.emc.2008.05.001

Despite recent advances, head and chest trauma remains the single greatest cause of death from injury. More than 50% of all trauma deaths occur within the first few hours after admission, and 75% occur within the first few days. A study of an estimated 20,000 injured patients identified age, pre-existing disease, non-white race, blunt injury type, and increased injury severity score as independent predictors of in-hospital mortality [11]. Another evaluation of 30,000 trauma patients found that increasing injury severity score corresponded to a 6- to 16-fold higher incidence of sepsis that resulted in significantly increased mortality and prolonged intensive care unit and hospital stays [12]. Bamvita and colleagues [13] investigated 463 blunt trauma deaths with regard to pre-existing comorbidities and concluded that incorporating information on premorbid conditions is essential for mortality analysis in an aging population. Data from Los Angeles County/USC Trauma Center on more than 4000 trauma deaths suggested that the classic "trimodal" distribution of deaths (first peak, at the scene; second peak, 1–4 hours after injury; third peak, in the intensive care unit weeks later) may no longer apply to patient care within a United States urban trauma system because of improvements in prehospital care, resuscitation, and intensive care. Instead, most injured patients die at the scene or within 4 hours of reaching the trauma center. Of note, in their patient population, 50% of trauma deaths were caused by penetrating injuries, and more than one third of admitted patients lacked vital signs [14,15].

With the knowledge that the first 24 hours are the most crucial in trauma care delivery, primary injury prevention, enforcement of protective mechanisms, early identification of injuries, improvement in emergent care, and early treatment of potentially lethal injuries should be the primary goals [16]. Alcohol and illicit drug abuse is directly linked to an increased risk of trauma, including motor vehicle collisions and interpersonal violence, particularly in adolescents [17]. Data from Louisville and Los Angeles clearly showed that intoxicated victims were more severely injured and had a higher risk of death [18,19]. With the increasing age of the American population, another recently recognized contributor to traumatic injury in elderly persons is the use of long-acting benzodiazepines [20]. This article focuses on recent changes in the epidemiology of trauma and summarizes new acute management strategies of these patients.

## Common injuries and their management

Despite its apparent simplicity and 30 years of advanced trauma life support courses, many injured patients still receive haphazard care without attention to airway, breathing, circulation, and neurological injury. No matter how trivial the mechanism of injury is reported to be, the initial evaluation of the injured patient must focus on the airway, respiratory, circulatory, and neurologic status of the patient to prevent the inevitable sequelae of missed or underestimated injuries. Table 1 shows the five entities and the

Table 1
The injured patient: initial assessment and therapy

| | Subjective | Physical examination | Imaging | Intervention |
|---|---|---|---|---|
| *Primary survey* (A, B, C, D, E) | Dyspnea? Altered mental status? | Protecting airway? Phonation? Breath sounds? Diminished pulses? JVD? | CXR FAST | Cervical collar, intubation, tube thoracostomy, IV access, hemorrhage control, exposure/warming |
| *Secondary survey* Head/face | Visual sx? Normal occlusion? Pain? | Following commands? Ocular trauma/visual acuity? Lateralizing signs? Wounds/lacerations? Facial instability? | CT scan | ICP, Monitor/ventriculostomy, Craniotomy ABX for facial fractures |
| Spine | Pain? | Midline tenderness? Neurologic deficits? | CT scan, Flexion/extension films, MRI/MRA | Cervical collar |
| Chest | Chest pain? Dyspnea? Symmetric breathing? | Subcutaneous emphysema? PTX/HTX? Hemorrhage? | CT scan | Tube thoracostomy, thoracotomy |
| Abdomen/pelvis | Pain? Nausea? | Seat-belt mark? Flank or periumbilical hematoma? GU hematoma or blood at urethral meatus or in vagina? Pelvic instability? | Pelvis radiograph, CT scan | Pelvic binder, laparotomy, angiography |
| Extremity | Pain? | Crepitus? Instability? Open wound? Arterial Pressure Index Asymetric extremity pulses | Radiograph, CT Scan/ CT angio | Consider blood pressure cuff above injury for hemorrhage ABX for open fractures, splints and dressings, angiography for potential vascular injury, shunt/vascular repair |

according goals of initial assessment and therapy and the diagnostic studies suggested by the advanced trauma life support curriculum. Table 2 demonstrates the clinical features and secondary complications for each group.

After primary and secondary surveys, including focused abdominal sonography for trauma (FAST) examination and plain films of the chest and pelvis, stable patients may undergo CT scanning to facilitate the decisions that must be made as to whether to admit the patient. If admission is needed, the decision must be made as to what unit, location, or service should receive the patient. In physiologically compensated severely injured patients with abdominal/pelvic injury, CT scanning is critical to decision making regarding whether one should take a patient to the intensive care unit, the operating room, or the interventional radiology suite for angiography with or without embolization. The total time for full imaging of the head, chest, and abdomen/pelvis is often less than 10 minutes, and images are available real-time for review. During this imaging process, rapid decision making is crucial. In an optimal setting, CT is available in close proximity to the emergency department, and a rapidly mobilized operating room for trauma patients should be available. In cases that involve hemorrhage and hypotension, imaging should be bypassed in favor of rapid transition to the operating room or rapid transfusion with simultaneous transfer to a trauma center if definitive surgical care is unavailable at the treating site. In general, unstable patients never should undergo CT imaging. One must be aware, however, that this decision can lead to delay in diagnosis of potentially fatal injuries and error in decision making.

For many injuries, conservative, interventional, and surgical therapies are competing entities [21]. In stable patients, CT angiography is an exciting tool that makes diagnosis of vascular injuries possible earlier in the resuscitation and evaluation phase [22]. For spinal cord injuries, the newest data emphasize that plain radiographs are (in general) not adequately accurate, and MRI or CT scan should be used evaluate patients with suspected injuries or severe mechanism of injury [23–25].

## End points of resuscitation

Data from the national trauma database, which includes almost 80,000 patients, were recently analyzed by Boulanger and colleagues [26]. They found that in blunt and penetrating trauma injuries, serious hemorrhage is significantly associated with excess mortality, longer hospital stays, and higher costs. In determining whether trauma patients are adequately resuscitated, the critical care of trauma patients does not differ greatly from the critical care of other patients from other populations, although some specialized differences do exist.

In treating actual (or potential) ongoing hemorrhage, one must remember that an ever-increasing number of trauma victims receive thrombocyte aggregation inhibitors or are anticoagulated; these patients seem to have

Table 2
The injured patient: initial assessment and therapy

| | Head trauma | Chest trauma | Abdominal trauma | Extremity trauma | Polytrauma |
|---|---|---|---|---|---|
| Incidence | 30% | 20% | 10% | 2% | 40% |
| Overall mortality | Highest | High | Moderately high | Lowest | Highest |
| Early mortality | Excessive | High | Low | Lowest | Highest |
| Prevalent injury | Hemorrhage, contusion | Hemorrhage, rib fracture, cardiac/pulmonary contusion | Hemorrhage, visceral perforation | Soft tissue necrosis, hemorrhage | Hemorrhage |
| Primary treatment goal | Evacuation of hematoma, prevention of cerebral edema | Hemostasis, decompression | Hemostasis/ contamination control | Hemostasis, stabilization, debridement, decompression | Resuscitation, control hemorrhage, |
| Imaging | Noncontrasted CT scan, CT angiography, MRI | Plain chest film, CT scan | Ultrasound, CT scan | Plain films, CT scan/CT angiography, MRI, angiography | CT head, chest, abdomen, pelvis; plain films, clear spine |
| Other test | EEG (status epilepticus) | ECG,l ECHO, bronchoscopy, EGD, angiography | Angiography, EGD, fluoroscopy, laparoscopy | Compartment pressures | Angiography |
| Compartment syndrome | Brain edema | Cardiac tamponade, pleural effusion, high airway pressures | Renal + respiratory failure + hypotension | Ischemia.hemorrhage | — |
| Therapy | Hypertonic saline/ mannitol, ventriculostomy craniectomy | Surgical decompression, thoracostomy | Decompressive laparotomy, evacuation of collections | Fasciotomy | — |
| Treatment of major vascular injuries | Anticoagulation ± stenting | Thoracic aorta stenting versus open repair | Surgical repair, excision of damaged organs, mechanical packing | Surgical reconstruction | Hybrid procedures |
| To be considered | Occult meningeal tear, | Arrythmia, bronchial, esophageal tear | Undetected viscus perforation, late hemorrhage from spleen or liver, pancreatitis | Overlooked compartment syndrome, nerve damage, vascular endothelial lesion | A, B, C, D, E (!) |

an increased mortality risk in particular when experiencing head injuries [27–29]. Activated factor VIIa (FVIIa) was developed to treat a subgroup of hemophiliacs, and two recent studies showed benefit in coagulopathic trauma victims [30,31]. Standard hemodynamic parameters do not seem to adequately differentiate which trauma patients require additional intervention. Initial lactate and base deficit correlate with severity of injury and provide valuable feedback regarding the predicted need for ongoing resuscitation [32,33].

The phenomenon of "occult hypoperfusion" describes a regional hypoperfusion syndrome that occurs in critically injured patients. When patients with multisystemic injury have serum lactates that remain at more than 2.5 mmol/L for longer than 12 hours after admission, they are at independent risk for in-hospital infectious complications. After 24 hours, elevations in serum lactate are predictive of mortality [32,34–39]. Elevated lactate measurements may serve as markers for more severely deranged physiology (in patients with multisystemic injury) and help to focus the attention of the physician on patients who need more intensive monitoring or who may have missed injuries. Alternatively, lactate-driven volume resuscitation may improve peripheral perfusion and limit immunologic activation. Persistent elevations in posttraumatic lactate measurements must not be neglected unless they can be attributed reliably to other factors, such as seizures or cocaine intoxication [40].

Finally, although not substantiated by more than level II evidence, the use of Swan-Ganz catheters seems to be associated with as much as a 33% reduction in mortality in the most severely injured patients—those with an injury severity score between 25 and 75 [41–43]. Routine use of transthoracic or transesophageal echocardiography has the potential to partially replace Swan-Ganz catheters, which may be particularly useful in cases of chest trauma and associated blunt myocardial injury [44].

## Damage control

The principle of performing the minimum necessary interventions to save life and limb acknowledges that meticulous attention to the details of what is maximally attainable for anatomic reconstruction often is counterproductive in the face of worsening metabolic and hemodynamic derangement. In critically injured patients, securing the airway and optimizing the respiratory system is followed by control of hemorrhage, assessment of neurologic deficit, and contamination control from enteric substances and embedded materials from the environment.

In the operating room, organ reconstruction, re-establishment of bowel continuity, and definitive closure of incisions occurs only if a patient is adequately resuscitated. If at any point a patient's clinical picture declines with hypothermia, acidosis, or coagulopathy, only life-threatening problems that require immediate therapy should be addressed before an expedient return to the intensive care unit for additional resuscitation. To facilitate expeditious departure from the operating room, external drainage with subsequent repair at a more advantageous time is a common, well-accepted principle. Occasional acceptance of external drainage of the biliary, urinary, and enteric stream is advisable if such options assist rapid operating room departure. Removal of damaged organs (eg, spleen or kidney) must be considered, especially if the injured organ adds uncertainty to the resuscitative (intensive care unit) phase of care and can be removed with minimal risk for morbidity. An example of this is low-grade spleen injury coexistent with severe closed head injury. Although most patients without head injury tolerate conservative (nonoperative) management of such solid organ injuries, patients with head injuries suffer greatly from a single episode of hypotension and should undergo expedient pre-emptive splenectomy or angiographic embolization. As a principle, emergency surgery should not last longer than 90 to 120 minutes because the outcome of extended procedures is poor [45,46]. In these cases, surgical procedures can be curtailed effectively after control of hemorrhage combined with a temporary abdominal closure, followed by intensive rewarming, resuscitation, and intravascular interventions.

The principles of damage control in critically injured patients have been appropriated by several supportive subspecialties. The term "damage control neurosurgery" describes focused attention toward expedient decompression of space-occupying posttraumatic hemorrhage, with or without ventriculostomy and craniectomy. Damage control orthopedics/extremity care involves vascular shunting and delayed definitive repair of bony injury. Damage control hematology/resuscitation is implemented through creation of massive transfusion protocols and normalizing fresh-frozen plasma to packed red blood cell unit ratios during massive transfusion toward a 1:1 ratio for transfusion [9]. Factor VIIa is being used with increasing frequency by military and trauma surgeons to stave bleeding in coagulopathic patients after exsanguinating hemorrhage. Despite anecdotal enthusiasm for its efficacy, the cost of Factor VIIa remains a significant barrier to more widespread use [30,31,47]. Although it may eventually emerge as a mainstream intervention in the resuscitation of critically injured patients, there remains a dearth of studies to support its efficacy for routine off-label use in posthemorrhagic resuscitation.

## Central nervous system trauma

Because the central nervous system is one of the most vulnerable systems to ischemic injury, the primary goal is assessment for and prevention of reversible sequelae secondary to the primary injury. Subdural or epidural hematomas [48], when associated with significant mass effect, are treated with invasive monitoring and often neurosurgical intervention and evacuation. Mitigation of secondary injury by maintaining intracranial pressure

(ICP) of less than 20 mm Hg and cerebral perfusion pressure (CPP) of more than 60 mm Hg can be achieved through a combination of volume and blood pressure management, ventriculostomy, osmotherapy, and even decompressive craniectomy.

Brain perfusion can be measured by several different means [49–52]. The extradural ICP monitoring probe ("bolt") can be placed by a neurosurgeon with infrequent complications through a small bur hole. Ventriculostomy catheters and intracerebral oximetric electrodes (Licox) require an experienced neurosurgeon for intracerebral placement. ICP and CPP monitoring via bolt or ventriculostomy and arterial pressure catheter remains the cornerstone of head injury management. Reports of using derived cardiac output and systemic vascular resistance estimates from a noninvasive cutaneous probe are appearing with increasing frequency in the literature. It is attractive to avoid invasive pressure-transducing catheters and their associated blood-stream infections, but there are inadequate data from noninvasive monitoring methods to modify the current monitoring and treatment of patients with severe head injury [53].

Osmotherapy with hypertonic saline infusion or mannitol is a useful means for reducing ICP and is thought to do so through mobilizing extracellular water from the interstitium of the brain into the vascular space, although this only happens in areas of the brain with an intact blood-brain barrier [54,55]. Mannitol can have undesirable secondary effects, such as slow diffusion into injured areas of the brain (with resultant late increases in ICP) and promotion of systemic hypotension through diuresis [56]. Hypertonic saline also decreases ICP with a theoretic lower potential for rebound elevation in ICP [54].

The use of some less commonly employed strategies, such as barbiturate coma and hemicraniectomy, is controversial [10,57,58]. Craniectomy is a therapeutic approach that acknowledges intracranial compartment syndrome [16,59]. In the pediatric population there may be a positive effect; however, thus far no definitive data from prospective trials are available [60].

Corticosteroids have been studied extensively for their application after traumatic brain injury, and they seem to render no benefit [61]. In large meta-analyses, the negative effects of immunosuppression, induction of diabetes mellitus, and delayed wound healing outweigh the benefits of inflammation prevention, associated vasodilatation, and subsequent brain swelling. Steroids may have a protective effect in spinal cord injuries, although this remains controversial and seems to be in an ever-increasing slide from the former position as the standard of care for spinal cord injury [62]. Barbiturate coma has been thought to be protective in terms of putting nerve cells to complete rest and preventing apoptosis and cell death [63]. Subgroups of patients with an intact carbon dioxide reactivity of the brain vessels may benefit, but a universal beneficial effect cannot be demonstrated clearly [64]. As such, prolonged barbiturate coma is not recommended.

Optimal analgesia and sedation for head trauma patients are still not well defined [65]. Currently, a trend toward rapid weaning can be observed, and new agents are increasingly used. No advantage has been found in the use of sufentanyl or remifentanil over other more commonly used opioids. In general, benzodiazepines are well tolerated, and propofol may decrease cerebral metabolism and volume [66,67]. Dexmedetomidine has some promising features, and preliminary studies show that the agent can be used safely, but its final place in the management of patients with head trauma has not yet been defined [68].

Hypothermia is a promising approach, because lowering central nervous system temperature has been shown in experimental models to protect against the detrimental effects of hypoxia and ischemia by reducing brain metabolism and energy consumption [59,69–72]. The protective effects of hypothermia have been demonstrated in experimental models of cerebral ischemia and in models of brain trauma. Jiang and colleagues [70,71] recently summarized more than 30 articles that investigated the effect of hypothermia in the management of brain trauma and reviewed their own center's experience. They concluded that systemic hypothermia may become an important asset in the management of children who have severe brain injury. On the other hand, Clifton and colleagues [59] found no protective effect of hypothermia to 33° C in a series of almost 400 patients with closed head trauma. There is no standardized approach on how to cool, when and how long to cool, and what temperature offers the best protective effect. Hypothermia is further limited by the fact that it can only be applied in isolated cases of central nervous system and spinal trauma. In polytraumatized patients, hypothermia may lead to aggravation of coagulopathy and other adverse effects. For spinal cord injuries, regionalized hypothermia after laminectomy has been suggested [69,72]. The temperature has been lowered to less than 30° C when using this technique. No final judgment with regard to patient outcome can be made currently, and use of hypothermia in injured patients should be restricted to application under the umbrella of an institutional review board–approved research protocol [73].

The sequelae of severe brain injury can be drastic, with death or permanent disability observed in more than half of all victims. Prevention of secondary complications is crucial for attaining optimal outcomes. Prevention of seizures is particularly important during the early phase after head trauma and can be achieved with several different agents, including phenytoin and carbamazepine [74]. Prophylactic antibiotics are indicated in open head trauma, and there may be a benefit in patients with ICP bolts [75–77]. May and colleagues [78] found an increase in the incidence of subsequent infections caused by multiresistant organisms when initially given broad-spectrum antibiotics for prophylaxis. Conflicting data exist on the use of standard heparin versus low molecular weight heparin or intermittent pneumatic compression devices in the setting of head injury [79]. The routine use of stress ulcer prophylaxis is an accepted strategy [80]. The questions surrounding the superiority of enteral feeding versus parenteral feeding and bolus feeds compared with continuous feeds remain unanswered [81,82]. It is common for most victims of head trauma to develop signs of malnutrition [81]. When favorable outcome becomes unlikely, referral of patients who have the most severe head injuries for potential organ donation must be considered.

## Thoracic trauma

Chest trauma is a common cause of morbidity and mortality in multiply injured patients and is thought to account for 20% to 25% of all trauma deaths [15]. Widespread training in advanced trauma life support has promoted the importance of rapid evaluation of the chest by auscultation and plain film chest radiography, promoting an enhanced awareness of expediently detecting and treating hemothorax and pneumothorax early.

The history and physical examination give important clues about the relative likelihood that a thoracic injury is present, and trauma to the great vessels and respiratory tree must be suspected in patients with high-energy mechanisms of injury. Examples of such mechanisms include high-speed motor vehicle collisions in which victims experience prolonged extrication or ejection, fall from a height, and any firearm injury. All patients with hypotension, shortness of breath, decreased breath sounds, an unstable chest wall, or subcutaneous emphysema should undergo rapid decompression of the chest by an experienced clinician. Needle thoracostomy with a 14- or 16-gauge angio catheter (in the second intercostal space) can temporize critically ill patients with suspected tension pneumothorax by rapid decompression of the chest. Needle decompression has mechanical limitations. One recent study found that a standard 14-gauge needle was too short for 10% to 33% of trauma patients, depending on age and gender [83]. Needle decompression is only an effective temporizing measure if the catheter is long enough to reach the thoracic cavity and should not be used in place of definitive tube thoracostomy. If there is any doubt as to whether needle thoracostomy has achieved adequate decompression of the thorax, it should be followed by emergent tube thoracostomy.

In stable patients, tube thoracostomy should be preceded by intravenous administration of appropriate antibiotics whenever feasible and conducted in a surgical field that has been appropriately prepared and draped by an experienced clinician who is appropriately attired in sterile surgical garb [84,85]. The more comfortable the patient, the easier the tube is to place, and generous administration of local anesthesia before and during the procedure facilitates placement. Intravenous sedation can be useful but should be avoided in unstable patients. A generous skin incision in the midaxillary fifth or sixth intercostal space facilitates assessment for pleural adhesions, accurate placement of the tube in the inferior aspect of the interspace, and eventual digital guidance of the tube into the apical-posterior position.

In critically ill trauma patients there is almost never a good reason to use a tube that is less than 32 Fr in diameter.

Emergent tube placement should precede interfacility transfer and moves between patient care areas. For placement of chest tubes and in evaluation of penetrating wounds, it is important to understand that diaphragmatic excursion reaches the level of the nipple during expiration. Penetrating injuries to the thorax with trajectories that extend below the tips of the scapula or nipple line may be associated with concomitant intra-abdominal injury. Intra-abdominal injuries frequently coexist with thoracic trauma and must be evaluated with laparoscopy or reconstructions of multi-slice CT scans. Finally, although most forms of blunt and penetrating trauma to the chest are adequately treated by tube thoracostomy alone, prompt surgical consultation should precede or accompany placement of all chest tubes whenever possible.

Plain film radiographs can give important clues to the presence of a thoracic injury, although some injuries, especially aortic tears, can be present despite apparently normal results on a film. High-energy mechanisms, especially when coexistent with fractures of the scapulae or the first or second ribs, should prompt the clinician to evaluate the thoracic aorta with CT or angiography. Sonography is a sensitive modality for early evaluation of the pericardium and is nearly a universal standard in the early evaluation of trauma patients. Sonography's only liability is its low sensitivity when applied to patients with coexistent pleural effusion or hemothorax [86,87]. CT is a sensitive imaging modality for all bony and soft tissue structures within the thorax but currently does not replace endoscopy or bronchoscopy for evaluation of suspected tracheal or esophageal injuries. Retained hemothorax, persistent atelectasis or air leak, empyema, and thoracic hemorrhage are common causes of preventable morbidity and mortality after trauma and must be treated expediently, preferably by a surgeon with extensive thoracic training and experience. Suspected tracheal or pulmonary aspiration should be evaluated bronchoscopically for the presence of foreign bodies and acquisition of a microbiologic sample for culture.

After the initial evaluation, patients with moderately severe but stable thoracic injuries (eg, isolated rib fractures with hemo- or pneumothorax) can be managed by observation, appropriate narcotic analgesia, and chest tube management strategies in the acute care setting if the patient is well compensated, has adequate analgesia, and is without significant comorbidities. Nearly all patients with substantial thoracic trauma (and especially patients with multiple rib fractures and pulmonary contusions) get worse in the initial 48 to 72 hours after injury, as measured by decrements in vital capacity, functional residual capacity, and compliance. If pain control and pulmonary toilet are neglected in elderly patients, they often decline precipitously, with progressive atelectasis, pneumonia, and the need for mechanical ventilation [88,89].

Ventilator management should follow the ARDSnet principles for patients with acute lung injury, with low tidal volume strategies ($< 6$ mL/kg) and limits in plateau pressure of less than 30 CM $H_2O$ [57,60,90]. Strict use of any single ventilator mode over another has not been demonstrated to change outcomes if patients are allowed a daily sedation holiday and spontaneous breathing trial [91]. High-frequency oscillating ventilation and airway pressure release ventilation/bilevel are useful modalities for ventilating decompensated patients who have atelectasis and acute respiratory distress syndrome [92]. In comparison to high-frequency oscillating ventilation, airway pressure release ventilation has the relative advantage of not requiring deep sedation or neuromuscular blockade to prevent ventilator-patient dysynchrony [91].

Emergency department thoracotomy with release of tamponade and cross-clamping of the thoracic aortic is associated with a low salvage rate, even when applied by the most experienced hands after witnessed cardiac arrest [93]. All other applications for the technique are unlikely to yield a change in patient outcome and unnecessarily subject members of the resuscitation team to needless risk of transmission of blood-borne communicable diseases [94]. Whether to apply these techniques to a patient for the sole purpose of salvaging a potential organ donor is controversial and up to the judgment of the individual trauma surgeon.

## Abdominal and pelvic trauma

The abdomen arguably presents the greatest diagnostic and therapeutic challenge among all the zones of injury because it requires an experienced surgical clinician and frequently advanced imaging or invasive procedures for accurate diagnosis and definitive therapy for traumatic injury. The first step in evaluating patients who are at risk for abdominal or pelvic trauma is to use the mechanism of injury and the vector of force to predict the most likely injury pattern to be seen. For example, knowing that a patient was the restrained driver of a motor vehicle hit on the driver's side with resultant heavy damage and entrapment of the victim should heighten the clinician's awareness of the possibility that the evaluation eventually will demonstrate left-sided rib fractures, a spleen injury, and renal laceration—an assessment that can be made even before the patient arrives at the trauma center.

Once the patient arrives in the emergency department and adequate attention has been given to the airway, thoracic cavity, and circulatory examination, the patient should undergo imaging of the chest and pelvis with plain film radiography. Ideally, the patient also should undergo simultaneous physical examination for abdominal pain and tenderness and FAST examination to evaluate the presence of free fluid. If intra-abdominal fluid is found within the abdomen of a hemodynamically unstable patient, priority should be placed on progressing toward laparotomy, even if it (infrequently) means that a patient with head injury goes to the operating room without preoperative CT imaging. Imaging of the head should occur whenever possible before operative therapy so that, if necessary, a simultaneous combined laparotomy/craniotomy or placement of an ICP-monitoring electrode can be performed. The presence of a pronounced seat belt sign or severe abdominal tenderness in should heighten suspicion of an intra-abdominal injury and mandate laparotomy, DPL, CT scanning of the abdomen, or serial examinations, even if the patient is normotensive and has no free fluid on the FAST examination [95,96].

If the initial pelvic radiograph demonstrates displaced fractures, especially of the pubic rami and sacroiliac joints, the possibility of pelvic hemorrhage or urethral, bladder, vaginal, or rectal injury must be considered and ruled out with a combination of digital rectal examination, vaginal examination, and retrograde urethrogram or cystogram. Placement of a pelvic binder can be useful for limiting the expansion of the pelvic ring in patients with an anterior compression injury and pubic diastasis but should be used with great caution (or not at all) in patients with lateral compression injuries and acetabular fractures [97].

Despite inherent limitations in its sensitivity to detect injuries in luminal structures, CT scanning has become the radiologic evaluation of choice after initial sonography. Injuries to the duodenum, small bowel, colon, and pancreas may be routinely overlooked [95]. Although diagnostic peritoneal lavage of the abdominal cavity has substantially lost its significance in diagnosing hemoperitoneum, this modality may be of great use in detecting bowel perforation [96,98,99]. Diagnostic laparoscopy is another rapidly evolving procedure in penetrating abdominal trauma and is an effective diagnostic modality in patients who clearly do not have penetration into the abdominal cavity after cross-sectional imaging or local wound exploration [100–102]. CT has limited diagnostic use in examining for the trajectory of low-velocity penetrating wounds, such as stab injuries, because of a relative lack of tissue destruction and gas dispersion. The maxim "accurate trajectory determination equals anatomic injury" holds true in firearm injuries, especially as determined by a combination of plain film radiography and cross-sectional imaging. Such an approach is difficult in the case of stab wounds, in which trajectory is often only determined accurately by wound exploration. In penetrating trauma of the abdomen, when laparoscopy detects penetration of the peritoneum, many surgeons perform the remainder of the exploration in open fashion rather than laparoscopically.

In addition to surgical therapy for life-threatening hemorrhage from a ruptured spleen, interventional radiology with embolization of the splenic artery may be a good option. In elderly and hemodynamically unstable patients, embolization (selective embolization especially) has the risk of rebleeding, and definitive care through splenectomy may be a safer option for such patients [58,103,104]. For extensive liver injuries (grades 3 and 4), angiography may be the best option for definitive treatment of bleeding but probably should be delayed (in patients who have hypotension) until after abdominal exploration and packing with laparotomy pads [105,106]. Pre- and retroperitoneal packing of pelvic fractures associated with pelvic hemorrhage is not widely practiced but holds promise for the future in what most clinicians find to be a dangerous and resource-consuming problem [107–109]. In general, any injury that remains packed after the operating room should have angiographic interrogation postoperatively for correctable sources of arterial hemorrhage.

## Extremity trauma

Life-threatening hemorrhage should be addressed during the primary survey. Direct pressure and elevation by bystanders, nurses, and technicians can be applied effectively to stem bleeding in trivial injuries but will not prevent exsanguination from named vessels in the upper or lower extremity. Field tourniquets are currently being used with considerable anecdotal efficacy by the United States military in the Iraq War but have not yet found their way into homeland emergency medical services. Injured patients who come to the emergency department with profuse bleeding from an extremity are rapidly and effectively treated with manual point pressure directly to the open orifice of the bleeding vessel. Alternatively, application of a blood pressure cuff above the site of injury can be sequentially inflated to a sufficient pressure to cause abatement of hemorrhage. This approach is substantially safer and more effective than blind application of hemostats.

The presence of profuse bleeding, expanding hematoma, loss of distal pulses, distal ischemia, and arterial bruit are hard signs of vascular injury and usually mandate immediate surgical exploration. In less severe injuries, when the diagnosis of vascular injury is uncertain, calculation of an arterial pressure index by comparing blood pressures between limbs can be useful. A difference in systolic blood pressure of more than 10% between ankles generally mandates CT or conventional arteriography when applied to patients with unilateral wounds of the lower extremities. Evaluation for vascular injury in the upper extremity is made somewhat more complicated by the presence of robust vascular collaterals around the shoulder and elbow. If the arterial pressure index differs between wrists, it nearly always signifies the presence of an injury. Absence of a difference in arterial pressure index between the upper extremities does not preclude the possibility that a vascular injury exists. Clinical suspicion and proximity to known vascular structures should impact the decision to perform CT or conventional angiography.

Suspected fractures should be splinted and imaged expediently. Potential open fractures should have sterile dressings applied along with splints, with simultaneous administration of appropriate intravenous antibiotics. Early consultation with an orthopedic surgeon is mandated. Delayed diagnosis of posttraumatic compartment syndrome of the extremity is an important source of preventable posttraumatic morbidity and medicolegal vulnerability. It should be suspected in all patients with multiple fractures, vascular injury, or prolonged ischemia of the leg or forearm. Pain upon passive flexion is a late sign of compartment syndrome–related ischemia. Ideally, the diagnosis of compartment syndrome is made by direct measurement of compartment pressures using a pressure transducer, usually by way of a handheld (Stryker) monitor. The best treatment strategy involves anticipating compartment syndrome before it develops and performing prophylactic fasciotomies or catching the syndrome early and enlisting the help of a surgeon to perform invasive monitoring and subsequent fasciotomies [110,111].

## The universal theory of compartment syndrome

Increased pressure within semi-rigid anatomic structures accounts for a substantial proportion of morbidity and mortality for injured patients. It is not coincidental that pathologic mean pressures within the head, thorax, abdomen, and extremities are tightly grouped within 5 to 10 mm Hg of 30 mm Hg, which is the upper limit of capillary pressure of normal human subjects [110,111]. When pressures in any compartment exceed the pressure of capillary perfusion, ischemic damage ensues and progresses in an uncontrolled fashion until perfusion is restored through release of compartment pressure or elevation of inflow pressure. A similar mechanism likely contributes to the pathophysiology of other surgical diseases that occur in confined spaces, despite the fact that that they are not commonly thought of as "compartment syndromes." Potential clinical correlates of compartment syndrome exist in appendicitis, bowel obstruction, and cholecystitis but remain unproven.

## Trauma in the elderly population

Trauma victims are not restricted to persons of younger age. As the population becomes more mobile, so do the members of the aging population. An increasing number of senior citizens are becoming trauma victims [112,113]. Because of the frailty of the aging body, severe injuries occur even in the setting of a seemingly trivial mechanism [114–116]. Postural instability and loss of protective reflexes may cause more severe injuries when experiencing equal force as compared to younger victims. Osteopenia and osteoporosis are much more prevalent in the aging population and result in more numerous and severe fractures [89,117,118]. Most importantly, elderly persons frequently take anticoagulant medications or platelet inhibitors, which can result in more severe intracranial bleeding after head injuries and visceral blood loss from blunt trauma. Other medications, such as benzodiazepines, psychotropic medications, and antiepileptic drugs, must be considered as potential causes of accidents [119–121]. Such drugs also should be taken into consideration during emergent care and may be responsible for the development of withdrawal symptoms or other complications, such as hypoglycemia and hypotension.

Comorbid conditions, such as arteriosclerosis, coronary artery disease, and chronic obstructive pulmonary disorder, lower the reserve capacity of patients to tolerate severe trauma. Mortality rates in elderly trauma victims are significantly elevated. In a recent study by Tornetta and colleagues [122], mortality rates were 18% in a cohort of 300 injured patients older than 60 years. If the acute phase can be overcome, it must be understood that elderly patients recover more slowly than younger patients with similar injuries and may have greater need for rehabilitation after discharge from the acute-care setting. Although specialized trauma centers for children produce better outcomes, such super-specialized care has not been attempted for the elderly population [123–125].

## Trauma in obese patients

Twenty-six percent of adults in the Unites States are obese, and trauma remains a major cause of death in this population. In this patient population, mortality after trauma is significantly increased [126–129]. Most studies have found a link to the comorbid conditions and the limited reserves of this patient population, whereas Brown and colleagues suggested that other demographic differences, such as age and pattern of injuries (particularly a higher rate of chest trauma) may be responsible for the worse outcomes [35,44,126]. Another study from Los Angeles even found no increased mortality in patients with a high body mass index [61]. Although under certain circumstances fat may function as a cushion to prevent injuries, survival of obese trauma victims is generally worse than that for the normal population. This finding is partially attributable to the significantly higher prevalence of observed comorbid conditions, such as diabetes mellitus, but obesity is also associated with a decreased pulmonary and cardiovascular reserve.

Most procedures (surgical or otherwise) are technically much more challenging and likely to be associated with marked increases in complications in morbidly obese patients. Many diagnostic tools routinely used for nonobese patients are not equipped or constructed to treat morbidly obese individuals. Examples extend beyond CT scan and MRI devices, which are frequently limited in their capacity to accommodate patients who weigh more than 400 lb. Standard tools for percutaneous procedures, such as tracheostomy or indwelling catheters, are of limited utility. Transport is more complicated and consumes increased resources. If obese patients are managed well and survive the acute phase of trauma, rehabilitation becomes another major challenge. During this period, many complications, including thrombosis, cardiovascular insufficiency, infectious complications, and pulmonary failure, can increase time in rehabilitative care or require rehospitalization.

## Care of the potential organ donor

Rapidly after brain death from trauma, the body of the potential organ donor undergoes dramatic changes in the physiologic, hemodynamic, and endocrinologic milieu [127]. The time course of brain death and dying varies and may be quick or last several days. Optimal potential donor management serves the individual who yet lives with a chance of recovery and serves the greater good of preventing irreversible organ dysfunction. Such essential care includes proper fluid and electrolyte management during the onset of posttraumatic diabetes insipidus, which is often followed by a rise in the serum sodium levels to more than 160 mmol/L and hypotension. This deadly combination is not only harmful to the individual who yet lives but is also known to cause significant damage to organs that are later procured for harvest. Dysregulation of the fundamental homeostatic/thermostatic functions of the hypothalamus frequently results in hypo- and hyperthermia in the setting of "cytokine storm" with massive release of tissue necrosis factor, interleukins, and other potentially harming agents [127].

Excessive use of vasopressors also is known to damage organs and should be avoided, if possible. When pressors are needed in potential organ donors, dopamine is favored because of its beneficial chronotropic effect in persons with relative bradycardia and its theoretic capacity to augment splanchnic perfusion. Unnecessary drugs that are toxic to the liver or kidneys should be avoided. Organ donors must be cared for in a most delicate way because failure of the transplanted grafts may cause death of several individuals. Currently, no clear special guidelines have been developed to optimize management.

The number of young donors who have died from head trauma seems to be continuously declining because of prevention and better treatment of patients with such injuries. Although previously considered unthinkable, it is currently common for individuals older than age 70 with massive strokes to be evaluated for possible organ donation [130,131]. Kidneys and livers from donors of advanced age have been used successfully. Such expanded criteria for donor suitability also must be considered for morbidly obese individuals and individuals who have extended stay on the intensive care unit with high-dose vasopressors. Traditionally, these individuals were not considered suitable for organ donation, but because of the shortage of available organs, nearly all individuals who experience in-hospital brain death are considered potential organ donors. A new development is donation after cardiac death [132]. In these cases, in patients without evidence of brain death but with an injury for which medical care is futile, ventilator support can be withdrawn with the consent of the family.

## The forgotten systems

Intensivist clinicians of various backgrounds, whether they are trained as emergency medicine clinicians, pediatricians, surgeons, anesthesiologists, or pulmonologists, are capable of providing outstanding care for injured patients. As trauma injury severity increases, involving secondary systems, or is associated with end-organ failure, however, a coordinated team approach with the trauma surgeon (in a designated trauma center) will likely

---

**Box 1. The forgotten systems: important critical care considerations in the trauma patient**

*Prophylaxis*
Is there a contraindication to low molecular weight heparin?
Is there an indication for a prophylactic inferior vena cava filter?
Does the patient have adequate prophylaxis against stress ulceration of the stomach?
Could withdrawal from recreational drugs or delirium tremens be an issue?
Have all home medications been considered?
Is a beta-blocker indicated?

*Surgical infections*
Can tubes, catheters, or drains be removed?
Do any of the tube, catheter, or drain sites have erythema or purulent discharge?
What is the appearance of the drain effluent?
Examine every wound every day.

*Missed injuries*
Has a tertiary survey been performed to detect missed injuries?
Have radiologic studies been performed of all sites at which the patient has pain, tenderness, external marks, or deficits?
Is there an unexplained failure to clear metabolic acidosis/lactate?

*Endocrine*
Have steroid needs been anticipated and addressed?
Was premorbid endocrinopathy present?
Has adequate glycemic control been achieved?

---

lead to lower mortality and decrements in morbidity. Meticulous attention to detail in the following secondary systems often picks up preventable sources of morbidity. Box 1 lists daily intensive care unit considerations that are particularly applicable to patients with injuries.

**Summary**

In terms of cost and years of potential lives lost, injury arguably remains the most important public health problem facing the United States. Care of traumatically injured patients depends on early surgical intervention and avoiding delays in the diagnosis of injuries that threaten life and limb. In the critical care phase, successful outcomes after injury depend almost solely on diligence, attention to detail, and surveillance for iatrogenic infections and complications.

## References

[1] Mackenzie EJ, Rivara FP, Jurkovich GJ, et al. The National Study on costs and outcomes of trauma. J Trauma 2007;63:S54.

[2] CDC. National estimates of the ten leading causes of nonfatal injuries. Atlanta (GA): Centers for Disease Control and Prevention; 2004.

[3] CDC. Ten leading causes of death. Atlanta (GA): Centers for Disease Control and Prevention; 2003.

[4] Corrada MM, Kawas CH, Mozaffar F, et al. Association of body mass index and weight change with all-cause mortality in the elderly. Am J Epidemiol 2006;163:938.

[5] Safar P. Critical care medicine: quo vadis? Crit Care Med 1974;2:1.

[6] MacKenzie EJ, Rivara FP, Jurkovich GJ, et al. A national evaluation of the effect of trauma-center care on mortality. N Engl J Med 2006;354:366.

[7] Sampalis JS, Denis R, Frechette P, et al. Direct transport to tertiary trauma centers versus transfer from lower level facilities: impact on mortality and morbidity among patients with major trauma. J Trauma 1997;43:288.

[8] Veenema KR, Rodewald LE. Stabilization of rural multiple-trauma patients at level III emergency departments before transfer to a level I regional trauma center. Ann Emerg Med 1995;25:175.

[9] Holcomb JB, Jenkins D, Rhee P, et al. Damage control resuscitation: directly addressing the early coagulopathy of trauma. J Trauma 2007;62:307.

[10] Spinella PC, Perkins JG, McLaughlin DF, et al. The effect of recombinant activated factor VII on mortality in combat-related casualties with severe trauma and massive transfusion. J Trauma 2008;64:286.

[11] Gannon CJ, Napolitano LM, Pasquale M, et al. A statewide population-based study of gender differences in trauma: validation of a prior single-institution study. J Am Coll Surg 2002;195:11.

[12] Osborn TM, Tracy JK, Dunne JR, et al. Epidemiology of sepsis in patients with traumatic injury. Crit Care Med 2004;32:2234.

[13] Bamvita JM, Bergeron E, Lavoie A, et al. The impact of premorbid conditions on temporal pattern and location of adult blunt trauma hospital deaths. J Trauma 2007;63:135.

[14] Demetriades D, Kimbrell B, Salim A, et al. Trauma deaths in a mature urban trauma system: is "trimodal" distribution a valid concept? J Am Coll Surg 2005;201:343.

[15] Demetriades D, Murray J, Charalambides K, et al. Trauma fatalities: time and location of hospital deaths. J Am Coll Surg 2004;198:20.

[16] Acosta JA, Yang JC, Winchell RJ, et al. Lethal injuries and time to death in a level I trauma center. J Am Coll Surg 1998;186:528.

[17] Madan A, Beech DJ, Flint L. Drugs, guns, and kids: the association between substance use and injury caused by interpersonal violence. J Pediatr Surg 2001;36:440.

[18] Demetriades D, Gkiokas G, Velmahos GC, et al. Alcohol and illicit drugs in traumatic deaths: prevalence and association with type and severity of injuries. J Am Coll Surg 2004;199:687.

[19] Draus JM Jr, Santos AP, Franklin GA, et al. Drug and alcohol use among adolescent blunt trauma patients: dying to get high? J Pediatr Surg 2008;43:208.

[20] Hemmelgarn B, Suissa S, Huang A, et al. Benzodiazepine use and the risk of motor vehicle crash in the elderly. JAMA 1997;278:27.

[21] Reuben BC, Whitten MG, Sarfati M, et al. Increasing use of endovascular therapy in acute arterial injuries: analysis of the National Trauma Data Bank. J Vasc Surg 2007; 46:1222.

[22] Anderson SW, Soto JA, Lucey BC, et al. Blunt trauma: feasibility and clinical utility of pelvic CT angiography performed with 64-detector row CT. Radiology 2008;246:410.

[23] Berry GE, Adams S, Harris MB, et al. Are plain radiographs of the spine necessary during evaluation after blunt trauma? Accuracy of screening torso computed tomography in thoracic/lumbar spine fracture diagnosis. J Trauma 2005;59:1410.

[24] Gale SC, Gracias VH, Reilly PM, et al. The inefficiency of plain radiography to evaluate the cervical spine after blunt trauma. J Trauma 2005;59:1121.

[25] Muchow RD, Resnick DK, Abdel MP, et al. Magnetic resonance imaging (MRI) in the clearance of the cervical spine in blunt trauma: a meta-analysis. J Trauma 2008; 64:179.

[26] Boulanger L, Joshi AV, Tortella BJ, et al. Excess mortality, length of stay, and costs associated with serious hemorrhage among trauma patients: findings from the National Trauma Data Bank. Am Surg 2007;73:1269.

[27] Inman DS, Michla Y, Partington PF. Perioperative management of trauma patients admitted on clopidogrel (Plavix): a survey of orthopaedic departments across the United Kingdom. Injury 2007;38:625.

[28] Jones K, Sharp C, Mangram AJ, et al. The effects of preinjury clopidogrel use on older trauma patients with head injuries. Am J Surg 2006;192:743.

[29] Ohm C, Mina A, Howells G, et al. Effects of antiplatelet agents on outcomes for elderly patients with traumatic intracranial hemorrhage. J Trauma 2005;58:518.

[30] Bartal C, Freedman J, Bowman K, et al. Coagulopathic patients with traumatic intracranial bleeding: defining the role of recombinant factor VIIa. J Trauma 2007;63:725.

[31] Dutton RP, McCunn M, Hyder M, et al. Factor VIIa for correction of traumatic coagulopathy. J Trauma 2004;57:709.

[32] Cerovic O, Golubovic V, Spec-Marn A, et al. Relationship between injury severity and lactate levels in severely injured patients. Intensive Care Med 2003;29:1300.

[33] Certo TF, Rogers FB, Pilcher DB. Review of care of fatally injured patients in a rural state: 5-year followup. J Trauma 1983;23:559.

[34] Blow O, Magliore L, Claridge JA, et al. The golden hour and the silver day: detection and correction of occult hypoperfusion within 24 hours improves outcome from major trauma. J Trauma 1999;47:964.

[35] Claridge JA, Crabtree TD, Pelletier SJ, et al. Persistent occult hypoperfusion is associated with a significant increase in infection rate and mortality in major trauma patients. J Trauma 2000;48:8.

[36] Claridge JA, Schulman AM, Young JS. Improved resuscitation minimizes respiratory dysfunction and blunts interleukin-6 and nuclear factor-kappa B activation after traumatic hemorrhage. Crit Care Med 2002;30:1815.

[37] Crowl AC, Young JS, Kahler DM, et al. Occult hypoperfusion is associated with increased morbidity in patients undergoing early femur fracture fixation. J Trauma 2000;48:260.

[38] Schulman AM, Claridge JA, Carr G, et al. Predictors of patients who will develop prolonged occult hypoperfusion following blunt trauma. J Trauma 2004;57:795.

[39] Schulman AM, Claridge JA, Young JS. Young versus old: factors affecting mortality after blunt traumatic injury. Am Surg 2002;68:942.

[40] Porter JM, Ivatury RR. In search of the optimal end points of resuscitation in trauma patients: a review. J Trauma 1998;44:908.

[41] Friese RS, Shafi S, Gentilello LM. Pulmonary artery catheter use is associated with reduced mortality in severely injured patients: a National Trauma Data Bank analysis of 53,312 patients. Crit Care Med 2006;34:1597.

[42] Kirton OC, Civetta JM. Do pulmonary artery catheters alter outcome in trauma patients? New Horiz 1997;5:222.

[43] Martin RS, Norris PR, Kilgo PD, et al. Validation of stroke work and ventricular arterial coupling as markers of cardiovascular performance during resuscitation. J Trauma 2006; 60:930.

[44] Chytra I, Pradl R, Bosman R, et al. Esophageal Doppler-guided fluid management decreases blood lactate levels in multiple-trauma patients: a randomized controlled trial. Crit Care 2007;11:R24.

[45] Ahmed JM, Tallon JM, Petrie DA. Trauma management outcomes associated with nonsurgeon versus surgeon trauma team leaders. Ann Emerg Med 2007;50:7.

[46] Higgins TL, McGee WT, Steingrub JS, et al. Early indicators of prolonged intensive care unit stay: impact of illness severity, physician staffing, and pre-intensive care unit length of stay. Crit Care Med 2003;31:45.

[47] Barletta JF, Ahrens CL, Tyburski JG, et al. A review of recombinant factor VII for refractory bleeding in nonhemophilic trauma patients. J Trauma 2005;58:646.

[48] Zweckberger K, Sakowitz OW, Unterberg AW, et al [Classification and therapy of craniocerebral injury (CCI)]. Laryngorhinootologie 2008;87:121 [in German].

[49] Czosnyka M, Smielewski P, Lavinio A, et al. A synopsis of brain pressures: Which? When? Are they all useful? Neurol Res 2007;29:672.

[50] Huang SJ, Hong WC, Han YY, et al. Clinical outcome of severe head injury using three different ICP and CPP protocol-driven therapies. J Clin Neurosci 2006;13:818.

[51] Stiefel MF, Heuer GG, Smith MJ, et al. Cerebral oxygenation following decompressive hemicraniectomy for the treatment of refractory intracranial hypertension. J Neurosurg 2004;101:241.

[52] Stiefel MF, Spiotta A, Gracias VH, et al. Reduced mortality rate in patients with severe traumatic brain injury treated with brain tissue oxygen monitoring. J Neurosurg 2005; 103:805.

[53] Newell DW, Aaslid R, Stooss R, et al. Evaluation of hemodynamic responses in head injury patients with transcranial Doppler monitoring. Acta Neurochir (Wien) 1997;139:804.

[54] Bhardwaj A, Ulatowski JA. Hypertonic saline solutions in brain injury. Curr Opin Crit Care 2004;10:126.

[55] White H, Cook D, Venkatesh B. The use of hypertonic saline for treating intracranial hypertension after traumatic brain injury. Anesth Analg 2006;102:1836.

[56] Wakai A, Roberts I, Schierhout G. Mannitol for acute traumatic brain injury. Cochrane Database Syst Rev 2007:CD001049.

[57] Petrucci N, Iacovelli W. Ventilation with smaller tidal volumes: a quantitative systematic review of randomized controlled trials. Anesth Analg 2004;99:193.

[58] Smith HE, Biffl WL, Majercik SD, et al. Splenic artery embolization: Have we gone too far? J Trauma 2006;61:541.

[59] Clifton GL, Miller ER, Choi SC, et al. Lack of effect of induction of hypothermia after acute brain injury. N Engl J Med 2001;344:556.

[60] Gillis RC, Weireter LJ Jr, Britt RC, et al. Lung protective ventilation strategies: have we applied them in trauma patients at risk for acute lung injury and acute respiratory distress syndrome? Am Surg 2007;73:347.

[61] Alderson P, Roberts I. Corticosteroids for acute traumatic brain injury. Cochrane Database Syst Rev 2005:CD000196.

[62] Sayer FT, Kronvall E, Nilsson OG. Methylprednisolone treatment in acute spinal cord injury: the myth challenged through a structured analysis of published literature. Spine J 2006;6:335.

[63] Roberts I. Barbiturates for acute traumatic brain injury. Cochrane Database Syst Rev 2000:CD000033.

[64] Moskopp D, Ries F, Wassmann H, et al. Barbiturates in severe head injuries? Neurosurg Rev 1991;14:195.

[65] Ghori KA, Harmon DC, Elashaal A, et al. Effect of midazolam versus propofol sedation on markers of neurological injury and outcome after isolated severe head injury: a pilot study. Crit Care Resusc 2007;9:166.

[66] Karabinis A, Mandragos K, Stergiopoulos S, et al. Safety and efficacy of analgesia-based sedation with remifentanil versus standard hypnotic-based regimens in intensive care unit

patients with brain injuries: a randomised, controlled trial [ISRCTN50308308]. Crit Care 2004;8:R268.

[67] Schmittner MD, Vajkoczy SL, Horn P, et al. Effects of fentanyl and S(+)-ketamine on cerebral hemodynamics, gastrointestinal motility, and need of vasopressors in patients with intracranial pathologies: a pilot study. J Neurosurg Anesthesiol 2007;19:257.

[68] Aryan HE, Box KW, Ibrahim D, et al. Safety and efficacy of dexmedetomidine in neurosurgical patients. Brain Inj 2006;20:791.

[69] Dimar JR II, Shields CB, Zhang YP, et al. The role of directly applied hypothermia in spinal cord injury. Spine 2000;25:2294.

[70] Jiang JY, Xu W, Li WP, et al. Effect of long-term mild hypothermia or short-term mild hypothermia on outcome of patients with severe traumatic brain injury. J Cereb Blood Flow Metab 2006;26:771.

[71] Jiang JY, Yang XF. Current status of cerebral protection with mild-to-moderate hypothermia after traumatic brain injury. Curr Opin Crit Care 2007;13:153.

[72] Martinez-Arizala A, Green BA. Hypothermia in spinal cord injury. J Neurotrauma 1992;(9 Suppl 2):S497.

[73] Alderson P, Gadkary C, Signorini DF. Therapeutic hypothermia for head injury. Cochrane Database Syst Rev 2004:CD001048.

[74] Schierhout G, Roberts I. Anti-epileptic drugs for preventing seizures following acute traumatic brain injury. Cochrane Database Syst Rev 2001:CD000173.

[75] Guidelines for the management of severe traumatic brain injury. IV: infection prophylaxis. J Neurotrauma 2007;24(Suppl 1):S26.

[76] Cosar A, Gonul E, Kurt E, et al. Craniocerebral gunshot wounds: results of less aggressive surgery and complications. Minim Invasive Neurosurg 2005;48:113.

[77] Eftekhar B, Ghodsi M, Nejat F, et al. Prophylactic administration of ceftriaxone for the prevention of meningitis after traumatic pneumocephalus: results of a clinical trial. J Neurosurg 2004;101:757.

[78] May AK, Fleming SB, Carpenter RO, et al. Influence of broad-spectrum antibiotic prophylaxis on intracranial pressure monitor infections and subsequent infectious complications in head-injured patients. Surg Infect (Larchmt) 2006;7:409.

[79] Kurtoglu M, Yanar H, Bilsel Y, et al. Venous thromboembolism prophylaxis after head and spinal trauma: intermittent pneumatic compression devices versus low molecular weight heparin. World J Surg 2004;28:807.

[80] Lu WY, Rhoney DH, Boling WB, et al. A review of stress ulcer prophylaxis in the neurosurgical intensive care unit. Neurosurgery 1997;41:416.

[81] Krakau K, Hansson A, Karlsson T, et al. Nutritional treatment of patients with severe traumatic brain injury during the first six months after injury. Nutrition 2007;23:308.

[82] Rhoney DH, Parker D Jr, Formea CM, et al. Tolerability of bolus versus continuous gastric feeding in brain-injured patients. Neurol Res 2002;24:613.

[83] Zengerink I, Brink PR, Laupland KB, et al. Needle thoracostomy in the treatment of a tension pneumothorax in trauma patients: what size needle? J Trauma 2008;64:111.

[84] Luchette FA, Barrie PS, Oswanski MF, et al. Practice management guidelines for prophylactic antibiotic use in tube thoracostomy for traumatic hemopneumothorax: the EAST Practice Management Guidelines Work Group. Eastern Association for Trauma. J Trauma 2000;48:753.

[85] Mandal AK, Thadepalli H, Chettipalli U. Posttraumatic empyema thoracis: a 24-year experience at a major trauma center. J Trauma 1997;43:764.

[86] Blaivas M, DeBehnke D, Phelan MB. Potential errors in the diagnosis of pericardial effusion on trauma ultrasound for penetrating injuries. Acad Emerg Med 2000;7:1261.

[87] Tayal VS, Beatty MA, Marx JA, et al. FAST (focused assessment with sonography in trauma) accurate for cardiac and intraperitoneal injury in penetrating anterior chest trauma. J Ultrasound Med 2004;23:467.

[88] Bakhos C, O'Connor J, Kyriakides T, et al. Vital capacity as a predictor of outcome in elderly patients with rib fractures. J Trauma 2006;61:131.

[89] Holcomb JB, McMullin NR, Kozar RA, et al. Morbidity from rib fractures increases after age 45. J Am Coll Surg 2003;196:549.

[90] Kallet RH, Jasmer RM, Pittet JF, et al. Clinical implementation of the ARDS network protocol is associated with reduced hospital mortality compared with historical controls. Crit Care Med 2005;33:925.

[91] Putensen C, Zech S, Wrigge H, et al. Long-term effects of spontaneous breathing during ventilatory support in patients with acute lung injury. Am J Respir Crit Care Med 2001; 164:43.

[92] Petsinger DE, Fernandez JD, Davies JD. What is the role of airway pressure release ventilation in the management of acute lung injury? Respir Care Clin N Am 2006;12:483.

[93] Branney SW, Moore EE, Feldhaus KM, et al. Critical analysis of two decades of experience with postinjury emergency department thoracotomy in a regional trauma center. J Trauma 1998;45:87.

[94] Weiss ES, Makary MA, Wang T, et al. Prevalence of blood-borne pathogens in an urban, university-based general surgical practice. Ann Surg 2005;241:803.

[95] Ng AK, Simons RK, Torreggiani WC, et al. Intra-abdominal free fluid without solid organ injury in blunt abdominal trauma: an indication for laparotomy. J Trauma 2002;52:1134.

[96] Ulman I, Avanoglu A, Ozcan C, et al. Gastrointestinal perforations in children: a continuing challenge to nonoperative treatment of blunt abdominal trauma. J Trauma 1996;41:110.

[97] Croce MA, Magnotti LJ, Savage SA, et al. Emergent pelvic fixation in patients with exsanguinating pelvic fractures. J Am Coll Surg 2007;204:935.

[98] Fang JF, Chen RJ, Lin BC. Cell count ratio: new criterion of diagnostic peritoneal lavage for detection of hollow organ perforation. J Trauma 1998;45:540.

[99] Talton DS, Craig MH, Hauser CJ, et al. Major gastroenteric injuries from blunt trauma. Am Surg 1995;61:69.

[100] Baldassarre E, Valenti G, Gambino M, et al. The role of laparoscopy in the diagnosis and the treatment of missed diaphragmatic hernia after penetrating trauma. J Laparoendosc Adv Surg Tech A 2007;17:302.

[101] Demetriades D, Hadjizacharia P, Constantinou C, et al. Selective nonoperative management of penetrating abdominal solid organ injuries. Ann Surg 2006;244:620.

[102] Weinberg JA, Magnotti LJ, Edwards NM, et al. "Awake" laparoscopy for the evaluation of equivocal penetrating abdominal wounds. Injury 2007;38:60.

[103] Galvan DA, Peitzman AB. Failure of nonoperative management of abdominal solid organ injuries. Curr Opin Crit Care 2006;12:590.

[104] McIntyre LK, Schiff M, Jurkovich GJ. Failure of nonoperative management of splenic injuries: causes and consequences. Arch Surg 2005;140:563.

[105] Gaarder C, Naess PA, Eken T, et al. Liver injuries: improved results with a formal protocol including angiography. Injury 2007;38:1075.

[106] Monnin V, Sengel C, Thony F, et al. Place of arterial embolization in severe blunt hepatic trauma: a multidisciplinary approach. Cardiovasc Intervent Radiol, 2008.

[107] Cothren CC, Osborn PM, Moore EE, et al. Preperitonal pelvic packing for hemodynamically unstable pelvic fractures: a paradigm shift. J Trauma 2007;62:834.

[108] Cowley RA. The resuscitation and stabilization of major multiple trauma patients in a trauma center environment. Clin Med 1976;83:14.

[109] Smith WR, Moore EE, Osborn P, et al. Retroperitoneal packing as a resuscitation technique for hemodynamically unstable patients with pelvic fractures: report of two representative cases and a description of technique. J Trauma 2005;59:1510.

[110] Olson SA, Glasgow RR. Acute compartment syndrome in lower extremity musculoskeletal trauma. J Am Acad Orthop Surg 2005;13:436.

[111] Weinmann M. Compartment syndrome. Emerg Med Serv 2003;32:36.

[112] Meldon SW, Reilly M, Drew BL, et al. Trauma in the very elderly: a community-based study of outcomes at trauma and nontrauma centers. J Trauma 2002;52:79.

[113] Taylor MD, Tracy JK, Meyer W, et al. Trauma in the elderly: intensive care unit resource use and outcome. J Trauma 2002;53:407.

[114] Demetriades D, Murray J, Brown C, et al. High-level falls: type and severity of injuries and survival outcome according to age. J Trauma 2005;58:342.

[115] Sterling DA, O'Connor JA, Bonadies J. Geriatric falls: injury severity is high and disproportionate to mechanism. J Trauma 2001;50:116.

[116] Stewart RM, Myers JG, Dent DL, et al. Seven hundred fifty-three consecutive deaths in a level I trauma center: the argument for injury prevention. J Trauma 2003;54:66.

[117] Bulger EM, Arneson MA, Mock CN, et al. Rib fractures in the elderly. J Trauma 2000;48:1040.

[118] Schrag SP, Toedter LJ, McQuay N Jr. Cervical spine fractures in geriatric blunt trauma patients with low-energy mechanism: are clinical predictors adequate? Am J Surg 2008;195:170.

[119] Hemmelgarn B, Levesque LE, Suissa S. Anti-diabetic drug use and the risk of motor vehicle crash in the elderly. Can J Clin Pharmacol 2006;13:e112.

[120] Landi F, Onder G, Cesari M, et al. Psychotropic medications and risk for falls among community-dwelling frail older people: an observational study. J Gerontol A Biol Sci Med Sci 2005;60:622.

[121] Pariente A, Dartigues JF, Benichou J, et al. Benzodiazepines and injurious falls in community dwelling elders. Drugs Aging 2008;25:61.

[122] Tornetta P III, Mostafavi H, Riina J, et al. Morbidity and mortality in elderly trauma patients. J Trauma 1999;46:702.

[123] Demetriades D, Karaiskakis M, Velmahos GC, et al. Pelvic fractures in pediatric and adult trauma patients: are they different injuries? J Trauma 2003;54:1146.

[124] Stylianos S, Egorova N, Guice KS, et al. Variation in treatment of pediatric spleen injury at trauma centers versus nontrauma centers: a call for dissemination of American Pediatric Surgical Association benchmarks and guidelines. J Am Coll Surg 2006;202:247.

[125] Stylianos S, Nathens AB. Comparing processes of pediatric trauma care at children's hospitals versus adult hospitals. J Trauma 2007;63:S96.

[126] Christmas AB, Reynolds J, Wilson AK, et al. Morbid obesity impacts mortality in blunt trauma. Am Surg 2007;73:1122.

[127] Amado JA, Lopez-Espadas F, Vazquez-Barquero A, et al. Blood levels of cytokines in brain-dead patients: relationship with circulating hormones and acute-phase reactants. Metabolism 1995;44:812.

[128] Duane TM, Dechert T, Aboutanos MB, et al. Obesity and outcomes after blunt trauma. J Trauma 2006;61:1218.

[129] Neville AL, Brown CV, Weng J, et al. Obesity is an independent risk factor of mortality in severely injured blunt trauma patients. Arch Surg 2004;139:983.

[130] Frei U, Noeldeke J, Machold-Fabrizii V, et al. Prospective age-matching in elderly kidney transplant recipients: a 5-year analysis of the Eurotransplant Senior Program. Am J Transplant 2008;8:50.

[131] Zapletal C, Faust D, Wullstein C, et al. Does the liver ever age? Results of liver transplantation with donors above 80 years of age. Transplant Proc 2005;37:1182.

[132] Doshi MD, Hunsicker LG. Short- and long-term outcomes with the use of kidneys and livers donated after cardiac death. Am J Transplant 2007;7:122.

ELSEVIER
SAUNDERS

Emerg Med Clin N Am
26 (2008) 649–683

EMERGENCY
MEDICINE
CLINICS OF
NORTH AMERICA

# Venothromboembolism

## J. Matthew Fields, MD, Munish Goyal, MD, FACEP*

*Department of Emergency Medicine, University of Pennsylvania School of Medicine,
3400 Spruce Street, Ground Ravdin Building, Philadelphia, PA 19104, USA*

Venothromboembolism (VTE) represents a spectrum of pathology from simple superficial thrombophlebitis to fatal pulmonary embolus (PE). It was first depicted in the thirteenth century, but was not described in the medical literature until the late 1600s [1,2]. In 1916, VTE became a treatable disease with the discovery of heparin. The presence of an effective therapy heightened the importance of diagnosing VTE, fueling a plethora of medical research and technologic developments over the next century. Despite advancements, VTE remains an elusive entity because of atypical presentations and associated diagnostic challenges.

In the mid to late twentieth century, autopsy and inpatient studies found PE was often deadly with an untreated mortality of 26% to 30% [3–5]. Up to 70% of PEs were diagnosed on autopsy that had not been suspected clinically [6]. The high frequency of missed diagnosis and mortality has since led clinicians aggressively to seek and treat this disorder. Recently, some authors suggest the incidence of VTE is lower in the emergency department (ED) population and may be less clinically significant than inpatient VTE [7]. Studies of ambulatory patients who did not receive anticoagulation for VTE failed to document negative outcomes of death or thrombus progression, challenging the idea that anticoagulation is beneficial to all patients with VTE [8,9]. Interestingly, heparin was accepted as the standard of care without studies validating its efficacy. A growing school of thought suggests that although PE is certainly fatal in some patients, it is a normal physiologic event in others that does not require treatment, and aggressive searches will likely identify patients with clinically insignificant VTE [7]. Unfortunately, no methods yet exist to identify patients who can safely be managed without anticoagulation.

Whether clinically significant or not, the occurrence of missed deep venous thrombosis (DVT) and PE is high [10,11], and when it is clinically

---

* Corresponding author.
*E-mail address:* munish.goyal@uphs.upenn.edu (M. Goyal).

suspected it is diagnosed only 20% to 35% of the time [12,13]. Classic presentations occur less frequently than atypical presentations and asymptomatic VTE is common. One recent study found 6.3% of cancer patients had asymptomatic VTE on routine imaging [14]. Furthermore, silent PE is present in approximately 40% to 60% of patients who present with DVT [8].

## Epidemiology

Because of the high rate of missed diagnosis, the true incidence of DVT and PE is unknown. In the United States, it is estimated that first-time VTE occurs in approximately 100 per 100,000 persons per year with approximately one third of cases caused by PE and two thirds of cases caused by DVT. There is no significant difference between men and women [15]. The incidence increases dramatically with age from less than 5 cases per 100,000 persons under the age of 15 to approximately 500 cases per 100,000 persons over the age of 80 [16,17]. The rate seems to increase sharply after age 45 [18]. Venous valve incompetence with increased venous stasis, sedentary lifestyle, and acquired comorbidities are some of the theoretic etiologies for the increased incidence with age. Other epidemiologic factors associated with increased incidence include white and African American race [19] and winter months [20].

## Pathophysiology

The spectrum of VTE begins with formation of a thrombus. In 1686, the surgeon Richard Wiseman suggested thrombus formation was related to coagulation of the serum, thickening of the blood, or venous obstruction, and recognized the high prevalence of VTE in both pregnancy and malignancy [2]. Rudolf Virchow [21] was later credited with the classic triad associated with VTE: stasis, endothelial injury, and hypercoagulability. When present, these factors disrupt the balance between endogenous fibrinolysis and fibrin formation contributing to the formation and propagation of thrombus. Vascular injury initiates release of tissue factor that activates factor Xa and leads to increased fibrin formation and deposition. Hypercoagulable states also offset the balance of the natural clotting cascade in favor of fibrin production and clot formation. Finally, venous stasis allows for increased fibrin cross-linking [22]. Clinical states that involve the presence of Virchow's triad result in a higher incidence of VTE (Box 1) [18,23,24].

## Deep vein thrombosis

Although thrombosis can occur anywhere in the venous system, it typically forms at locations of injury or stasis, particularly in the valve cusps in the venous sinuses of the calf veins [25]. Approximately 90% of DVTs

---

**Box 1. Risk factors for venous thromboembolism**

History of VTE
Major surgery
Trauma
Immobility
  Travel, paralysis, hospital or nursing home resident
Cancer
Increased estrogen states
  Pregnancy or puerperium, oral contraceptive pills, hormonal
    therapy
Indwelling central venous access devices
Age >45
Smoking
Medical comorbidities
  Congestive heart failure, chronic obstructive pulmonary
    disease, stroke
Obesity
Inherited coagulopathy
  Factor V Leiden mutation, antithrombin III deficiency, protein C
    deficiency, protein S deficiency, dysfibrinogenemia

---

occur in the lower extremities, but only thrombus from deeper and more proximal vessels are believed to embolize to the lungs. For this reason, the venous system is divided by proximity and depth. In the lower extremity, the superficial system is comprised of the greater and short saphenous veins (Fig. 1). The deep veins are divided into proximal and distal. The distal deep veins include the anterior tibial, posterior tibial, and peroneal veins (collectively called the calf veins). The proximal deep veins include the popliteal, superficial femoral, deep femoral, common femoral, and external iliac veins. A DVT is classified as distal if it is below the knee (also called a calf DVT) and proximal if it is located in the popliteal vein or above. Although distal DVTs are generally not thought to pose an immediate threat to embolization, there is a 20% to 30% incidence of propagation to the proximal venous system [26]. Clinically significant thrombosis can also involve pelvic veins, upper extremity veins, and venous sinuses of the skull.

*Clinical presentation*

The history and physical examination are helpful in suggesting thediagnosis, but no one sign or symptom in isolation maintains significant sensitivity or specificity for DVT [27]. Symptoms can include a sense of fullness, paresthesia, or pain in the calf or thigh. Physical examination may show unilateral leg edema, erythema, warmth, tenderness, or a palpable cord.

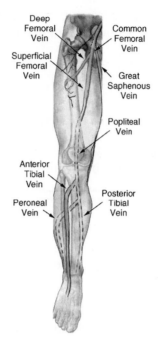

Fig. 1. Normal venous anatomy of the leg. (*From* Tracy JA, Edlow JA. Ultrasound diagnosis of deep venous thrombosis. Emerg Med Clin North Am 2004;22:776; with permission.)

The classic Homan's sign (sharp calf pain on passive dorsiflexion of the foot) has proved to be insensitive and nonspecific [28]. Although symptoms are less frequent with smaller and more distal clots, large proximal clots may also be asymptomatic in the presence of adequate collateral veins and patency of vessels [24]. The clinical signs and symptoms of DVT are often found in many other conditions affecting the lower extremity including musculoskeletal injuries, cellulitis, ruptured Baker's cyst, vasculitis, congestive heart failure, lymphedema, and other nonthrombotic conditions. Laboratory and radiologic testing are fundamental in the diagnosis of DVT.

*Ultrasound*

Ultrasound is the test of choice for diagnosis of DVT. It is fast, accurate, and readily available in most EDs. Since the 1990s, ultrasound has replaced venography as the gold standard for DVT evaluation. Ultrasound provides nearly equal diagnostic information while avoiding the risks of invasive venography, which has a 2% chance of inducing DVT [29].

The two methods of ultrasound commonly used when assessing DVT are compression and duplex. Compression ultrasound works by the principle that normal veins collapse when extrinsic pressure is applied by the sonographer. When a vein fails to collapse, it indicates the presence of an intravascular mass (thrombus by default) (Figs. 2–4).

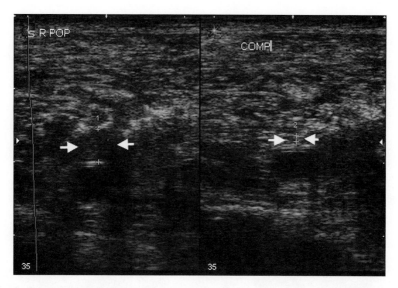

Fig. 2. Compression ultrasonography in normal lower extremity. Popliteal vein (*arrows*) collapses with compression (*right*). (*Courtesy of* Anthony J. Dean, MD, Philadelphia, PA.)

Duplex ultrasound is compression ultrasound with the addition of spectral and color flow Doppler to assess respiratory variation and augmentation. In contrast to compression ultrasonography that is easily learned and can be quickly performed by clinicians in the ED, duplex is relatively complicated, time consuming, and expensive. Despite these characteristics, it adds little to compression ultrasonography in the diagnosis of DVT (Table 1) [30–39].

When performing compression ultrasonography, assessment of the entire proximal venous system is unnecessary to rule out proximal DVT. In a study of 562 venograms performed on patients with DVT, no cases of isolated superficial femoral or pelvic vein thrombosis were identified. All DVTs

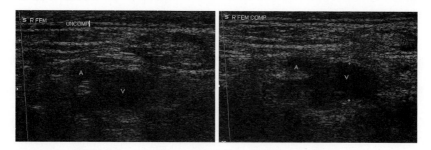

Fig. 3. Compression ultrasonography of DVT in the common femoral vein. Vein (V) does not collapse with compression (*right*) indicating presence of DVT. (*Courtesy of* Anthony J. Dean, MD, Philadelphia, PA.)

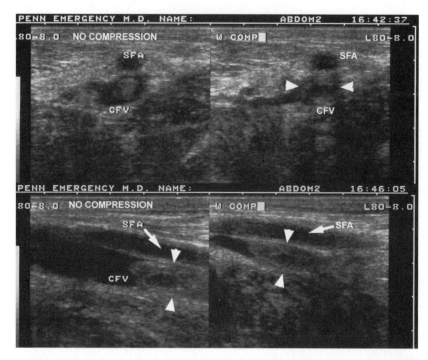

Fig. 4. Compression ultrasonography in axial (*top*) and longitudinal (*bottom*) views of DVT located in the common femoral vein (CFV). In addition to lack of compressibility (*right*), thrombus is visualized (*arrowheads and arrows*). SFA, superficial femoral artery. (*Courtesy of* Anthony J. Dean, MD, Philadelphia, PA.)

involved either the popliteal, common femoral, or both veins [40]. This has led to the development of limited compression ultrasonography (LCUS). LCUS is compression ultrasonography focused on the common femoral and popliteal veins. Despite rare case reports of isolated superficial femoral DVTs, studies have demonstrated the safety of withholding anticoagulation after negative LCUS [41,42]. It should be noted that LCUS is insensitive for calf DVTs and repeat ultrasonography in 7 days is recommended in certain high-risk patients (see later).

Many clinicians, including emergency physicians (EPs), are performing bedside ultrasonography to evaluate for DVTs. Jolly and colleagues [43] were the first to demonstrate the ability of EPs to perform color Doppler

Table 1
Performances of various ultrasonography methods for proximal deep venous thrombosis

| Ultrasonography method | % Sensitivity | % Specificity | % PPV | % NPV |
|---|---|---|---|---|
| Duplex [31–33] | 95–100 | 91–100 | 96–100 | 97–100 |
| Compression [34–36] | 93–100 | 96–100 | 99–100 | 92–100 |
| Limited compression [37–39] | 95–100 | 96–97 | 96–98 | 90–100 |

*Abbreviations:* NPV, negative predictive value; PPV, positive predictive value.

ultrasonography successfully in a retrospective observational analysis in 1994. Two EPs performed ultrasounds in the ED after training in a vascular laboratory (performing 25–30 studies each). The sensitivity and specificity of their color Doppler ultrasounds for acute DVTs were 100% (seven of seven) and 75% (six of eight), respectively. The two false-positives were patients with old DVT. In 1999, Frazee and colleagues [44] prospectively demonstrated a 95.7% negative predictive value (NPV) of EP-performed LCUS.

Although accurate, EPs can also maintain their goal of rapid throughput by performing LCUS. Blaivas and colleagues [45] demonstrated a median examination time of 3 minutes and 28 seconds of EP-performed LCUS, while maintaining a 98% correlation with vascular laboratory–performed studies on the same patients. Another study by Theodoro and colleagues [46] observed a 125-minute reduction in time to patient disposition with EP-performed US compared with radiology-performed US while also maintaining good correlation. Jang and colleagues [47] prospectively studied the ability of eight emergency medicine residents with minimal training in LCUS and found a sensitivity and specificity of 100% and 91.8%, respectively, with an average scan time of 11.7 minutes.

Recently, Maggazini and colleagues [48] demonstrated that full duplex scanning can also be performed effectively by EPs. After a 30-hour training course, five EPs performed duplex ultrasound on 399 patients who then had formal vascular scanning within 24 hours. EPs achieved a NPV of 100% and a positive predictive value of 95%. Although average study time was longer at approximately 10 minutes, the authors suggest that this is still more efficient than having the patient return for a repeat examination in 7 days (as recommended with LCUS) and avoids issues of failure to follow-up. Regardless of full versus limited studies, EP-performed ultrasonography may be particularly valuable in EDs without around-the-clock access to trained ultrasound technicians. Criticisms of ultrasonography include its inability to distinguish acute versus chronic DVT, decreased accuracy in obese patients, and lack of availability in some institutions.

*Other imaging modalities*

The traditional gold standard diagnostic modality for DVT was contrast venography, which yields a 99% to 100% sensitivity and specificity [49]. This invasive test is rarely performed because of high demand of resources and associated complications [50].

CT venography (CTV) is a diagnostic modality that evaluates the pelvis, thighs, and calves after injection of venous phase contrast material. It has near equal sensitivity and specificity to ultrasound for diagnosing proximal DVT [51]. Because CT angiography (CTA) of the pulmonary vessels and CTV can be performed simultaneously, CTA-CTV is an attractive option for patients with concern for both DVT and PE. Furthermore, CTV can diagnose pelvic and calf DVTs. Cost, radiation exposure (particularly through the reproductive organs), intravenous contrast exposure, and need for intravenous access are ongoing concerns about the use of CTV.

Magnetic resonance venography is another attractive alternative for diagnosis of DVT. It is highly accurate with a sensitivity of 100% and specificity of 98% to 99% for pelvic and proximal DVTs. It is less reliable for calf DVTs (sensitivity 68%), but often provides an alternative nonthrombotic diagnosis [52]. MRI is able to distinguish between acute and chronic DVTs. As opposed to CT, pelvic and lower-extremity MRI is considered safe in pregnancy. Cost and availability have limited the use of magnetic resonance venography in clinical practice.

Impedance plethysmography is a noninvasive test that estimates blood volume by measuring changes in electrical resistance in a targeted area of the body. Although it can be used to diagnose DVT, impedance plethysmography is less favorable in the ED and other clinical settings because of lower sensitivity when compared with LCUS, common interobserver disagreements, and lack of availability [35,53].

## D-dimer

D-dimer is an end product of clot lysis. Its presence signifies the existence of thrombus with an active deposition and degradation of cross-linked fibrin by plasmin [22]. Small amounts of D-dimer are normally present in the serum; however, elevated D-dimer levels correlate with increased thrombus volume. The D-dimer test does not discriminate between physiologic (eg, postoperative or posttrauma) and pathologic (eg, deep vein) thrombus. D-dimer levels may also be elevated in cancer, late pregnancy, recent trauma or surgery, sepsis, and many other medical conditions, limiting its use [54]. For these reasons the D-dimer is a sensitive, but nonspecific test. Many clinical algorithms have incorporated D-dimer testing as a way to rule out DVT and prevent the need for further imaging [55–59].

There are currently three main ways of detecting D-dimer levels in the bloodstream: (1) ELISA, (2) latex-agglutination, and (3) whole-blood agglutination. The ELISA test is the gold standard, yielding 95% sensitivity and 45% specificity for PE and a 94% sensitivity and 43% specificity for DVT. A typical 4-hour turnaround time, however, hinders the use of ELISA in the ED [60]. Rapid ELISA tests, however, are suitable for ED use. They perform similarly to standard ELISA and can be run in 35 minutes [60].

First-generation latex-agglutination tests are inexpensive and rapid, but lack adequate sensitivity for ED testing [61]. Newer second-generation latex-agglutination tests use immunoturbidimetric techniques and demonstrate sensitivity profiles similar to ELISA. Studies of second-generation latex-agglutination D-dimer tests have been used in low- and intermediate-risk patients to exclude VTE [56,57].

Whole-blood agglutination tests are qualitative tests that change color when D-dimer is bound by a monoclonal antibody that is linked to another monoclonal antibody, binding red blood cells. Whole-blood agglutination is rapid and inexpensive, but is criticized for being operator dependent. Sensitivity and specificity are approximately 87% and 68%, respectively, but it has been combined with low pretest probability scores to achieve high NPVs successfully for VTE [58].

Appropriate use of D-dimer testing in VTE hinges on understanding the concepts of pretest probability, likelihood ratio, and posttest probability. In the example of VTE and D-dimer, the pretest probability is the chance that the patient has VTE before D-dimer testing. The posttest probability is the chance of disease after testing. The negative likelihood ratio (NLR) is a factor that when applied to the pretest probability yields the posttest probability given a negative D-dimer. Each D-dimer test has a different NLR and yields different posttest probabilities for a given pretest probability (Table 2).

Before obtaining a D-dimer test, the clinician should determine whether a negative result yields a posttest probability acceptable for excluding VTE. This requires an understanding of the patient's pretest probability and the NLR of the D-dimer test being used. Most studies that validate D-dimer testing focus on patients with a low pretest probability and implement a D-dimer test with a strong NLR [55,57–59,62–65]. D-dimer tests maintain a higher specificity if used in appropriate patient populations, such as younger, otherwise healthy people, without comorbid conditions or late pregnancy.

Causes for a false-negative D-dimer test include small amounts of thrombus, old thrombus, and impaired fibrinolysis. D-dimer levels correlate with the amount of thrombus surface area participating in active fibrinolysis. For this reason, D-dimer testing is often negative with smaller thrombi, as is seen with distal DVTs [66,67]. Older clots tend to stabilize with cross-linked fibrin and may produce little or no D-dimer. D-dimer levels may normalize as early as 7 days after clot formation [68]. Finally, acute thrombus may not generate D-dimer in patients with impaired endogenous fibrinolysis [69].

## Clinical pathways

Although the diagnosis of DVT by physical examination alone is inadequate, performing radiologic testing on all patients is unnecessary. Furthermore, performing serial ultrasonography on all patients is inefficient because only 1% to 2% of patients have proximal DVT on repeat imaging after initial negative ultrasound [70,71]. In 1995, Wells and colleagues [36] discovered that implementation of clinical prediction rules to assess a patient's pretest probability could reduce the need for formal radiologic studies to rule out DVT. In 1997, Wells and colleagues [72] demonstrated that a single negative LCUS was sufficient to rule out DVT in low-risk patients. In 2003, Wells and colleagues [58] showed that a negative whole-blood agglutination or immunoturbidimetric D-dimer test eliminated the need for ultrasound in low- and intermediate-risk patients. Although a negative D-dimer test does not eliminate the need for ultrasound in the high-risk population, it did predict

Table 2
Negative likelihood ratios of various D-dimer tests

| D-dimer | Deep vein thrombosis | | | Pulmonary embolus | | |
|---|---|---|---|---|---|---|
| | NLR (95% CI) | Post-test probability Given (-) D-dimer | | NLR (95% CI) | Post-test probability Given (-) D-dimer | |
| | | PTP 20% | PTP 40% | | PTP 20% | PTP 40% |
| ELISA | 0.15 (0.07–0.30) | 3.6 | 9.1 | 0.11 (0.03–0.39) | 2.7 | 6.8 |
| Quantitative rapid ELISA | 0.08 (0.02–0.38) | 2 | 5.1 | 0.05 (0.00–4.15) | 1.2 | 3.2 |
| Semiquantitative rapid ELISA | 0.21 (0.10–0.42) | 5 | 12.3 | 0.15 (0.02–1.13) | 3.6 | 9.1 |
| Qualitative rapid ELISA | 0.13 (0.06–0.32) | 3.1 | 8 | 0.11 (0.01–1.45) | 2.7 | 6.8 |
| Quantitative latex | 0.21 (0.12–0.38) | 5 | 12.3 | 0.21 (0.09–0.49) | 5 | 12.3 |
| Semiquantitative latex | 0.31 (0.21–0.47) | 7.2 | 17.1 | 0.29 (0.14–0.58) | 6.8 | 16.2 |
| Whole-blood agglutination | 0.25 (0.18–0.36) | 5.9 | 14.3 | 0.28 (0.18–0.43) | 6.5 | 15.7 |

*Abbreviations:* NLR, negative likelihood ratio; PTP, pretest probability.

*Data from* Stein PD, Hull RD, Patel KC, et al. D-dimer for the exclusion of acute venous thrombosis and pulmonary embolism: a systematic review. Ann Intern Med 2004;140(8):596.

which patients required repeat ultrasonography for the possibility of a missed distal DVT on LCUS. In this latter study, the Wells' criteria were simplified (Table 3) into a dichotomous outcome of pretest probability ("DVT likely" or "DVT unlikely") [58,72]. Although other prediction rules exist, the modified Wells' criteria are the most validated in the literature [36,55,73–75].

Studies by Wells and others can be assimilated into a simple clinical pathway to approach the diagnosis of DVT (Fig. 5) [36,55,65,74,76,77]. A negative D-dimer test or a negative LCUS in the "DVT unlikely" group rules out DVT and these patients do not require serial ultrasonography. All patients in the "DVT likely" group should undergo ultrasonography. In patients with a negative LCUS and positive D-dimer test, repeat ultrasonography is recommended to exclude the possibility of distal DVT, which have a 20% to 30% incidence of propagation [24].

When ultrasound is unavailable, other diagnostic modalities including CTV, magnetic resonance venography, and contrast venography may be used. Another approach is to administer one dose of low-molecular-weight heparin (LMWH) and arrange an outpatient ultrasound within 24 hours. Anderson and colleagues [74] validated the safety of this approach in low- and intermediate-risk patients. In this study, low-risk patients were given no treatment, whereas intermediate-risk patients were given one dose of LMWH before ED discharge. No patients developed PE or major bleeding within 48 hours of initial ED presentation.

Table 3
Clinical model for predicting the pretest probability of deep vein thrombosis

| Clinical characteristic | Score |
| --- | --- |
| Active cancer (treatment ongoing, administered within previous 6 mo or palliative) | 1 |
| Paralysis, paresis, or recent plaster immobilization of the lower extremities | 1 |
| Recently bedridden >3 d or major surgery within previous 12 wk requiring general or regional anesthesia | 1 |
| Localized tenderness along the distribution of the deep venous system | 1 |
| Swelling of the entire leg | 1 |
| Calf swelling >3 cm larger than asymptomatic side (measured 10 cm below tibial tuberosity) | 1 |
| Pitting edema confined to the symptomatic leg | 1 |
| Collateral superficial veins (nonvaricose) | 1 |
| Previously documented DVT | 1 |
| Alternative diagnosis at least as likely as DVT | −2 |

In patients who have symptoms in both legs, the more symptomatic leg is used.

A score of 2 or higher indicates that the probability of DVT is "likely"; a score of less than 2 indicates that the probability is "unlikely."

*Abbreviation:* DVT, deep venous thrombosis.

*From* Wells PS, Anderson DR, Rodger M, et al. Evaluation of D-Dimer in the diagnosis of suspected deep vein thrombosis. N Engl J Med 2003;349:1230 with permission. Copyright © 2003, Massachusetts Medical Society.

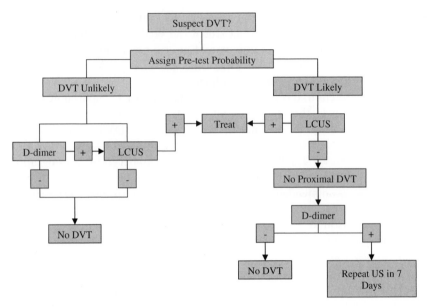

Fig. 5. Clinical algorithm for the diagnosis of suspected DVT. DVT, deep vein thrombosis; LCUS, limited compression ultrasonography.

## Treatment and management

VTE occurs from an imbalance in endogenous fibrin formation and fibrinolysis. The cornerstone of VTE treatment is pharmacologic anticoagulation. Anticoagulants work by inhibiting the clotting cascade and shifting the imbalance back in favor of endogenous fibrinolysis. No randomized controlled trial has ever been performed proving the usefulness of heparin, and it was accepted as standard therapy before the widespread use of current diagnostic modalities. Treatment with either fixed-dosing LMWH or adjusted-dosing unfractionated heparin (UH) is acceptable. Benefits of LMWH include easier dosing, no required serial laboratory studies, and easier transition to the outpatient setting potentially decreasing hospital length of stay. A meta-analysis of LMWH versus UH found LMWH more efficacious with significantly less complications including major bleeding events and death, suggesting superiority of LMWH [78].

One major limitation of LMWH is cost. Two studies have now demonstrated that subcutaneous UH can be used alone to treat VTE with similar efficacy and safety as LMWH [79,80]. Furthermore, Kearon and colleagues [79] validated a safe and effective method of fixed-dosing subcutaneous UH that does not require following activated partial thromboplastin times. Pending further studies, subcutaneous UH may provide a significantly cheaper and promising alternative to LMWH.

Outpatient management of proximal DVT can be achieved with LMWH [81]. Although this is possible from the ED it requires a clinical pathway in place that can ensure patient teaching, safety, and follow-up. Unfortunately, studies attempting to validate outpatient treatment from the ED suffer from such issues as prolonged ED stays and high patient exclusion rates [81,82].

Generalized fibrinolysis (commonly referred to as "thrombolysis") is a less frequently used therapeutic intervention. Unlike heparin's reliance on endogenous fibrinolysis, the administration of recombinant or bacterial tissue plasminogen activators increase circulating plasmin and accelerate fibrin breakdown. Although it has been shown to improve speed of clot resolution and a decreased incidence of postthrombotic complications [83], generalized fibrinolysis is associated with an increased risk of bleeding, including intracranial hemorrhage, and is generally not used in the management of DVT. Catheter-directed fibrinolysis and surgical thrombectomy are reserved for special situations including phlegmasia cerulea dolens and some cases of catheter-related upper-extremity DVT [26,84].

*Special cases*

Upper-extremity DVT includes thrombosis in the internal jugular, innominate, subclavian, or axillary veins. It occurs in approximately 16 per 100,000 persons in the United States [85]. Central access devices represent the largest risk factor and are associated with 80% of all upper-extremity DVTs [86]. Peripherally inserted central catheters, frequently used for their lower incidence of infectious complications, have a 10% to 40% incidence of upper-extremity DVT [87,88]. It is unclear why some patients form spontaneous (noncatheter associated) upper-extremity DVTs. An analysis of one large registry found younger age, lower body mass index, non-white race, and smoking to be factors more common in spontaneous upper-extremity DVTs, suggesting this entity has a different pathophysiology from other forms of VTE [89]. Although the incidences of PE and postthrombotic syndrome are poorly defined, upper-extremity DVTs warrant anticoagulation therapy [85,90].

Phlegmasia cerulea dolens is a severe form of DVT in which venous obstruction of the major deep veins and collateral veins leads to a sharp rise in venous pressure, massive interstitial fluid shifts, decreased arterial perfusion, compartment syndrome, and gangrene. Recognition of phlegmasia cerulea dolens (Fig. 6) is important in the ED for consideration of time-sensitive interventions, including anticoagulation, catheter-directed thrombolysis, and vascular surgical consultation [91–93].

Previously, it was believed that isolated calf DVTs did not pose a thromboembolic risk. Longitudinal studies have since shown a 20% to 30% incidence of clot propagation to the proximal venous system with a 20% incidence of embolization [94]. In symptomatic patients, LCUS provides only 73% sensitivity for distal DVTs [70]. High-risk patients with a negative LCUS and positive D-dimer test should undergo repeat ultrasound in 7 days to exclude propagation of a distal clot [56]. In addition to clot propagation

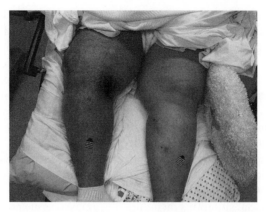

Fig. 6. Phlegmasia cerulea dolens. (*Courtesy of* Anthony J. Dean, MD, Philadelphia, PA.)

and PE, distal DVTs result in postthrombotic complications, such as pain, edema, and hyperpigmentation, in 10% to 38% of patients [24,94,95]. Treatment of distal DVT is controversial and either aspirin or low-dose LMWH therapy is currently acceptable. Given the incidence of clot propagation and postthrombotic complications, many clinicians recommend treating distal DVTs the same as proximal DVTs with full anticoagulation therapy [94]. When aspirin therapy is used alone, serial ultrasonography is recommended to ensure lack of propagation to proximal vessels.

Superficial thrombophlebitis in the absence of proximal DVT is not known directly to lead to PE. Approximately 8% of superficial thrombophlebitis can extend into the deep venous system, however, usually at the site of the proximal greater saphenous vein, and potentially embolize to the lung [96]. The main concern in the ED is to rule out superficial thrombophlebitis extension into the deep venous system by ultrasonography. Isolated superficial thrombophlebitis does not require admission, but treatment should be initiated to prevent propagation to deeper veins. Aspirin and LMWH both decrease superficial thrombophlebitis propagation and recurrence with similar efficacy and safety, and either is an acceptable option for superficial thrombophlebitis of the legs [97]. Graded compression stockings, heat pads, and elevation of the affected extremity may help provide symptomatic relief.

## Pulmonary embolism

### Pathophysiology

PE occurs when a thrombus breaks free from the endothelial wall, travels through the right side of the heart, and lodges into the narrowing pulmonary arteries. Depending on the size and shape of the clot, it may come to rest in the main pulmonary artery, in a tiny subsegmental artery, or anywhere in between. The shape may allow for normal blood flow or it may obstruct an entire vessel. Minute differences within the vasculature can lead to a myriad of pathophysiologic consequences resulting in a wide range of clinical signs and symptoms.

PE causes mismatching of ventilation and perfusion (V/Q). Alveoli with obstructed pulmonary capillaries become overventilated relative to the decreased blood flow, increasing functional dead space. Increased blood flow to unaffected pulmonary capillaries, despite unchanged alveolar ventilation, causes transpulmonary shunting. Pulmonary vascular resistance also increases by both the physical obstruction from the clot and inflammatory cytokine-mediated pulmonary vasoconstriction. The increase in pulmonary vascular resistance leads to increased right heart pressures, which can induce right heart failure or open previously closed atrial septal defects, leading to intracardiac shunting. In patients with normal lungs, the degree of pulmonary vascular resistance correlates with the degree of obstruction on pulmonary angiogram [98]. Pleural effusions develop from venous congestion and increased interstitial fluid secondary to ischemia and the release of inflammatory cytokines [99]. Pulmonary infarction is thought to be an uncommon occurrence from VTE because of the redundant oxygen sources including the pulmonary arteries, airways, and bronchial arteries. When thrombus obstructs smaller pulmonary arteries, blood can extravasate into alveoli preventing oxygenation from the airways. When this blood cannot be cleared quickly, as in left ventricular failure, pulmonary infarction can occur [98].

*Clinical presentation*

Symptoms associated with PE depend on the degree of vascular obstruction, the magnitude of inflammatory response, and the patient's physiologic reserve. V/Q mismatch manifests as dyspnea, hypoxemia, and increased A-a gradient. Extravasation of blood into alveoli can cause pleuritic pain, cough, or hemoptysis. Increased pulmonary vascular resistance can lead to strain patterns on EKG; pleural effusions; right ventricular dilatation or hypokinesis; or severe right heart outflow obstruction manifesting as hypotension, syncope, or pulseless electrical activity cardiac arrest. It may also manifest as hypoxia if previously closed atrial septal defects open and cause significant transcardiac shunting. The natural history of PE is to present atypically and can include any combination of these findings or none at all.

Multiple studies have demonstrated the variability in clinical manifestations of PE (Table 4) [13,100]. The most common finding is dyspnea with 79% of patients with PE having dyspnea at rest or on exertion [13]. In PIOPED II, when PE was suspected and diagnosed, 97% to 98% of patients had at least one of the following: dyspnea, tachypnea, pleuritic pain, or signs of a DVT. Dyspnea or tachypnea was less frequent in elderly patients and at least one patient manifested circulatory collapse in the absence of dyspnea.

Table 4
Frequency of symptoms and signs in pulmonary embolus

| | No prior CPD | | All patients | |
|---|---|---|---|---|
| Symptoms of pulmonary embolism | % PE | % No PE | % PE | % No PE |
| Dyspnea | | | | |
|   Dyspnea (rest or exertion) | 73 | 68 | 79 | 73 |
|   Dyspnea (at rest) | 55 | 46 | 61 | 54 |
|   Dyspnea (exertion only) | 16 | 20 | 16 | 18 |
|   Orthopnea (>1-pillow) | 28 | 24 | 36 | 35 |
| Pleuritic chest pain | | | | |
| Chest pain (not pleuritic) | 44 | 57[a] | 47 | 59[a] |
| Cough | 19 | 22 | 17 | 21 |
|   Hemoptysis | 34 | 28 | 43 | 39 |
| Wheezing | 5 | 3 | 6 | 4 |
| Calf or thigh | 21 | 18 | 31 | 31 |
|   Swelling | 41 | 17[b] | 39 | 20[b] |
|   Pain | 44 | 23[b] | 42 | 25[a] |
| Calf and thigh | | | | |
|   Swelling | 7 | 4 | 8 | 6 |
|   Pain | 17 | 7[b] | 16 | 10[a] |

| | No prior CPD | | All patients | |
|---|---|---|---|---|
| Signs of pulmonary embolism | % PE | % No PE | % PE | % No PE |
| General | | | | |
|   Tachypnea ($\geq$20/min) | 54 | 43[a] | 57 | 47[a] |
|   Tachycardia ($\geq$100/min) | 24 | 14[a] | 26 | 16[a] |
|   Diaphoresis | 2 | 7[a] | 4 | 6 |
|   Cyanosis | 0 | 0.003 | 1 | 0 |
|   Temperature $\geq$38.5°C ($\geq$101.3°F) | 1 | 3 | 2 | 2 |
| Cardiac examination (abnormal) | 21 | 11[a] | 22 | 12[b] |
|   Increased P2 | 15 | 5[b] | 15 | 5[b] |
|   Right ventricular lift | 4 | 2 | 5 | 2[a] |
|   Jugular venous distention | 14 | 8%[a] | 13 | 8[a] |
| Lung examination (abnormal) | 29 | 26 | 37 | 36 |
|   Rales (crackles) | 18 | 14 | 21 | 18 |
|   Wheezes | 2 | 3 | 3 | 9 |
|   Rhonchi | 2 | 2 | 5 | 5 |
|   Decreased breath sounds | 17 | 12 | 21 | 17 |
|   Pleural friction rub | 0 | 1 | 1 | 1 |
| DVT signs[c] | | | | |
|   Calf or thigh | 47 | 21[b] | 47 | 23[b] |
|   Calf and thigh | 14 | 4[b] | 12 | 5[b] |

*Abbreviations:* CPD, cardiopulmonary disease; DVT, deep venous thrombosis; PE, pulmonary embolism; P2, pulmonary component of second sound.

[a] $P<.05$

[b] $P<.01$

[c] Edema, erythema, tenderness, or palpable cord.

*Data from* Stein PD, Beemath A, Matta F, et al. Clinical characteristics of patients with acute pulmonary embolism: data from PIOPED II. Am J Med 2007;120:875–6.

*Nondiagnostic tests*

Similar to clinical signs and symptoms, most tests used in the ED have poor sensitivity and specificity for PE and are nondiagnostic. Nondiagnostic tests that may be abnormal in PE include electrocardiogram, chest radiograph, arterial blood gas, echocardiography, brain natriuretic peptide, and troponin-T. Nondiagnostic tests help suggest PE, but are inconclusive.

*Electrocardiogram*

The EKG occasionally reveals manifestations of right heart strain, usually in patients with massive PE. The most common finding in patients with non-massive PE is normal sinus rhythm. In patients with massive PE, anterior T-wave inversions were found more frequently (68%) than sinus tachycardia (28%) or S1Q3T3 (50%) (Fig. 7) [101]. The number of inverted T-waves in the anterior and inferior distribution seems to increase with severity of cor pulmonale and resulting subepicardial ischemia and predicts early complications from PE [102]. In a population of patients with confirmed PE studied by Kosuge and colleagues [103], T-wave inversions in both leads V1 and III had 99% specificity. Some authors suggest that the finding of simultaneous T-wave inversions in the anterior and inferior leads should prompt consideration of PE even when it had not been previously suspected.

Other EKG findings are less helpful. Sinus tachycardia is present in less than half of cases [13]. The classic S1Q3T3 pattern sometimes found in the subset of patients with right heart strain has low sensitivity and specificity. Atrial fibrillation, right bundle branch block, and axis change occur with considerable variability and are less clinically useful [104].

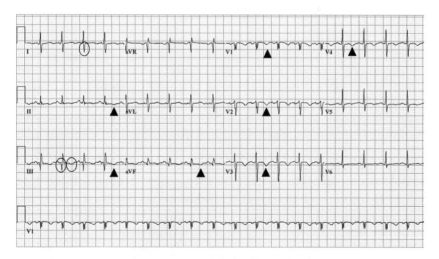

Fig. 7. EKG findings in a patient with massive PE. Sinus tachycardia, S1Q3T3 (*circles*), and anterior-inferior T-wave inversions (*triangles*).

## Chest radiography

Manifestations of PE on chest radiograph include cardiomegaly, pleural effusions, elevated hemidiaphragm, pulmonary artery enlargement, atelectasis, infiltrate, pulmonary congestion, and the rarely described Hampton's hump and Westermark's sign. One study found that 76% of patients with PE have some abnormality on chest radiograph, but these abnormalities were nonspecific [105].

## Arterial blood gas and pulse oximetry

The arterial blood gas and pulse oximetry do not reliably predict the presence of PE and 25% to 35% of patients with diagnosed PE have a normal arterial blood gas, pulse oximetry, and A-a gradient [106–108]. Obtaining arterial blood is relatively invasive and its inability to affect management makes it a less favored test among clinicians [108]. Furthermore, if fibrinolytics are being considered as a treatment option, arterial puncture should be limited.

## Alveolar dead space measurements

When a PE obstructs blood flow to alveoli that are still ventilated, the amount of dead space is increased. An increase in dead space is indirect evidence of PE. Studies of alveolar dead space measurements combined with other clinical factors have shown promise in ruling out PE quickly and without imaging in the ED [109–111]. These measurements have not gained widespread acceptance in the ED because it requires obtaining an arterial blood gas and the presence of a respiratory therapist with specialized equipment to perform capnography.

## Echocardiography

Echocardiography (echo) is a useful adjunct in the diagnosis of PE. Its application in the ED is most pertinent in patients presenting in extremis when rapid diagnosis is essential and fibrinolysis may be indicated. Furthermore, echo has the ability to rule out other conditions, such as pericardial effusion and tamponade, which also cause hypotension, but present a contraindication to fibrinolysis. Findings can include right ventricular dilatation (Fig. 8), right ventricular hypokinesis, intracardiac thrombus, abnormal septal wall motion, and loss of the normal inferior vena cava collapse index [112,113]. Grifoni and colleagues [113] demonstrated 51% sensitivity and 87% specificity of echo for PE, but when applied to patients with massive PE, sensitivity and NPV were 97% and 98%, respectively. Studies have demonstrated the ability of nonexpert sonographers to identify cardiac abnormalities associated with PE [114,115]. When echo is performed, ultrasound of the legs can easily be performed also to assess for DVT. Grifoni

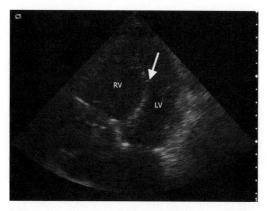

Fig. 8. Bedside echo in patient with massive PE causing right ventricular (RV) dilatation and bowing of interventricular septum (*arrow*) into left ventricle (LV). (Courtesy of Anthony J. Dean, MD, Philadelphia, PA.)

and colleagues [113] also found that when two of three of the following clinical parameters were present (high clinical probability, right ventricular dilatation, or DVT) massive PE was present in 97% of patients with a NPV of 98%.

## Diagnostic tests

Diagnostic tests are tests that maintain good clinical use in diagnosis of PE with either high sensitivity, specificity, or both. Diagnostic tests are often found in clinical algorithms and include D-dimer and various radiologic studies (CTA, CTV, CTA-CTV, V/Q scan, magnetic resonance angiography [MRA], pulmonary angiography).

## D-dimer

The same principles apply to D-dimer in PE as in DVT. D-dimer tests have been combined with clinical prediction rules successfully and safely to reduce imaging. The use of the test depends on the likelihood ratio and acceptable posttest probability, which some claim less than 2% for PE. Generally, as in DVT, its use in PE is reserved for low probability patients, because it is only in this group that a negative D-dimer test acceptably rules out PE. There are multiple types of D-dimer and one must be familiar with the operating characteristics, specifically the NLR, of the D-dimer test in one's own institution.

## CT

CTA has become the imaging test of choice to diagnose PE [116]. It is quick, widely available, relatively noninvasive, and performs similarly to formal pulmonary MRA [117]. Studies of multidetector row CTA (MDR-CTA) show an 82% to 100% sensitivity and 89% to 98% specificity for diagnosing PE [117–120]. CTA provides a diagnostic binary outcome ("PE" or "no PE") in 95% of cases, making it preferred over other imaging modalities, such as V/Q scan, which may provide indeterminate results [121]. Furthermore, CTA often offers alternative diagnoses when PE is absent.

Data from PIOPED II shows that CTA follows the rules of Bayes' theorem similarly to other diagnostic tests in VTE, in that the positive and negative predictive values of CTA are affected by the pretest probability of disease. A negative CTA is more likely a true-negative in the low-risk group, and a positive CTA is most likely a true-positive in the high-risk group (Table 5) [118]. In high-risk patients, the NPV is a disappointing 60%. In this group, the addition of CTV to CTA augments the NPV to 82% and is recommended [116,122–124].

The weakness of CTA is its poor ability to detect small peripheral PEs. Despite improved visualization of segmental and subsegmental PEs with MDR-CTA over single-detector row CTA, these emboli are still imaged poorly with CT [117,120,125]. In addition, MDR-CTA often overrepresents subsegmental PEs when they are not present. In PIOPED II, a subsegmental PE in a low clinical probability patient was most often a false-positive with a positive predictive value of only 25% [118]. Furthermore, there is poor interobserver agreement between radiologists when diagnosing subsegmental PE on CT scan [120,125].

The dilemma in diagnosing smaller peripheral PEs is underscored by the uncertainty of their clinical significance. Studies comparing MDR-CTA with single-detector row CTA show a higher diagnosis rate of subsegmental PEs with MDR-CTA [120,126]. Some argue that these subsegmental emboli are significant, because MDR-CTA does not increase the overall diagnosis rate of PE when compared with previous studies, such as PIOPED I,

Table 5
Positive predictive values and negative predictive values of computed tomographic angiography and venography compared with previous clinical assessment

| | Clinical probability | | |
| | High value (95% CI) | Intermediate value (95% CI) | Low value (95% CI) |
| Variable | | | |
|---|---|---|---|
| PPV CTA | 96 (78–99) | 92 (84–96) | 58 (40–73) |
| PPV CTA or CTV | 96 (81–99) | 90 (82–94) | 57 (40–72) |
| NPV CTA | 60 (32–83) | 89 (82–93) | 96 (92–98) |
| NPV of both CTA and CTV | 82 (48–97) | 92 (85–96) | 97 (92–98) |

*Abbreviations:* CTA, computed tomographic angiography; CTV, computed tomographic venography; NPV, negative predictive value; PPV, positive predictive value.

*Data from* Stein PD, Fowler SE, Goodman LR, et al. Multidetector computed tomography for acute pulmonary embolism. N Engl J Med 2006;354:2325.

suggesting these subsegmental PEs were also picked up on V/Q scan and pulmonary angiography [12]. A recent randomized controlled trial of MDR-CTA versus V/Q scan, however, proves otherwise. In this study MDR-CTA increased the diagnosis rate of PE (19%) compared with V/Q scan (14.2%) [127]. In patients in whom PE was excluded, 0.4% of the MDR-CTA group and 1% of the V/Q scan group developed VTE in follow-up. Despite the superior detection of PE with MDR-CTA, withholding anticoagulation based on a negative single-detector row CTA scan seems to be safe with less than 1% of patients developing VTE after 3 months [128,129]. These findings prompt the question whether these additional subsegmental PEs found on MDR-CTA are clinically relevant. No study has demonstrated safety in withholding anticoagulation to patients with diagnosed isolated subsegmental PEs, but some authors liken them to distal DVTs that do not necessarily warrant full anticoagulation. Given the dynamic balance of fibrin formation and breakdown in the body, some believe that one of the natural functions of the lung vasculature is to filter the blood and prevent clots from traveling to other end-organs. Others believe, however, that diagnosis of subsegmental PE is evidence of a prothrombotic state and increased risk for further VTE.

Drawbacks to CTA are mainly radiation exposure and possible untoward effects of intravenous contrast including anaphylactoid reactions, contrast extravasation, and contrast nephropathy. Additionally, renal insufficiency, prior contrast allergy, and hemodynamic instability are relative contraindications, or require preparation.

## Ventilation-perfusion scanning

Before single and MDR-CT, the V/Q scan was the first-line imaging modality for PE. It is a nuclear imaging test that assesses for areas of ventilation without perfusion as evidence of PE. Scan results include normal, low probability, intermediate probability, or high probability. The appropriate interpretation of results depends on assessment of pretest probability. In the original PIOPED study, a high probability scan was 96% accurate when the clinical probability was high, but only 56% accurate when clinical probability was low [12]. Furthermore, 57% of patients with PE had low- or intermediate-probability V/Q scans. Because of frequent indeterminate results, V/Q scans do not affect management 40% to 60% of the time, making it a less popular test in the ED [130].

Patients who have structurally abnormal lungs from chronic lung disease, mass, cavitation or other pathology usually have an abnormal V/Q scan despite the absence of PE. A normal chest radiograph increases the likelihood of a diagnostic V/Q scan, whereas patients with abnormal chest radiographs have diagnostic scintigraphy only 9% of the time in one report [131]. Still, the V/Q scan is useful and needed in a subset of patients with a contraindication to CT. Data from PIOPED II are more promising for V/Q scan than

PIOPED I, finding a determinate result of "PE" or "no PE" in 77.4% of patients [121].

## Pulmonary angiography

Pulmonary angiography is the gold standard for PE diagnosis, but its many disadvantages make it less useful in the ED. It is invasive, expensive, and generally not readily available. Furthermore, CTA now provides a modality with near identical detection rates. In a comparison of digital subtraction pulmonary angiography with MDR-CTA, MDR-CTA demonstrated 100% sensitivity and specificity of 89% with digital subtraction pulmonary angiography as the reference standard. More proximal clots were detected with MDR-CTA, whereas digital subtraction pulmonary angiography picked up more distal clots. There were three false-positives on MDR-CTA, which when reviewed had characteristic appearances of PE. Even though they were not seen on digital subtraction pulmonary angiography, the authors suggested that these were probably true-positives and the digital subtraction pulmonary angiography was incorrect. If MDR-CTA was used as the reference standard, pulmonary angiography would have a sensitivity, specificity, and accuracy of 86%, 100%, and 97%, respectively [117].

## Magnetic resonance angiography

MRA provides another diagnostic choice in PE diagnosis. Multiple MRA techniques exist with varying degrees of accuracy. The most common is gadolinium-enhanced MRA, which accurately identifies proximal clots, but poorly detects subsegmental emboli. Oudkerk and colleagues [132] found a sensitivity of 77% and specificity of 98% of gadolinium-enhanced MRA for PE. Real-time MRI improves on gadolinium-enhanced MRA by timing MRI scanning with patient breathing. Its sensitivity and specificity was 85% and 98% in a study by Kluge and colleagues [133]. Neither gadolinium-enhanced MRA nor real-time MRI achieves sensitivity to function as a single diagnostic test. Recently, MR perfusion scanning was developed, which uses signals from gadolinium to estimate blood volume in regions of the lung. Identification of decreased blood volume represents indirect evidence of PE. Although studies are few, one study found a sensitivity and specificity of 100% and 91%, respectively, when perfusion MRI was compared with MDR-CTA [133].

Advantages of MRA include elimination of ionizing radiation, safety in pregnancy, and decreased nephrotoxicity from contrast enhancing agents. Still, failure to demonstrate adequate sensitivity, costs, and lack of availability makes this modality not a standardized test in diagnosing PE. Many studies are underway including one by PIOPED investigators comparing MRA with CT, which will further define the role of MRA in VTE diagnosis.

## Clinical pathway

As with DVT, optimal work-up of PE begins with an assessment of pre-test probability. Multiple scoring systems exist to aid clinicians, but perform no better than experienced clinical judgment [134]. The most studied and accessible scoring systems are the simplified Well's criteria and revised Geneva score (Table 6). Objective scoring systems have the advantage of being able successfully to stratify patients into appropriate risk categories even with little physician experience [135].

Because PE presents atypically, it should be considered often in the ED. Overuse of D-dimer testing is problematic, however, leading to overtesting and more false-positives. To avoid this problem, Kline and colleagues [136] developed the pulmonary embolus rule out criteria rule to identify which low-risk patients do not need D-dimer or other testing, essentially a close to no-risk group (Box 2). When all eight pulmonary embolus rule out

Table 6
Prediction rules for suspected pulmonary embolus

| Revised Geneva score | Points | Simplified Wells' score | Points |
|---|---|---|---|
| Age >65 y | 1 | Clinical signs or symptoms of DVT (leg swelling and pain with palpation of deep veins of leg) | 3 |
| Previous DVT or PE | 3 | No alternate diagnosis as likely or more likely than PE | 3 |
| Surgery (under general anesthesia) or fracture (of the lower limbs) within 1 mo | 2 | Heart rate >100 beats per min | 1.5 |
| Active malignant condition (solid or hematologic malignant condition, currently active or considered cured <1 y) | 2 | Immobilization or surgery in last 4 wk | 1.5 |
| Unilateral lower-limb pain | 3 | Previous history of DVT or PE | 1.5 |
| Hemoptysis | 2 | Hemoptysis | 1 |
| Heart rate | | Cancer actively treated in last 6 mo | 1 |
| 75–94 | 3 | | |
| ≥95 | 4 | | |
| Pain on lower-limb deep venous palpation and unilateral edema | 4 | | |
| Clinical probability | | Clinical probability | |
| Low | 0–3 | Low | 0–1 |
| Intermediate | 4–10 | Intermediate | 2–6 |
| High | ≥11 | High | ≥7 |

*Abbreviations:* DVT, deep venous thrombosis, PE, pulmonary embolism.

*Data from* Le Gal G, Righini M, Roy PM, et al. Prediction of pulmonary embolism in the emergency department: the revised Geneva Score. Ann Intern Med 2006;144:168; and Wells PS, Anderson DR, Rodger M, et al. Derivation of a simple clinical model to categorize patient's probability of pulmonary embolism: increasing the models utility with the SimpliRED D-dimer. Thromb Haemost 2000;83:416–20.

---

**Box 2. Pulmonary embolism rule out criteria rule**

Age <50
Pulse <100
Oxygen saturation >94%
No unilateral leg swelling
No hemoptysis
No recent surgery or trauma
No prior PE or DVT
No hormone use

_____

If all present <2% risk of PE in low-risk groups.
*Data from* Kline JA, Mitchell AM, Kabrhel C, et al. Clinical criteria to prevent unnecessary diagnostic testing in emergency department patients with suspected pulmonary embolism. J Thromb Haemost 2004;2:1247–55.

---

criteria are present there is less than 2% possibility of PE. The pulmonary embolus rule out criteria have been validated in two separate patient populations.

When testing is needed, clinical judgment or clinical prediction rules, such as the simplified Wells' or revised Geneva score, should be implemented to stratify patients into risk categories.

Low-probability patients should undergo testing with a rapid ELISA or an equivalent highly sensitive D-dimer test. A positive result prompts further testing, generally with CTA (Fig. 9). There is some debate to the use of D-dimer in the intermediate probability group. Although some studies have demonstrated that a single D-dimer may safely be used in the intermediate-risk group, the clinician must be aware that the posttest probability from a negative D-dimer in this group was still 5% (assuming a pretest probability of 30% and a NLR of 0.1) [62,118]. The use of D-dimer testing in the intermediate-risk group should depend on the NLR of the D-dimer test and the comfort of the EP. Intermediate-risk patients with a positive D-dimer test should undergo CTA. High-risk patients should undergo CTA-CTV because the addition of CTV to CTA increases the NPV from 60% to 82% in this group [118].

*Treatment and management*

On diagnosis or high suspicion of PE, rapid initiation of therapy can be lifesaving. Treatment with either UH or LMWH is acceptable and the principles are similar to treatment of DVT.

When PE is strongly suspected (ie, high probability), initiation of heparin therapy before radiologic confirmation likely provides more benefit than risk. Clots can enlarge at an exponential rate. Furthermore, normotensive patients who die from PE do so within the first 24 hours, underscoring

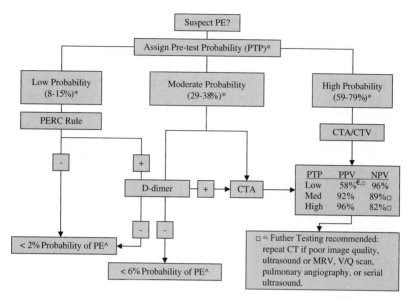

Fig. 9. Clinical algorithm for the diagnosis of suspected PE. CTA, computed tomography angiography; CTV, computed tomography venography; MRV, magnetic resonance venography; NLR, negative likelihood ratio; NPV, negative predictive value; PERC, pulmonary embolus rule-out criteria; PPV, positive predictive value; PTP, pretest probability. *Prevalence rates of PE for each pretest probability group based on multiple clinical prediction rules (Empiric, Wells' Extended, Wells' Simplified, Geneva, Geneva Revised) from PIOPED II. Calculations assume D-dimer with NLR of 0.1. € Low PTP CTA: main or primary lobar PE PPV 97%, segmental PPV 68%, subsegmental PPV 25%. (*Adapted from* Stein PD, Woodard PK, Weg JG, et al. Diagnostic pathways in acute pulmonary embolism: recommendations of the PIOPED II investigators [see comment]. Am J Med 2006;119:1048–55; with permission.)

the importance of rapid assessment and treatment. In patients with PE and an absolute contraindication to anticoagulation or patients already on full anticoagulation, an emergent inferior vena cava filter should be considered.

Fibrinolytics rapidly dissolve clot by active breakdown of fibrin, but they are nonselective and can cause severe bleeding. Fibrinolysis involves the administration of recombinant or bacterial tissue plasminogen activators that increase circulating plasmin and accelerate fibrin breakdown. Their use is generally recommended for massive PE with hemodynamic instability where the risk of bleeding is overshadowed by the potential benefits, but the benefit is unclear. Multiple case reports and small case series suggest potential improved outcomes and return of spontaneous circulation following fibrinolytic administration [137–140]. In a study by Kucher and colleagues [141], fibrinolytic therapy did not decrease 90-day mortality or recurrence of PE in patients with massive PE. The data are equally as unimpressive in patients with submassive PE [142,143]. Still, fibrinolysis should be considered in patients who show signs of clinical deterioration with worsening respiratory distress or hypotension because PE-related cardiac arrest has a dismal prognosis.

In patients with massive PE refractory to fibrinolysis, surgical embolectomy performs better than repeat fibrinolysis [144]. Embolectomy provides a reasonable and potentially lifesaving final therapeutic pathway in massive PE. When successful, patients have excellent long-term results [145].

In addition to selection of appropriate therapies, the EP must also determine appropriate triage of patients with PE. Patients with massive PE deserve ICU level care because they have the poorest prognosis. Normotensive patients with submassive PE and cor pulmonale evidenced by anterior and inferior T-wave inversions on EKG, elevated brain natriuretic peptide, elevate troponin-T, or right heart dilatation or hypokinesis on echocardiography have poorer clinical outcomes and may benefit from a higher level of care [102,146–148]. Normotensive patients without right heart strain generally have excellent clinical outcomes [148] and can likely be admitted to hospital ward beds.

## Considerations for special populations

### Pregnancy

VTE is the most frequent cause of death in pregnancy with the highest risk in the postpartum period [149,150]. As with nonpregnant patients, symptoms and signs of VTE can be highly variable. Because many trials exclude pregnant patients, questions arise as to the correct usage of diagnostic testing in this population.

Use of D-dimer testing in pregnancy is controversial. As in nonpregnant patients, D-dimer tests provide good sensitivity, but specificity decreases as gestational age increases [151]. Lower specificity means D-dimer tests increase the number of negative diagnostic VTE tests. When signs of DVT are present, ultrasound is the recommended diagnostic strategy because it poses no known risk to the fetus. When PE is suspected, presence of DVT clinches the diagnosis, but when symptoms of DVT are absent, ultrasound is rarely positive [152].

Previously, V/Q scan was recommended over CTA as the initial diagnostic study for PE in pregnant patients because of decreased radiation exposure. Newer-age CT scanners have significantly less radiation delivered to the fetus to near equal or even lower doses of radiation from V/Q scanning [153]. Because V/Q scanning frequently produces indeterminate results, CTA is preferred. MRA or venography may be promising for VTE diagnosis in pregnancy, but clinical studies have yet to be performed in this population precluding its recommendation at this time. Treatment of VTE in pregnancy is the same as VTE in other populations with the exception that warfarin, a known teratogen, cannot be used.

### Comorbid conditions

Various comorbid conditions, such as congestive heart failure and chronic obstructive pulmonary disease, may commonly present with symptoms similar to VTE. When VTE is present in these patients, it is often not recognized. This is worsened by the fact that debilitating conditions place patients at increased risk for PE from immobility and sedentary lifestyle and are often associated with other risk factors, such as obesity and smoking.

Autopsy studies suggest that patients with chronic obstructive pulmonary disease have a high rate of missed PE [154]. Two prospective studies evaluated all patients presenting with chronic obstructive pulmonary disease exacerbations for PE and found very different prevalence rates. Tillie-Leblond and colleagues [155] found a prevalence of 25% of PE (49 of 197), whereas Rutschmann and colleagues [155,156] found a prevalence rate of only 3.3% (4 of 123). The explanation for the difference in prevalence rates is unclear. Further studies need to clarify the prevalence of PE in this population. Still, a high index of suspicion in patients with chronic obstructive pulmonary disease, congestive heart failure, and other comorbid conditions that may mask symptoms of PE is appropriate, particularly because of the worse outcomes associated with these patients.

## Summary

The approach to VTE in the ED has evolved tremendously over the last 20 years. Pretest probability scores and clinical pathways using highly sensitive rapid D-dimer tests have been established and validated. This has safely reduced costly and invasive radiographic evaluation, improving the diagnosis of DVT and PE. Furthermore, EP-performed ultrasound is now a well-established, fast, and accurate method of ruling out DVT. The advent of MDR-CTA has increased the detection rate of PE, but recent data have revealed that, like V/Q scans, predictive values of CTA depend on pretest probability. Treatment of VTE with intravenous UH or subcutaneous LMWH is well-established, with the latter preferred because of ease of administration and lower rates of adverse events. Subcutaneous UH may play a future role, however, as sole treatment of VTE. Fibrinolysis has had disappointing results and its appropriate role in VTE is yet to be determined. Use of fibrinolysis should be limited to patients with massive PE in cardiopulmonary extremis until further clinical trials are performed. Many issues still exist including underdiagnosis in some patients and concerns of possible overdiagnosis in others. It is unclear whether all patients with proximal DVT or subsegmental PE benefit from anticoagulation, and perhaps future studies will elucidate this further. Current studies are under way to research other modalities, such as MRA, to diagnose PE better.

## Acknowledgment

The authors thank Anthony J. Dean, MD, for providing many of the figures used in this review article.

# References

[1] Dexter L, Folch-Pi W. Venous thrombosis: an account of the first documented case. JAMA 1974;228(2):195–6.

[2] Wiseman R. Several chirurgical treatises. 2nd edition. London: Norton and Macock; 1686.

[3] Barritt DW, Jordan SC. Anticoagulant drugs in the treatment of pulmonary embolism: a controlled trial. Lancet 1960;1:1309–12.

[4] Alpert JS, Smith R, Carlson J, et al. Mortality in patients treated for pulmonary embolism. JAMA 1976;236(13):1477–80.

[5] Horlander KT, Mannino DM, Leeper KV. Pulmonary embolism mortality in the United States, 1979–1998: an analysis using multiple-cause mortality data. Arch Intern Med 2003;163(14):1711–7.

[6] Rubinstein I, Murray D, Hoffstein V. Fatal pulmonary emboli in hospitalized patients: an autopsy study. Arch Intern Med 1988;148(6):1425–6.

[7] Calder KK, Herbert M, Henderson SO. The mortality of untreated pulmonary embolism in emergency department patients. Ann Emerg Med 2005;45(3):302–10.

[8] Nielsen HK, Husted SE, Krusell LR, et al. Silent pulmonary embolism in patients with deep venous thrombosis: incidence and fate in a randomized, controlled trial of anticoagulation versus no anticoagulation. J Intern Med 1994;235(5):457–61.

[9] Stein PD, Henry JW, Relyea B. Untreated patients with pulmonary embolism: outcome, clinical, and laboratory assessment. Chest 1995;107(4):931–5.

[10] Pulido T, Aranda A, Zevallos MA, et al. Pulmonary embolism as a cause of death in patients with heart disease: an autopsy study. Chest 2006;129(5):1282–7.

[11] Stein PD, Henry JW. Prevalence of acute pulmonary embolism among patients in a general hospital and at autopsy. Chest 1995;108(4):978–81.

[12] PIOPED. Value of the ventilation/perfusion scan in acute pulmonary embolism. Results of the prospective investigation of pulmonary embolism diagnosis (PIOPED). The PIOPED Investigators. JAMA 1990;263(20):2753–9.

[13] Stein PD, Beemath A, Matta F, et al. Clinical characteristics of patients with acute pulmonary embolism: data from PIOPED II. Am J Med 2007;120(10):871–9.

[14] Cronin CG, Lohan DG, Keane M, et al. Prevalence and significance of asymptomatic venous thromboembolic disease found on oncologic staging CT. AJR Am J Roentgenol 2007; 189(1):162–70.

[15] White RH. The epidemiology of venous thromboembolism. Circulation 2003;107(23 Suppl 1): I4–8.

[16] Anderson FA Jr, Wheeler HB, Goldberg RJ, et al. A population-based perspective of the hospital incidence and case-fatality rates of deep vein thrombosis and pulmonary embolism. The Worcester DVT Study. Arch Intern Med 1991;151(5):933–8.

[17] Silverstein MD, Heit JA, Mohr DN, et al. Trends in the incidence of deep vein thrombosis and pulmonary embolism: a 25-year population-based study. Arch Intern Med 1998;158(6): 585–93.

[18] Cushman M. Epidemiology and risk factors for venous thrombosis. Semin Hematol 2007; 44(2):62–9.

[19] White RH, Zhou H, Romano PS. Incidence of idiopathic deep venous thrombosis and secondary thromboembolism among ethnic groups in California. Ann Intern Med 1998; 128(9):737–40.

[20] Fink AM, Mayer W, Steiner A. Seasonal variations of deep vein thrombosis and its influence on the location of the thrombus. Thromb Res 2002;106(2):97–100.

[21] Virchow R. Abhandlungen zur wissenschaftlichen medicin. Frankfurt (Germany): Meidinger Sohn & Co.; 1856.

[22] Bockenstedt P. D-Dimer in venous thromboembolism. N Engl J Med 2003;349(13): 1203–4.

[23] James AH. Prevention and management of venous thromboembolism in pregnancy. Am J Med 2007;120(10 Suppl 2):S26–34.

[24] Kearon C. Natural history of venous thromboembolism. Circulation 2003;107(23 Suppl 1): I22–30.

[25] Ouriel K, Green RM, Greenberg RK, et al. The anatomy of deep venous thrombosis of the lower extremity. J Vasc Surg 2000;31(5):895–900.

[26] Scarvelis D, Wells PS. Diagnosis and treatment of deep-vein thrombosis. CMAJ 2006; 175(9):1087–92.

[27] Barnes RW, Wu KK, Hoak JC. Fallibility of the clinical diagnosis of venous thrombosis. JAMA 1975;234(6):605–7.

[28] Vaccaro P, Van Aman M, Miller S, et al. Shortcomings of physical examination and impedance plethysmography in the diagnosis of lower extremity deep venous thrombosis. Angiology 1987;38(3):232–5.

[29] Fraser JD, Anderson DR. Deep venous thrombosis: recent advances and optimal investigation with US. Radiology 1999;211(1):9–24.

[30] Poppiti R, Papanicolaou G, Perese S, et al. Limited B-mode venous imaging versus complete color-flow duplex venous scanning for detection of proximal deep venous thrombosis. J Vasc Surg 1995;22(5):553–7.

[31] Elias A, Le Corff G, Bouvier JL, et al. Value of real time B mode ultrasound imaging in the diagnosis of deep vein thrombosis of the lower limbs. Int Angiol 1987;6(2):175–82.

[32] Vogel P, Laing FC, Jeffrey RB Jr, et al. Deep venous thrombosis of the lower extremity: US evaluation. Radiology 1987;163(3):747–51.

[33] Mitchell DC, Grasty MS, Stebbings WS, et al. Comparison of duplex ultrasonography and venography in the diagnosis of deep venous thrombosis. Br J Surg 1991;78(5):611–3.

[34] Cronan JJ, Dorfman GS, Scola FH, et al. Deep venous thrombosis: US assessment using vein compression. Radiology 1987;162(1 Pt 1):191–4.

[35] Heijboer H, Buller HR, Lensing AW, et al. A comparison of real-time compression ultrasonography with impedance plethysmography for the diagnosis of deep-vein thrombosis in symptomatic outpatients. N Engl J Med 1993;329(19):1365–9.

[36] Wells PS, Hirsh J, Anderson DR, et al. Accuracy of clinical assessment of deep-vein thrombosis. Lancet 1995;345(8961):1326–30.

[37] Monreal M, Montserrat E, Salvador R, et al. Real-time ultrasound for diagnosis of symptomatic venous thrombosis and for screening of patients at risk: correlation with ascending conventional venography. Angiology 1989;40(6):527–33.

[38] Lensing AW, Prandoni P, Brandjes D, et al. Detection of deep-vein thrombosis by real-time B-mode ultrasonography. N Engl J Med 1989;320(6):342–5.

[39] Appelman PT, De Jong TE, Lampmann LE. Deep venous thrombosis of the leg: US findings. Radiology 1987;163(3):743–6.

[40] Cogo A, Lensing AW, Prandoni P, et al. Distribution of thrombosis in patients with symptomatic deep vein thrombosis: implications for simplifying the diagnostic process with compression ultrasound. Arch Intern Med 1993;153(24):2777–80.

[41] Birdwell BG, Raskob GE, Whitsett TL, et al. The clinical validity of normal compression ultrasonography in outpatients suspected of having deep venous thrombosis. Ann Intern Med 1998;128(1):1–7.

[42] Cogo A, Lensing AW, Koopman MM, et al. Compression ultrasonography for diagnostic management of patients with clinically suspected deep vein thrombosis: prospective cohort study. BMJ 1998;316(7124):17–20.

[43] Jolly BT, Massarin E, Pigman EC. Color Doppler ultrasonography by emergency physicians for the diagnosis of acute deep venous thrombosis. Acad Emerg Med 1997;4(2): 129–32.

[44] Frazee BW, Snoey ER, Levitt A. Emergency department compression ultrasound to diagnose proximal deep vein thrombosis. J Emerg Med 2001;20(2):107–12.

[45] Blaivas M, Lambert MJ, Harwood RA, et al. Lower-extremity Doppler for deep venous thrombosis: can emergency physicians be accurate and fast? Acad Emerg Med 2000;7(2): 120–6.

[46] Theodoro D, Blaivas M, Duggal S, et al. Real-time B-mode ultrasound in the ED saves time in the diagnosis of deep vein thrombosis (DVT). Am J Emerg Med 2004;22(3):197–200.

[47] Jang T, Docherty M, Aubin C, et al. Resident-performed compression ultrasonography for the detection of proximal deep vein thrombosis: fast and accurate. Acad Emerg Med 2004; 11(3):319–22.

[48] Magazzini S, Vanni S, Toccafondi S, et al. Duplex ultrasound in the emergency department for the diagnostic management of clinically suspected deep vein thrombosis. Acad Emerg Med 2007;14(3):216–20.

[49] Rabinov K, Paulin S. Roentgen diagnosis of venous thrombosis in the leg. Arch Surg 1972; 104(2):134–44.

[50] Tapson VF, Carroll BA, Davidson BL, et al. The diagnostic approach to acute venous thromboembolism. Clinical practice guideline. American Thoracic Society. Am J Respir Crit Care Med 1999;160(3):1043–66.

[51] Goodman LR, Stein PD, Matta F, et al. CT venography and compression sonography are diagnostically equivalent: data from PIOPED II. AJR Am J Roentgenol 2007;189(5): 1071–6.

[52] Cantwell CP, Cradock A, Bruzzi J, et al. MR venography with true fast imaging with steady-state precession for suspected lower-limb deep vein thrombosis. J Vasc Interv Radiol 2006;17(11 Pt 1):1763–9.

[53] Wells PS, Hirsh J, Anderson DR, et al. Comparison of the accuracy of impedance plethysmography and compression ultrasonography in outpatients with clinically suspected deep vein thrombosis: a two centre paired-design prospective trial. Thromb Haemost 1995;74(6): 1423–7.

[54] Kelly J, Rudd A, Lewis RR, et al. Plasma D-dimers in the diagnosis of venous thromboembolism. Arch Intern Med 2002;162(7):747–56.

[55] Dryjski M, O'Brien-Irr MS, Harris LM, et al. Evaluation of a screening protocol to exclude the diagnosis of deep venous thrombosis among emergency department patients. J Vasc Surg 2001;34(6):1010–5.

[56] Bates SM, Kearon C, Crowther M, et al. A diagnostic strategy involving a quantitative latex D-dimer assay reliably excludes deep venous thrombosis. Ann Intern Med 2003;138(10): 787–94.

[57] Schutgens RE, Ackermark P, Haas FJ, et al. Combination of a normal D-dimer concentration and a non-high pretest clinical probability score is a safe strategy to exclude deep venous thrombosis. Circulation 2003;107(4):593–7.

[58] Wells PS, Anderson DR, Rodger M, et al. Evaluation of D-Dimer in the diagnosis of suspected deep-vein thrombosis. N Engl J Med 2003;349(13):1227–35.

[59] Subramaniam RM, Snyder B, Heath R, et al. Diagnosis of lower limb deep venous thrombosis in emergency department patients: performance of Hamilton and modified Wells scores. Ann Emerg Med 2006;48(6):678–85.

[60] Stein PD, Hull RD, Patel KC, et al. D-dimer for the exclusion of acute venous thrombosis and pulmonary embolism: a systematic review. Ann Intern Med 2004;140(8):589–602.

[61] van Beek EJ, van den Ende B, Berckmans RJ, et al. A comparative analysis of D-dimer assays in patients with clinically suspected pulmonary embolism. Thromb Haemost 1993; 70(3):408–13.

[62] Mountain D, Jacobs I, Haig A. The VIDAS D-dimer test for venous thromboembolism: a prospective surveillance study shows maintenance of sensitivity and specificity when used in normal clinical practice. Am J Emerg Med 2007;25(4):464–71.

[63] van Belle A, Buller HR, Huisman MV, et al. Effectiveness of managing suspected pulmonary embolism using an algorithm combining clinical probability, D-dimer testing, and computed tomography. JAMA 2006;295(2):172–9.

[64] Anderson DR, Wells PS, Stiell I, et al. Management of patients with suspected deep vein thrombosis in the emergency department: combining use of a clinical diagnosis model with D-dimer testing. J Emerg Med 2000;19(3):225–30.

[65] Anderson DR, Kovacs MJ, Kovacs G, et al. Combined use of clinical assessment and d-dimer to improve the management of patients presenting to the emergency department with suspected deep vein thrombosis (the EDITED Study). J Thromb Haemost 2003;1(4):645–51.

[66] Jennersjo CM, Fagerberg IH, Karlander SG, et al. Normal D-dimer concentration is a common finding in symptomatic outpatients with distal deep vein thrombosis. Blood Coagul Fibrinolysis 2005;16(7):517–23.

[67] Goodacre S, Sampson FC, Sutton AJ, et al. Variation in the diagnostic performance of D-dimer for suspected deep vein thrombosis. QJM 2005;98(7):513–27.

[68] Sadosty AT, Goyal DG, Boie ET, et al. Emergency department D-dimer testing. J Emerg Med 2001;21(4):423–9.

[69] Becker DM, Philbrick JT, Bachhuber TL, et al. D-dimer testing and acute venous thromboembolism: a shortcut to accurate diagnosis? Arch Intern Med 1996;156(9):939–46.

[70] Kearon C, Julian JA, Newman TE, et al. Noninvasive diagnosis of deep venous thrombosis. McMaster diagnostic imaging practice guidelines initiative. Ann Intern Med 1998;128(8): 663–77.

[71] Wells PS, Lensing AW, Davidson BL, et al. Accuracy of ultrasound for the diagnosis of deep venous thrombosis in asymptomatic patients after orthopedic surgery: a meta-analysis. Ann Intern Med 1995;122(1):47–53.

[72] Wells PS, Anderson DR, Bormanis J, et al. Value of assessment of pretest probability of deep-vein thrombosis in clinical management. Lancet 1997;350(9094):1795–8.

[73] Anderson DR, Kovacs MJ, Dennie C, et al. Use of spiral computed tomography contrast angiography and ultrasonography to exclude the diagnosis of pulmonary embolism in the emergency department. J Emerg Med 2005;29(4):399–404.

[74] Anderson DR, Wells PS, Stiell I, et al. Thrombosis in the emergency department: use of a clinical diagnosis model to safely avoid the need for urgent radiological investigation. Arch Intern Med 1999;159(5):477–82.

[75] Shields GP, Turnipseed S, Panacek EA, et al. Validation of the Canadian clinical probability model for acute venous thrombosis. Acad Emerg Med 2002;9(6):561–6.

[76] Arnason T, Wells PS, Forster AJ. Appropriateness of diagnostic strategies for evaluating suspected venous thromboembolism. Thromb Haemost 2007;97(2):195–201.

[77] Hogg K, Dawson D, Mackway-Jones K. The emergency department utility of simplify D-dimer to exclude pulmonary embolism in patients with pleuritic chest pain. Ann Emerg Med 2005;46(4):305–10.

[78] van Dongen CJ, van den Belt AG, Prins MH, et al. Fixed dose subcutaneous low molecular weight heparins versus adjusted dose unfractionated heparin for venous thromboembolism. Cochrane Database Syst Rev 2004;(4):CD001100.

[79] Kearon C, Ginsberg JS, Julian JA, et al. Comparison of fixed-dose weight-adjusted unfractionated heparin and low-molecular-weight heparin for acute treatment of venous thromboembolism. JAMA 2006;296(8):935–42.

[80] Prandoni P, Carnovali M, Marchiori A. Subcutaneous adjusted-dose unfractionated heparin vs fixed-dose low-molecular-weight heparin in the initial treatment of venous thromboembolism. Arch Intern Med 2004;164(10):1077–83.

[81] Othieno R, Abu Affan M, Okpo E. Home versus in-patient treatment for deep vein thrombosis. Cochrane Database Syst Rev 2007;(3):CD003076.

[82] Vinson DR, Berman DA. Outpatient treatment of deep venous thrombosis: a clinical care pathway managed by the emergency department. Ann Emerg Med 2001;37(3):251–8.

[83] Watson LI, Armon MP. Thrombolysis for acute deep vein thrombosis. Cochrane Database Syst Rev 2004;(4):CD002783.

[84] Wells PS, Forster AJ. Thrombolysis in deep vein thrombosis: is there still an indication? Thromb Haemost 2001;86(1):499–508.

[85] Spencer FA, Emery C, Lessard D, et al. Upper extremity deep vein thrombosis: a community-based perspective. Am J Med 2007;120(8):678–84.

[86] Bernardi E, Piccioli A, Marchiori A, et al. Upper extremity deep vein thrombosis: risk factors, diagnosis, and management. Semin Vasc Med 2001;1(1):105–10.

[87] Martin C, Viviand X, Saux P, et al. Upper-extremity deep vein thrombosis after central venous catheterization via the axillary vein. Crit Care Med 1999;27(12):2626–9.

[88] Abdullah BJ, Mohammad N, Sangkar JV, et al. Incidence of upper limb venous thrombosis associated with peripherally inserted central catheters (PICC). Br J Radiol 2005;78(931): 596–600.

[89] Joffe HV, Kucher N, Tapson VF, et al. Upper-extremity deep vein thrombosis: a prospective registry of 592 patients. Circulation 2004;110(12):1605–11.

[90] Monreal M, Raventos A, Lerma R, et al. Pulmonary embolism in patients with upper extremity DVT associated to venous central lines–a prospective study. Thromb Haemost 1994;72(4):548–50.

[91] Patel NH, Plorde JJ, Meissner M. Catheter-directed thrombolysis in the treatment of phlegmasia cerulea dolens. Ann Vasc Surg 1998;12(5):471–5.

[92] Hood DB, Weaver FA, Modrall JG, et al. Advances in the treatment of phlegmasia cerulea dolens. Am J Surg 1993;166(2):206–10.

[93] Oguzkurt L, Tercan F, Ozkan U. Manual aspiration thrombectomy with stent placement: rapid and effective treatment for phlegmasia cerulea dolens with impending venous gangrene. Cardiovasc Intervent Radiol 2008;31(1):205–8.

[94] Meissner MH, Caps MT, Bergelin RO, et al. Early outcome after isolated calf vein thrombosis. J Vasc Surg 1997;26(5):749–56.

[95] Saarinen J, Domonyi K, Zeitlin R, et al. Post-thrombotic symptoms after an isolated calf deep venous thrombosis. J Cardiovasc Surg (Torino) 2002;43(5):687–91.

[96] Blumenberg RM, Barton E, Gelfand ML, et al. Occult deep venous thrombosis complicating superficial thrombophlebitis. J Vasc Surg 1998;27(2):338–43.

[97] Di Nisio M, Wichers IM, Middeldorp S. Treatment for superficial thrombophlebitis of the leg. Cochrane Database Syst Rev 2007;(2):CD004982.

[98] Elliott CG. Pulmonary physiology during pulmonary embolism. Chest 1992;101(Suppl 4): 163S–71S.

[99] Light RW. Pleural effusion due to pulmonary emboli. Curr Opin Pulm Med 2001;7(4): 198–201.

[100] Miniati M, Prediletto R, Formichi B, et al. Accuracy of clinical assessment in the diagnosis of pulmonary embolism. Am J Respir Crit Care Med 1999;159(3):864–71.

[101] Ferrari E, Imbert A, Chevalier T, et al. The ECG in pulmonary embolism: predictive value of negative T waves in precordial leads–80 case reports. Chest 1997;111(3):537–43.

[102] Kosuge M, Kimura K, Ishikawa T, et al. Prognostic significance of inverted T waves in patients with acute pulmonary embolism. Circ J 2006;70(6):750–5.

[103] Kosuge M, Kimura K, Ishikawa T, et al. Electrocardiographic differentiation between acute pulmonary embolism and acute coronary syndromes on the basis of negative T waves. Am J Cardiol 2007;99(6):817–21.

[104] Pollack ML. ECG manifestations of selected extracardiac diseases. Emerg Med Clin North Am 2006;24(1):133–43.

[105] Elliott CG, Goldhaber SZ, Visani L, et al. Chest radiographs in acute pulmonary embolism. Results from the International Cooperative Pulmonary Embolism Registry. Chest 2000; 118(1):33–8.

[106] Jones JS, Neff TL, Carlson SA. Use of the alveolar-arterial oxygen gradient in the assessment of acute pulmonary embolism. Am J Emerg Med 1998;16(4):333–7.

[107] Stein PD, Goldhaber SZ, Henry JW. Alveolar-arterial oxygen gradient in the assessment of acute pulmonary embolism. Chest 1995;107(1):139–43.

[108] Stein PD, Goldhaber SZ, Henry JW, et al. Arterial blood gas analysis in the assessment of suspected acute pulmonary embolism. Chest 1996;109(1):78–81.

[109] Kline JA, Wells PS. Methodology for a rapid protocol to rule out pulmonary embolism in the emergency department. Ann Emerg Med 2003;42(2):266–75.

[110] Kline JA, Webb WB, Jones AE, et al. Impact of a rapid rule-out protocol for pulmonary embolism on the rate of screening, missed cases, and pulmonary vascular imaging in an urban US emergency department. Ann Emerg Med 2004;44(5):490–502.

[111] Rodger MA, Bredeson CN, Jones G, et al. The bedside investigation of pulmonary embolism diagnosis study: a double-blind randomized controlled trial comparing combinations of 3 bedside tests vs ventilation-perfusion scan for the initial investigation of suspected pulmonary embolism. Arch Intern Med 2006;166(2):181–7.

[112] Miniati M, Monti S, Pratali L, et al. Value of transthoracic echocardiography in the diagnosis of pulmonary embolism: results of a prospective study in unselected patients. Am J Med 2001;110(7):528–35.

[113] Grifoni S, Olivotto I, Cecchini P, et al. Utility of an integrated clinical, echocardiographic, and venous ultrasonographic approach for triage of patients with suspected pulmonary embolism. Am J Cardiol 1998;82(10):1230–5.

[114] Niendorff DF, Rassias AJ, Palac R, et al. Rapid cardiac ultrasound of inpatients suffering PEA arrest performed by nonexpert sonographers. Resuscitation 2005;67(1):81–7.

[115] Jones AE, Tayal VS, Kline JA. Focused training of emergency medicine residents in goal-directed echocardiography: a prospective study. Acad Emerg Med 2003;10(10):1054–8.

[116] Stein PD, Woodard PK, Weg JG, et al. Diagnostic pathways in acute pulmonary embolism: recommendations of the PIOPED II investigators [see comment]. Am J Med 2006;119(12): 1048–55.

[117] Winer-Muram HT, Rydberg J, Johnson MS, et al. Suspected acute pulmonary embolism: evaluation with multi-detector row CT versus digital subtraction pulmonary arteriography. Radiology 2004;233(3):806–15.

[118] Stein PD, Fowler SE, Goodman LR, et al. Multidetector computed tomography for acute pulmonary embolism. N Engl J Med 2006;354(22):2317–27.

[119] Perrier A, Roy PM, Sanchez O, et al. Multidetector-row computed tomography in suspected pulmonary embolism. N Engl J Med 2005;352(17):1760–8.

[120] Patel S, Kazerooni EA, Cascade PN. Pulmonary embolism: optimization of small pulmonary artery visualization at multi-detector row CT. Radiology 2003;227(2):455–60.

[121] Sostman HD, Stein PD, Gottschalk A, et al. Acute pulmonary embolism: sensitivity and specificity of ventilation-perfusion scintigraphy in PIOPED II study. Radiology 2008; 246(3):941–6.

[122] Lim KE, Hsu YY, Hsu WC, et al. Combined computed tomography venography and pulmonary angiography for the diagnosis PE and DVT in the ED. Am J Emerg Med 2004; 22(4):301–6.

[123] Cham MD, Yankelevitz DF, Henschke CI. Thromboembolic disease detection at indirect CT venography versus CT pulmonary angiography. Radiology 2005;234(2):591–4.

[124] Loud PA, Katz DS, Bruce DA, et al. Deep venous thrombosis with suspected pulmonary embolism: detection with combined CT venography and pulmonary angiography. Radiology 2001;219(2):498–502.

[125] Revel MP, Petrover D, Hernigou A, et al. Diagnosing pulmonary embolism with four-detector row helical CT: prospective evaluation of 216 outpatients and inpatients. Radiology 2005;234(1):265–73.

[126] Raptopoulos V, Boiselle PM. Multi-detector row spiral CT pulmonary angiography: comparison with single-detector row spiral CT. Radiology 2001;221(3):606–13.

[127] Anderson DR, Kahn SR, Rodger MA, et al. Computed tomographic pulmonary angiography vs ventilation-perfusion lung scanning in patients with suspected pulmonary embolism: a randomized controlled trial. JAMA 2007;298(23):2743–53.

[128] Donato AA, Scheirer JJ, Atwell MS, et al. Clinical outcomes in patients with suspected acute pulmonary embolism and negative helical computed tomographic results in whom anticoagulation was withheld. Arch Intern Med 2003;163(17):2033–8.

[129] van Strijen MJ, de Monye W, Schiereck J, et al. Single-detector helical computed tomography as the primary diagnostic test in suspected pulmonary embolism: a multicenter clinical management study of 510 patients. Ann Intern Med 2003;138(4):307–14.

[130] Perrier A, Howarth N, Didier D, et al. Performance of helical computed tomography in unselected outpatients with suspected pulmonary embolism. Ann Intern Med 2001; 135(2):88–97.

[131] Forbes KP, Reid JH, Murchison JT. Do preliminary chest X-ray findings define the optimum role of pulmonary scintigraphy in suspected pulmonary embolism? Clin Radiol 2001;56(5):397–400.

[132] Oudkerk M, van Beek EJ, Wielopolski P, et al. Comparison of contrast-enhanced magnetic resonance angiography and conventional pulmonary angiography for the diagnosis of pulmonary embolism: a prospective study. Lancet 2002;359(9318):1643–7.

[133] Kluge A, Luboldt W, Bachmann G. Acute pulmonary embolism to the subsegmental level: diagnostic accuracy of three MRI techniques compared with 16-MDCT. AJR Am J Roentgenol 2006;187(1):W7–14.

[134] Chunilal SD, Eikelboom JW, Attia J, et al. Does this patient have pulmonary embolism? JAMA 2003;290(21):2849–58.

[135] Chagnon I, Bounameaux H, Aujesky D, et al. Comparison of two clinical prediction rules and implicit assessment among patients with suspected pulmonary embolism. Am J Med 2002;113(4):269–75.

[136] Kline JA, Mitchell AM, Kabrhel C, et al. Clinical criteria to prevent unnecessary diagnostic testing in emergency department patients with suspected pulmonary embolism. J Thromb Haemost 2004;2(8):1247–55.

[137] Bottiger BW, Bode C, Kern S, et al. Efficacy and safety of thrombolytic therapy after initially unsuccessful cardiopulmonary resuscitation: a prospective clinical trial. Lancet 2001;357(9268):1583–5.

[138] Langdon RW, Swicegood WR, Schwartz DA. Thrombolytic therapy of massive pulmonary embolism during prolonged cardiac arrest using recombinant tissue-type plasminogen activator. Ann Emerg Med 1989;18(6):678–80.

[139] Sheth A, Cullinan P, Vachharajani V, et al. Bolus thrombolytic infusion during prolonged refractory cardiac arrest of undiagnosed cause. Emerg Med J 2006;23(3):e19.

[140] Tiffany PA, Schultz M, Stueven H. Bolus thrombolytic infusions during CPR for patients with refractory arrest rhythms: outcome of a case series. Ann Emerg Med 1998;31(1): 124–6.

[141] Kucher N, Rossi E, De Rosa M, et al. Massive pulmonary embolism. Circulation 2006; 113(4):577–82.

[142] Ramakrishnan N. Thrombolysis is not warranted in submassive pulmonary embolism: a systematic review and meta-analysis. Crit Care Resusc 2007;9(4):357–63.

[143] Hamel E, Pacouret G, Vincentelli D, et al. Thrombolysis or heparin therapy in massive pulmonary embolism with right ventricular dilation: results from a 128-patient monocenter registry. Chest 2001;120(1):120–5.

[144] Meneveau N, Seronde MF, Blonde MC, et al. Management of unsuccessful thrombolysis in acute massive pulmonary embolism. Chest 2006;129(4):1043–50.

[145] Dauphine C, Omari B. Pulmonary embolectomy for acute massive pulmonary embolism. Ann Thorac Surg 2005;79(4):1240–4.

[146] Kucher N, Printzen G, Goldhaber SZ. Prognostic role of brain natriuretic peptide in acute pulmonary embolism. Circulation 2003;107(20):2545–7.

[147] Pruszczyk P, Bochowicz A, Torbicki A, et al. Cardiac troponin T monitoring identifies high-risk group of normotensive patients with acute pulmonary embolism. Chest 2003; 123(6):1947–52.

[148] Grifoni S, Olivotto I, Cecchini P, et al. Short-term clinical outcome of patients with acute pulmonary embolism, normal blood pressure, and echocardiographic right ventricular dysfunction. Circulation 2000;101(24):2817–22.

[149] Chang J, Elam-Evans LD, Berg CJ, et al. Pregnancy-related mortality surveillance—United States, 1991–1999. MMWR Surveill Summ 2003;52(2):1–8.

[150] McColl MD, Ramsay JE, Tait RC, et al. Risk factors for pregnancy associated venous thromboembolism. Thromb Haemost 1997;78(4):1183–8.

[151] Rosenberg VA, Lockwood CJ. Thromboembolism in pregnancy. Obstet Gynecol Clin North Am 2007;34(3):481–500, xi.

[152] Daniel KR, Jackson RE, Kline JA. Utility of lower extremity venous ultrasound scanning in the diagnosis and exclusion of pulmonary embolism in outpatients. Ann Emerg Med 2000;35(6):547–54.

[153] Winer-Muram HT, Boone JM, Brown HL, et al. Pulmonary embolism in pregnant patients: fetal radiation dose with helical CT. Radiology 2002;224(2):487–92.

[154] Pineda LA, Hathwar VS, Grant BJ. Clinical suspicion of fatal pulmonary embolism. Chest 2001;120(3):791–5.

[155] Tillie-Leblond I, Marquette CH, Perez T, et al. Pulmonary embolism in patients with unexplained exacerbation of chronic obstructive pulmonary disease: prevalence and risk factors. Ann Intern Med 2006;144(6):390–6.

[156] Rutschmann OT, Cornuz J, Poletti PA, et al. Should pulmonary embolism be suspected in exacerbation of chronic obstructive pulmonary disease? Thorax 2007;62(2):121–5.

ELSEVIER
SAUNDERS

Emerg Med Clin N Am
26 (2008) 685–702

EMERGENCY
MEDICINE
CLINICS OF
NORTH AMERICA

# Critical Care Aspects in the Management of Patients with Acute Coronary Syndromes

Robin M. Naples, MD[a], James W. Harris, MD[b],
Chris A. Ghaemmaghami, MD[a,c,*]

[a]Department of Emergency Medicine, University of Virginia School of Medicine,
Charlottesville, VA 22908–0699, USA
[b]Department of Emergency Medicine, University of Virginia Health System, University
of Virginia School of Medicine, Charlottesville, VA 22908–0699, USA
[c]Chest Pain Center, University of Virginia Health System, PO Box 800699,
Charlottesville, VA, USA

Coronary heart disease is an especially prevalent disease in the United States with an estimated more than 13 million persons affected. Worldwide prevalence of coronary heart disease has been increasing at an alarming rate as western diets and industrialization reaches developing countries with large populations (eg, India and China). Of individuals with coronary heart disease, approximately half eventually have acute myocardial infarctions (AMIs), whereas the other half suffer from angina [1]. There are almost 1.7 million distinct acute coronary syndrome (ACS) discharges from American hospitals annually including approximately 500,000 ST-elevation myocardial infarctions (STEMI) [2]. Additionally, coronary heart disease is the leading cause of death in the United States among both men and women [3].

The critical care aspects of treatment of the ACS patient are the focus of this article. The American Heart Association (AHA) and American College of Cardiology (ACC) maintain comprehensive evidence-based guidelines for the diagnosis and treatment of ACS. Much of the emphasis of these guidelines is related to early recognition, diagnosis, and treatment of ACS based on principles of prevention of major complications caused by ACS and improvements in survival. Pharmacologic and reperfusion therapies designed to improve myocardial blood flow are the primary focus of the sections

* Corresponding author. Department of Emergency Medicine, University of Virginia School of Medicine, Charlottesville, VA 22908–0699.
*E-mail address:* cg3n@virginia.edu (C.A. Ghaemmaghami).

0733-8627/08/$ - see front matter © 2008 Elsevier Inc. All rights reserved.
doi:10.1016/j.emc.2008.04.002                                    *emed.theclinics.com*

dedicated to therapeutics. In contrast to these broad guidelines, this article discusses specific situations that may arise during the care of the patient experiencing an ACS that may result in patient instability and require critical care management.

Contained in this article are discussions of common complicating features of ACS with an emphasis on those occurring during AMI. Hemodynamic and electrophysiologic problems are the most common and serious immediate complications faced by providers treating ACS patients. Reperfusion therapy is the widespread standard for the treatment of STEMI. Complications specifically related to fibrinolytic therapy, including major hemorrhages and failure to reperfuse, are also included in this discussion.

## Cardiogenic shock

### Background

Cardiogenic shock represents a state of end-organ hypoperfusion and dysfunction secondary to low cardiac output. With the development of coronary care units, cardiogenic shock has surpassed arrhythmias as the leading cause of in-hospital mortality after AMI [4,5]. The incidence of cardiogenic shock complicating MI has remained relatively constant despite marked improvements in revascularization over the past few decades [6–8].

### Epidemiology

Cardiogenic shock complicates approximately 7% of ACS cases [6,8–10]. Although it is commonly perceived that only a small subset of AMI patients have an initial presentation of cardiogenic shock, the incidence has been reported to be as high as 28% [8,9,11]. Most ACS patients who develop cardiogenic shock during their hospitalizations are experiencing a STEMI. A small percentage patients with non-STEMI also suffer from cardiogenic shock as described in the GUSTO II-B and PURSUIT trials (2.5% and 2.9%, respectively) [7,12]. The onset of cardiogenic shock has been shown to occur later in the course of the AMI in non-STEMI versus STEMI [7,12,13]. Fifty percent of the overall mortality in cardiogenic shock is within the first 10 hours of symptom onset [14,15]. This fact demonstrates the importance of early recognition and intervention by the treating physician. The etiologies of cardiogenic shock from the *SH*ould we emergently revascularize *O*ccluded *C*oronaries for cardiogenic shoc*K* (SHOCK) Registry are represented in Fig. 1 and are discussed in more detail next.

### Mechanism

#### Left ventricle failure

Severe left ventricle (LV) dysfunction is responsible for nearly 80% of cases of cardiogenic shock after MI [16–18]. LV dysfunction occurs when greater than 40% of the LV myocardium is affected [19,20]. It is more

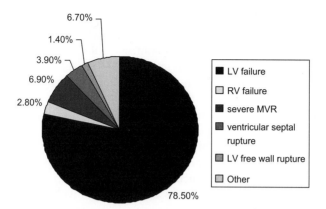

Fig. 1. Etiologies of cardiogenic shock complicating myocardial infarction from the SHOCK Trial registry. LV, left ventricle; MVR, mitral valve regurgitation; RV, right ventricle. (*Data from* Hochman JS, Buller CE, Sleeper LA, et al. Cardiogenic shock complicating acute myocardial infarction: etiologies, management and outcome. A report from the SHOCK trial registry. J Am Coll Cardiol 2000;36:1063–70.)

commonly associated with large anterior MIs, although it can be seen in other distributions or secondary to recurrent infarction or extension of previous damage [19,21]. Hochman and colleagues [18] found that patients were more likely to develop severe LV dysfunction with cardiogenic shock if they had a prior MI (40.1% versus 29.5%). In the SHOCK trial, 60% of patients with cardiogenic shock were found to have triple-vessel disease and 20% had left main disease as the culprit lesion; the group with left main disease had the highest in-hospital mortality [21].

The myocardial pathology involved in ischemia and infarction helps to explain why patients with multivessel disease or previous infarction are at increased risk for dysfunction and failure. Myocytes adjacent to the infarct are susceptible to expanding ischemia because of decreased coronary perfusion pressure, increased oxygen demand, or propagation of thrombus [22]. Sites remote to the initial infarct may develop systolic dysfunction because of impaired autoregulation, limited vasodilatation, hypotension, or metabolic derangement resulting from the original insult [23]. Myocardial stunning and hibernation are both additional components of nonfunctional myocardium during cardiogenic shock. Myocardial stunning is dysfunction that occurs postinfarction and is eventually reversible with restoration of normal coronary flow [24,25]. The severity of stunning is dependent on the degree of preceding ischemia and is thought to occur because of oxidative stress, disruption of calcium homeostasis, and decreased myocardial calcium responsiveness [25]. Myocardial hibernation does not result from the ischemic insult itself, but from chronically reduced coronary blood flow to an area. This hypoperfused myocardium has reduced contractility that may be recovered with revascularization allowing for overall improved cardiac output [26–28].

*Right ventricle failure*

Right ventricle (RV) infarction complicates anywhere from 30% to 50% of ACS cases, although it only clinically manifests as RV failure in 10% of cases [29]. It is commonly associated with inferior MI, but also it can be found in posterior and anterior distributions, usually to much lesser degrees. Isolated RV failure is a rare cause of cardiogenic shock after MI, occurring in less than 3% of patients [18,30]. These patients are preload dependent and often require judicious intravenous resuscitation with crystalloid to improve hemodynamics. Patients with RV failure are also reliant on atrial filling and the atrial kick for right-sided cardiac output. Ironically, patients with RV involvement after inferior wall MI are much more likely to develop high-degree atrioventricular (AV) block (48%) than those without RV involvement (13%) [31].

*Acute mitral valve regurgitation*

Acute mitral valve regurgitation (MVR) is found commonly in patients with AMI. Almost 40% of patients have mild to moderate regurgitation seen on echocardiogram 24 hours after infarction [32,33]. A total of 6% to 7% of patients have severe MVR resulting in hemodynamic compromise and pulmonary edema [33]. Acute MVR is associated more with inferior and posterior MI than in anterior distributions [34]. Acute MVR occurs by several mechanisms [35,36]:

1. Systolic tenting or tethering of the valve
2. Mitral annulus dilation from severe left ventricular dysfunction
3. Ischemia of papillary muscle
4. Ruptured papillary muscle
5. Ruptured chordae tendinae
6. Worsening pre-existing mitral regurgitation

In the setting of acute MVR, afterload reduction improves cardiac output by allowing greater forward flow. Development of severe MVR has been found to have significant prognostic implication with higher prevalence of long-standing heart failure and death [33].

Papillary muscle rupture is a distinct entity causing acute MVR. It is usually seen 2 to 7 days postinfarction. Often the posterior papillary muscle is the site of rupture because of a typical, singular blood supply from the posterior descending branch of a dominant right coronary artery [37]. Immediate surgical repair or valve replacement is indicated in papillary muscle rupture with a mortality rate of 50% within the first 24 hours in patients who do not undergo surgical intervention [38]. Risk factors for the development of acute MVR and papillary muscle rupture are listed previously.

*Left ventricle free wall rupture*

Incidence of free wall rupture has significantly decreased from 6% to around 1% with the use of angioplasty for AMI [18,39,40]. Rupture occurs within the first 24 hours after infarction in 40% of cases and within 1 week

85% of the time [41]. Patients often complain of persistent or recurrent chest pain, intractable nausea or repeated emesis, or present with syncope or agitation [39]. Paradoxical bradycardia is seen in up to 20% of cases [42,43]. Risk factors for free wall rupture are listed along with the other mechanical causes in Table 1.

*Ventricular septal rupture*

The reported incidence of ventricular septal rupture varies from 0.4% in the GUSTO-I trial to as high as 4% seen in the SHOCK trail [18,44]. Rupture usually occurs within a thin, akinetic area of septal myocardium. Interestingly, ventricular septal rupture more commonly occurs in patients without a history for MI who have complete occlusion of a single vessel [45]. It is thought that chronic stenosis is protective against rupture by allowing scarring and remodeling of the damaged myocardium, which produces a more durable fibrinous architecture [45]. The left anterior descending artery is most frequently the causative vessel. Table 2 lists the risk factors for ventricular septal rupture.

*Diagnostic evaluation*

Clinically, the patient with cardiogenic shock has a systolic blood pressure less than 90 mm Hg; evidence of hypoperfusion (decreased urine output; decreased mental status; cool, clammy skin); cardiac index less than 2.2 L/min/m$^2$; and LV end diastolic pressure or pulmonary capillary wedge pressure greater than 15 mm Hg [17]. Patients with LV failure often have extra heart sounds and rales on lung examination, whereas patients with RV failure often have clear lung fields with jugular venous distention or Kussmaul's sign (paradoxical increase in jugular venous distention with inspiration). Mechanical etiologies of shock may produce their own discrete physical findings. In the case of LV free wall rupture, the patient has signs

Table 1
Risk factors for mechanical causes of cardiogenic shock complicating acute myocardial infarction

|  | Acute mitral valve regurgitation | Papillary muscle rupture | Left ventricle free wall rupture | Ventricular septal rupture |
|---|---|---|---|---|
| Age | >65 y | >65 y | >65 y | >65 y |
| Gender | Female | Female | Female | Female |
| Multivessel versus single-vessel | Multivessel | Single-vessel | Single-vessel | ? |
| Location | Inferior-posterior | Inferior-posterior | Anterior | Anterior |
| History of previous myocardial infarction | Yes | No | No | No |

*Data from* Bates ER, Topol EJ. Limitations of thrombolytic therapy for acute myocardial infarction complicated by congestive heart failure and cardiogenic shock. J Am Coll Cardiol 1991;18:1077–84.

Table 2
Hemodynamic profiles in various states of cardiogenic shock

| | |
|---|---|
| Left ventricle failure | ↑PCWP, ↓cardiac output, ↑systemic vascular resistance |
| Right ventricle failure | ↑RAP, RAP/PCWP >0.8, exaggerated RA $y$ descent, RV square root sign |
| Mitral valve regurgitation | Large PCWP $v$ wave |
| Ventricular free wall rupture, tamponade | Equalization of diastolic pressures (approximately 20 mm Hg) |
| Ventricular septal rupture | Large PCWP $v$ wave, oxygen saturation step-up (>5%) from RA to RV |

*Abbreviations:* PCWP, pulmonary capillary wedge pressure; RA, atrium; RAP, right atrial pressure; RV, right ventricle.

*Data from* Hollenberg SM, Kavinsky CJ, Pairillo JE. Cardiogenic shock. Ann Intern Med 1999;131:47–59.

of cardiac tamponade with distended neck veins; hypotension with a narrow pulse pressure; and distant, muffled heart sounds. Patients with acute MVR and ventricular septal rupture may have an audible murmur, although they may be clinically silent because of low cardiac output [46].

Ideally, an ECG should be performed expeditiously on all patients with suspected cardiogenic shock. Depending on the etiology, different ECG patterns may be expected. Patients may have tracings consistent with an acute STEMI, Q waves consistent with areas of previous damage, or diffuse ST-depression representing ischemia. Right precordial leads may be useful in patients with clinical signs of right heart failure. Arrhythmias, atrioventricular dissociation, and left bundle branch block may be noted and present additional complications that worsen the patient's cardiac output.

Echocardiography and right heart catheterization are excellent tools to guide therapy. According to the 2003 guidelines of the ACC, AHA, and American Society of Echocardiography, the use of echocardiography to

Table 3
Arterial supply to the cardiac conducting system

| Conduction system component | Vascular supply |
|---|---|
| SA node | RCA in 60% |
| | Left circumflex in 40% |
| AV node | RCA 90% |
| | Left circumflex 10% |
| His-bundle | Primarily RCA with some septal perforators from the LAD |
| Proximal left bundle branch | LAD predominates |
| Left anterior fascicle | Proximally AV nodal branch of RCA |
| | Distal dual supplied by anterior and posterior septal perforating arteries |
| Left posterior fascicle | Septal perforators ± AV nodal |
| Right bundle branch | LAD perforators ± collateral from RCA/LCX |

*Abbreviations:* AV, atrioventricular; LAD, left anterior descending; LCX, left circumflex; RCA, right coronary artery; SA, sinoatrial.

*Data from* Zimetbaum PJ, Josephson ME. Use of the electrocardiogram in acute myocardial infarction. N Engl J Med 2003;348:933.

diagnosis mechanical complications of MI receives a class I recommendation [47]. Echocardiography allows for rapid assessment of myocardial and valvular function, and presence of pericardial effusion from free wall rupture. It also provides an assessment of the RV in possible cases of RV infarction. Subset analysis of the SHOCK trial demonstrated that echocardiographic evaluation of left ventricular ejection fraction and mitral regurgitation performed within 24 hours of infarction could provide more detailed information on prognosis and mortality [32].

Right heart catheterization allows for central hemodynamic monitoring. The patient's volume status and pulmonary capillary wedge pressure can be evaluated. Table 3 illustrates the hemodynamic profiles associated with each specific clinical scenario [48]. This objective information may be critical in guiding treatment with vasopressors, vasodilators, and inotropes.

*Treatment*

*Inotropes and vasopressors*

The goal of treating patients with cardiogenic shock is tissue perfusion stabilization and optimization, with a goal systolic blood pressure greater than 90, mean arterial pressure greater than 65, and urine output of 0.5 mL/kg/h. Initial intervention may include fluid resuscitation, unless the patient is in frank pulmonary edema. Judicious use of intravenous fluid boluses allows for optimizing preload and filling pressures so that cardiac output is maximized. Patients with RV failure have great dependence on preload and may require more aggressive fluid resuscitation. If hypotension persists despite adequate filling pressures achieved with fluid resuscitation, then inotropes and vasopressors may be necessary. Dobutamine, a selective $\beta_1$-adrenergic receptor agonist, improves myocardial contractility and cardiac output with less effect on heart rate and systemic vascular resistance and is the inotrope of choice in patients with systolic blood pressure greater than 80 mm Hg. Dopamine also acts directly on $\beta_1$-adrenergic receptors and indirectly through norepinephrine. It causes increases in vasoconstriction, heart rate, and myocardial contractility. Because it may increase myocardial demand, dopamine is the inotrope of choice in patients with systolic blood pressure less than 80 mm Hg. If hypoperfusion persists despite the use of dobutamine and dopamine, norepinephrine or phenylephrine may be necessary. Phenylephrine, a pure $\alpha_1$-adrenergic agonist, is useful when tachyarrhythmias limit the use of vasopressors. Care must be taken with the addition of vasopressors because there is a delicate balance between improved coronary perfusion pressures and increasing myocardial demand. Phosphodiesterase inhibitors, such as milrinone, have inotropic actions but also cause vasodilatation. Although they are less arrhythmogenic and chronotropic, they have prolonged half-lives and may cause hypotension, so one must be cautious when using them in patients with acute cardiogenic shock in the setting of ischemia.

*Intra-aortic balloon pump counterpulsation*

Intra-aortic balloon pump couterpulsation increases diastolic coronary artery perfusion pressures and decreases afterload without increasing myocardial demand. The Thrombolysis and Counterpulsation to Improve Cardiogenic Shock Survival trial randomized patients to thrombolysis with or without intra-aortic balloon pump use and found improved 6-month mortality in patients with Killip class III or IV failure (39% versus 80%, respectively) [49]. Intra-aortic balloon pump use is advocated as a Class IB recommendation in the ACC-AHA guideline as a stabilizing measure when mechanical complications of MI result in cardiogenic shock or when hypotension persists despite other interventions [50]. It should be noted that the placement of an intra-aortic balloon pump by emergency physicians does not represent the standard of care in most communities and that this procedure is usually performed by an interventional cardiologist or a cardiothoracic surgeon.

*Fibrinolysis versus revascularization*

There are limited data to support the efficacy of fibrinolysis in patients with cardiogenic shock. Thrombolysis has been shown to decrease the incidence of cardiogenic shock in patients with STEMI, but not to improve outcomes in patients presenting with AMI and cardiogenic shock [35,51,52,]. It is presumed that decreased coronary perfusion pressures limit the effectiveness of fibrinolytics and that use of intra-aortic balloon pump counterpulsation may improve their efficacy [36].

Revascularization by percutaneous coronary intervention (PCI) or coronary artery bypass grafting allows for improved coronary flow after infarction. In the Primary Angioplasty in Myocardial Infarction trial, PCI was compared with fibrinolysis in high-risk patients (>70 years, large anterior MI, heart rate >100) and was found to have significant mortality benefit (2% versus 10.4%, respectively) [53]. GUSTO-1 showed a significant decrease in 30-day mortality in patients who underwent aggressive revascularization within 24 hours of shock onset (38%) versus fibrinolysis alone (62%) [9]. Additionally, the SHOCK study showed a nonsignificant decrease in 30-day all-cause mortality between the group undergoing early revascularization versus medical management (46.7% versus 56%) [5]. There was a significant absolute risk reduction for morality of 13% at 6 months in the early revascularization group, which persisted at 12 months [5]. Based on these data, the ACC-AHA guidelines recommend patients younger than 75 years of age undergo early revascularization as a Class I indication [50].

## Complications of fibrinolysis

Fibrinolytic therapy remains a common treatment for STEMI both in the Unites States and abroad. Severe hemorrhage, specifically intracranial hemorrhage (ICH), is the most feared complication of fibrinolytic therapy for

AMI. The failure to re-establish coronary perfusion after administration of a fibrinolytic agent is also a common scenario. These topics are discussed in the following section.

## Hemorrhage

Hemorrhagic complications after fibrinolytic therapy can range from minor gingival bleeding to ICH. Bleeding after fibrinolysis most frequently occurs at venous access or vascular puncture sites [54–56]. Invasive procedures should be limited after fibrinolysis is given. If bleeding occurs at a compressible site, then direct pressure should be used to minimize bleeding. Gastrointestinal bleeding has been shown in studies to be the most common form of severe spontaneous bleeding [54,56,57]. Blood transfusions should be given to patients with hemodynamic compromise with gastrointestinal bleeding. Only a minority of patients, less than 1% in most studies, who receive fibrinolytic therapy develop ICH [54,58–62]. Several studies have examined patient factors that may indicate a higher risk for ICH after fibrinolysis. Patient characteristics associated with increased rates of ICH after fibrinolytic therapy are as follows [56,59–62]:

Age >75 years
Female gender
Black race
History of cerebrovascular accident
Systolic blood pressure >160 mm Hg on presentation
Dyastolic blood pressure >100 mm Hg on presentation
Low body weight
Tissue plasminogen activator dose >1.5 mg/kg.

Although these risk factors are not contraindications for fibrinolysis, the recognition of their presence allows the emergency department physician to estimate better the risk of ICH.

Any change in neurologic status including focal deficits, seizure activity, or change in mental status occurring during or after fibrinolytic therapy should be presumed to be from ICH until proved otherwise. Fibrinolytic, antiplatelet, and anticoagulant therapy should be discontinued until neuroimaging is performed. If ICH is present, fresh frozen plasma and cryoprecipitate can be used to restore fibrinogen levels. Protamine should be given to reverse the effect of heparin, and platelet transfusions may be necessary if bleeding times are prolonged. ε-Aminocaproic acid is an option for fibrinolysis reversal by inhibiting activation of plasminogen to plasmin. Much consideration must be taken before administration because its use may cause significant systemic thrombosis.

In addition to the management of the fibrinolytic-induced coagulopathy, patients with ICH may also require other medical interventions and neurosurgical consultation. If there are concerns for increased intracranial pressure, then such methods as elevating the head of bed, optimizing blood pressure, administration of mannitol, and endotracheal intubation with hyperventilation may be necessary.

## Failure of fibrinolysis

Failure to reperfuse has been defined by the ACC-AHA as absence of at least some normalization of ST-segment elevation 60 to 90 minutes after initiation of fibrinolytic therapy; persistent symptoms (eg, chest pain, diaphoresis, shortness of breath); or electrical or hemodynamic instability [63]. There have been several randomized studies performed to evaluate the benefit of rescue PCI versus conservative therapy or repeat fibrinolysis [64–67]. The largest and most comprehensive trial was the Rescue Angioplasty versus Conservative Treatment or Repeat Thrombolysis trial that showed significantly higher rate of event-free survival with PCI compared with both conservative therapy and repeat fibrinolysis [67]. Results of three meta-analyses performed on rescue PCI trials have shown decreased rates of mortality and decreased need for revascularization, but they have also shown increased rates of thromboembolic stroke [68–70]. At facilities that do not have PCI capabilities, the potential benefits of rescue PCI should be countered with the risk of emergency transportation of a patient with presumed failed fibrinolysis. Patients at higher risk for complications from their AMI, such as those with large anterior infarctions or inferior infarctions with RV involvement, may benefit more from rescue PCI than their lower-risk counterparts. As for risk factors that predispose patients to fibrinolytic failure, a small study by Deepa and Mishra [71], found that patients with more than three risk factors for coronary artery disease were at higher risk of failing fibrinolysis than those with fewer than three risk factors. This was a limited study, but may serve as a catalyst for additional research into high-risk characteristics for failure of fibrinolysis.

## Arrhythmias in acute coronary syndrome

### Background

Arrhythmias occur in anywhere from 3% to 40% of patients with AMI [72–75]. Onset of arrhythmias may occur during the acute phase of an ACS or later after AMI. There are multiple mechanisms for the development of arrhythmia in ACS. The interruption of normal electrical impulse transmission through the myocardium creates areas of tissue that are supersensitive to sympathetic stimulation, rendering them more arrhythmogenic [76]. At the cellular level, decreased function of the energy-dependent sodium-potassium-ATPase pump and increased permeability of myocardial cell walls lead to metabolic derangement of the myocardium [77]. These changes affect the resting membrane potential of the myocardium causing increased arrhythmogenicity. Increased levels of metabolic by-products can also adversely affect the heart raising the risk of arrhythmias [78]. Ischemia can also have significant effects on the action potential of cardiac myocytes to varying degrees depending on their proximity to the area of infarction, and this heterogenic conduction provides further arrhythmogenicity [79]. The categories of arrhythmias seen in ACS can be broken down into bradyarrhythmias, tachyarrhythmias, and reperfusion rhythms.

*Bradyarrhythmias*

Bradyarrhythmias at the simplest level can be divided into sinus bradycardia and heart blocks. Sinus bradycardia is defined as a heart rate less than 60 beats per minute with each QRS complex preceded by a P wave and is seen in up to 40% of patients with AMI. The blood supply to the heart's conduction system plays a significant role in certain arrhythmias seen in AMI (Table 3). Sinus bradycardia is seen most commonly with inferior MI because of the blood supply of the sinoatrial node [73]. Loss of blood supply to the normal pacemakers of the heart can cause bradycardia secondary to ischemia and relatively increased vagal tone. Sinus bradycardia in the setting of AMI is usually transient and typically resolves within 24 hours. Treatment with vagolytics, such as atropine, is reserved for patients who are suffering from hypotension or ischemia secondary to bradycardia. Temporary pacing can be used if the patient fails to respond to atropine, but permanent pacing is rarely required in these patients [73].

Multiple types of heart block can be seen in the setting of AMI [80]. The basic underlying pathology of these conduction disturbances is caused by decreased upstroke velocity of the action potential in the cardiac myocytes secondary to ischemia [81]. The type of block seen depends on the coronary artery creating ischemia and the portion of the conduction pathway that it supplies. For instance, the right coronary artery supplies the AV node in approximately 90% of patients and either a first-degree AV block, a second-degree type I, or a complete heart block with a narrow QRS complex indicates an infranodal lesion associated in patients with acute right coronary artery infarction. For this same reason, second-degree type 2 AV block, complete heart block with a wide QRS complex, or new bundle branch blocks may be present in a patient suffering from acute left anterior descending occlusion because it supplies most of the blood to the conduction system distal to the AV node.

Atropine should be considered as a first-line agent for use in patients who are symptomatic with signs of hypoperfusion and either second-degree type one or complete heart block with a narrow QRS (ie, lesions at the level of the AV node). The use of atropine is discouraged in patients with high-degree AV block (ie, infranodal block), and asymptomatic patients [82]. In some cases of second-degree heart block, the use of atropine has been reported to cause progression to complete heart block, although conflicting evidence in the literature exists [83].

In cases where atropine is not used or is unsuccessful, temporary pacing may be indicated for symptomatic bradycardia. Transcutaneous pacing is easily done in most emergency department cases, but occasionally transvenous pacing wires may need to be placed. Optimally, this procedure is performed under fluoroscopy, and possibly done in coordination with rapid coronary catheterization for diagnostic and potentially therapeutic purposes.

## Tachyarrhythmias

Tachyarrhythmias fall into two major groups: atrial and ventricular tachyarrhythmias. Atrial tachyarrhythmias are commonly associated with AMI and are seen in approximately 6% to 20% of these patients [75]. These arrhythmias are most often seen 3 to 72 hours after an infarction occurs. Atrial fibrillation or atrial flutter associated with rapid ventricular responses in the setting of AMI can significantly increase oxygen demands, exacerbating the already ischemic myocardium. Atrial fibrillation in the setting of AMI does impart a significantly higher short- and long-term mortality demonstrated by the GUSTO-I and III trials and the PURSUIT and TRACE trials [84–87]. In GUSTO-I, the unadjusted mortality rate at 30 days was 14.3% in patients with atrial fibrillation versus 6.2% in those with sinus rhythm [84].

The presence of hemodynamic compromise and ongoing ischemia must be assessed to determine the appropriate intervention in patients with tachycardic atrial fibrillation and atrial flutter. Heart rate control with an AV nodal blocker (eg, β-adrenergic antagonists and nondihydropyridine-type calcium channel blockers) is appropriate in patients without hypotension or cardiogenic shock. Amiodarone is also a reasonable option for slowing or chemically cardioverting rapid atrial fibrillation and atrial flutter. β-Blockers are generally preferred as a first-line agent for rate control because there is the added benefit of decreasing sympathetic stimulation to the heart, further decreasing ischemia. Care must be taken to avoid hypotension in all ACS patients to avoid extending the ischemic penumbra of an AMI.

In those patients with both hemodynamic compromise and ongoing ischemia, synchronized cardioversion should be attempted to treat atrial fibrillation or atrial flutter. Repeated shocks with escalating energy may be required, but the danger of ventricular arrhythmia induction or asystole increases with multiple shocks. Combinations of pharmacologic agents and cardioversion may be effective in recalcitrant cases.

Paroxysmal supraventricular tachycardia is also seen in the setting of AMI, although with a lower frequency. As in atrial fibrillation with a rapid ventricular response, rate-induced ischemia in the ACS patient mandates rapid treatment. Reentrant mechanisms and increased automaticity are the primary mechanisms involved, so the administration of a vagal maneuver including carotid massage, Valsalva, or coughing is initially indicated

and advanced cardiac life support algorithms suggest the use of adenosine bolus therapy if simple vagal maneuvers fail. Electrical cardioversion is indicated for hemodynamically unstable patients and in those in whom pharmacologic treatment has failed [82].

Ventricular arrhythmias can range from premature ventricular contractions to ventricular fibrillation. Ventricular arrhythmias are common in the setting of AMI with incidence ranging as high as 20% for ventricular fibrillation, up to 40% for ventricular tachycardia, and as high as 90% for premature ventricular contractions [72], although more recent studies in the era of fibrinolysis indicate significantly lower incidence. Premature ventricular contractions are typically asymptomatic and acutely have no bearing on short- or long-term morbidity and mortality. Treatment aimed at suppression of these beats is not helpful and in some cases may even be harmful [88]. Nonsustained ventricular tachycardia is defined as ventricular tachycardia that spontaneously resolves in less than 30 seconds. The significance of nonsustained ventricular tachycardia depends on its temporal relationship to AMI. Specifically, nonsustained ventricular tachycardia early in course of AMI defined as within 48 hours of AMI onset was relatively benign and did not require treatment unless associated with concurrent hemodynamic decompensation. If a patient becomes hypotensive or has angina during recurrent nonsustained ventricular tachycardia, then a rate-controlling medication, such as intravenous amiodarone or a β-blocker, may be used [82]. Sustained ventricular tachycardia is divided into two distinct categories: stable or unstable. The unstable varieties are further subdivided into polymorphic or pulseless monomorphic, which are treated with unsynchronized electrical defibrillation, and monomorphic ventricular tachycardia with hemodynamic instability, which is treated with synchronized cardioversion [82]. Stable ventricular tachycardia may be treated initially medically with amiodarone, or procainamide before cardioversion if a patient can temporarily tolerate the increased heart rate of the ventricular tachycardia. The final ventricular tachydysrrhythmia is ventricular fibrillation. This rhythm is almost universally terminal if left untreated and usually deteriorates into asystole within a few minutes time. Prompt recognition and intervention in the form of electrical defibrillation is crucial. Ventricular fibrillation that does not respond to initial defibrillation should be treated following current ACLS guidelines.

## Reperfusion arrhythmias

Ventricular arrhythmia and ectopy following the administration of fibrinolytic therapy in the setting of STEMI are termed "reperfusion arrhythmias." Premature ventricular contractions, ventricular tachycardia, ventricular fibrillation, and accelerated idioventricular rhythms all may be observed when reperfusion occurs. The hypothesized etiologies underlying the development of reperfusion are numerous and include cell injury, swelling, and necrosis, and myocardial stunning [89]. Accelerated idioventricular rhythms is seen in up to 50% of patients with AMI, but is not considered a sensitive or specific marker for reperfusion [89–91]. Pulse rates with accelerated idioventricular rhythms in the 60 to 100 range are usually associated with improved cardiac output and systemic perfusion. Accelerated idioventricular rhythms should be observed unless the patient becomes hemodynamically compromised and it generally resolves spontaneously. The use of antiarrhythmic agents in stable patients with accelerated idioventricular rhythms may present risk of harm without significant benefit.

## Summary

ACS and associated ACS complications are highly prevalent among emergency department patients. The spectrum of ACS and ACS complications are very treatable diseases and modern aggressive therapy has greatly reduced patient morbidity and mortality. The maintenance of specific critical care management skills in the recognition and treatment of ACS complications is essential for the practicing emergency physician.

## References

[1] American Heart Association. Heart and stroke facts: 1995 statistical supplement. Dallas (TX): American Heart Association; 1994.

[2] Wiviott SD, Morrow DA, Giugliano RP, et al. Performance of the thrombolysis in myocardial infarction risk index for early acute coronary syndrome in the National Registry of Myocardial Infarction: a simple risk index predicts mortality in both ST and non-ST elevation myocardial infarction. J Am Coll Cardiol 2003;41:365A–6A.

[3] Thom TJ, Kannel WB, Silbershatz S, et al. Incidence, prevalence, and mortality of cardiovascular diseases in the United States. In: Alexander RW, Schlant RC, Fuster V, et al, editors. Hurst's the heart. 9th edition. New York: McGraw Hill; 1998. p. 3.

[4] Hochman JS. Cardiogenic shock complicating acute myocardial infarction: expanding the paradigm. Circulation 2003;107(24):2998–3002.

[5] Hocman JS, Boland J, Sleeper LA, et al. Current spectrum of cardiogenic shock and effect of early revascularization on mortality. Results of an International Registry. SHOCK Registry Investigators. Circulation 1995;91:873–81.

[6] Goldberg RJ, Samad NA, Yarzebski J, et al. Temporal trends in cardiogenic shock complicating acute myocardial infarction. N Engl J Med 1999;340:1162–8.

[7] Holmes DR Jr, Berger PB, Hochman JS, et al. Cardiogenic shock in patients with acute ischemic syndromes with and without ST-segment elevation. Circulation 1999;100:2067–73.

[8] Babaev A, Fedrick PD, Pasta DJ, et al. Trends in management and outcomes of patients with acute myocardial infarction complicated by cardiogenic shock. JAMA 2005;294:448–54.

[9] Holmes DR Jr, Bates ER, Kleiman NS, et al. Contemporary reperfusion therapy in cardiogenic shock: the GUSTO-I trial experience. The GUSTO-I Investigators. J Am Coll Cardiol 1995;26:668–74.

[10] Hands ME, Rutherford JD, Muller JE, et al. The in-hospital development of cardiogenic shock after myocardial infarction: incidence, predictors of occurrence, outcome and prognostic factors. J Am Coll Cardiol 1989;14:40–6.

[11] Webb JG, Sleeper LA, Buller CE, et al. Implication of the timing of onset of cardiogenic shock after acute myocardial infarction: a report from the SHOCK trial registry. J Am Coll Cardiol 2000;36:1084–90.

[12] Hasdai D, Harrington RA, Hochman JS, et al. Platelet glycoprotein IIb/IIIa blockade and outcome of cardiogenic shock complicating acute coronary syndrome without persistent ST-segment elevation. J Am Coll Cardiol 2000;36:685–92.

[13] Jacobs AK, French JK, Col J, et al. Cardiogenic shock with non ST-segment elevation myocardial infarction. A report from the SHOCK Trial Registry. J Am Coll Cardiol 2000;36:1091–6.

[14] Hasdai D, Topol EJ, Califf RM, et al. Cardiogenic shock complicating acute coronary syndromes. Lancet 2000;356:749–56.

[15] Scheidt S, Ascheim R, Killip T. Shock after acute myocardial infarction. Am J Cardiol 1970; 26:556–64.

[16] Duvernoy CS, Bates ER. Management of cardiogenic shock attributable to acute myocardial infarction in the reperfusion era. J Intensive Care Med 2005;20(4):188–98.

[17] Hollenberg SM, Kavinsky CJ, Parrillo JE. Cardiogenic shock. Ann Intern Med 1999;131: 47–59.

[18] Hochman JS, Buller CE, Sleeper LA, et al. Cardiogenic shock complicating acute myocardial infarction-etiologies, management and outcome: a report from the SHOCK trial registry. J Am Coll Cardiol 2000;36:1063–70.

[19] Alonso DR, Scheidt S, Post M, et al. Pathophysiology of cardiogenic shock: quantification of myocardial necrosis, clinical and pathologic and electrocardiographic correlations. Circulation 1973;48:588–96.

[20] Quigley RL, Milano CAD, Smith LR, et al. Prognosis and management of anterolateral myocardial infarction in patients with severe left main disease and cardiogenic shock: the left main shock syndrome. Circulation 1993;88:65–70.

[21] Wong SC, Sanborn T, Sleeper LA, et al. Angiographic findings and clinical correlates in patients with cardiogenic shock complicating acute myocardial infarction: a report for the SHOCK Trial Registry. J Am Coll Cardiol 2000;36(3 Suppl A):1077–83.

[22] Olivetti G, Quaini F, Sala R, et al. Acute myocardial infarction in humans is associated with activation of programmed myocyte cell death in the surviving portion of the heart. J Mol Cell Cardiol 1996;28:2005–16.

[23] Grines CL, Topol EJ, Califf RM, et al. Prognostic implications and predictors of enhanced regional wall motion of the noninfarct zone after thrombolysis and angioplasty therapy of acute myocardial infarction. The TAMI Study Groups. Circulation 1989;80:245–53.

[24] Bolli R. Myocardial stunning in man. Circulation 1992;86:1671–91.

[25] Bolli R. Basic and clinical aspects of myocardial stunning. Prog Cardiovasc Dis 1998;40: 477–516.

[26] Wijns W, Vatner SF, Camici PG. Hibernating myocardium. N Engl J Med 1998;339:173–81.

[27] Topol EJ, Weiss JL, Guzman PA, et al. Immediate improvement of dysfunctional myocardial segments after coronary revascularization: detection by intraoperative transesophageal echocardiography. J Am Coll Cardiol 1984;4:1123–34.

[28] Bonow RO. The hibernating myocardium: implications for management of congestive heart failure. Am J Cardiol 1995;75:17A–25A.

[29] Zehender M, Kasper W, Kauder E, et al. Right ventricular infarction as an independent predictor of prognosis after acute inferior myocardial infarction. N Engl J Med 1993;328:981–8.

[30] Kinch JW, Ryan TJ. Right ventricular infarction. N Engl J Med 1994;330:1211–7.

[31] Braat SH, deZwaan C, Brugada P, et al. Right ventricular involvement with acute inferior wall myocardial infarction identifies high risk developing atrioventricular nodal conduction disturbances. Am Heart J 1984;107(6):1183–7.

[32] Picard MH, Davidoff R, Sleeper LA, et al. Echocardiographic predictors of survival and response to early revascularization in cardiogenic shock. Circulation 2003;107:279–84.

[33] Aronson D, Goldsher N, Zukermann R, et al. Ischemic mitral regurgitation and risk of heart failure after myocardial infarction. Arch Intern Med 2006;166(21):2362–8.

[34] Thompson CR, Buller CE, Sleeper LA, et al. Cardiogenic shock due to acute severe mitral regurgitation complicating acute myocardial infarction: a report from the SHOCK Trial Registry. J Am Coll Cardiol 2000;36:1104–9.

[35] Voci P, Bilotta F, Caretta Q, et al. Papillary muscle perfusion pattern: a hypothesis for ischemic papillary muscle dysfunction. Circulation 1995;91:1714–8.

[36] Nishimura RA, Gersh B, Schaff HV. The case from an aggressive surgical approach to papillary muscle rupture following myocardial infarction: from paradise lost to paradise regained. Heart 2000;83:611–3.

[37] Lopez-Sendon JG, Gonzalez A, Lopez de Sa E, et al. Diagnosis of subacute ventricular wall rupture after acute myocardial infarction: sensitivity and specificity of clinical, hemodynamic and echogradiographic criteria. J Am Coll Cardiol 1992;19:1145–53.

[38] Becker R, Gore JM, Lanbrew C, et al. A composite view of cardiac rupture in the United States National Registry of Myocardial Infarction. J Am Coll Cardiol 1996;27:1321–6.

[39] Raitt MH, Kraft CD, Gardner CJ, et al. Subacute ventricular free wall rupture complicating acute myocardial infarction. Am Heart J 1993;126:946–55.

[40] Oliva P, Hamill SC, Edwards WD, et al. Cardiac rupture, a clinically predictable complication of myocardial infarction: report of 70 cases with clinicopathologic correlations. J Am Coll Cardiol 1993;22:720–6.

[41] Wehrens XH, Doevendans PA. Cardiac rupture complicating myocardial infarction. Int J Cardiol 2004;95:285–92.

[42] Birnbaum Y, Wagner GS, Gates KB, et al. Clinical and electrocardiographic variables associated with increased risk of ventricular septal defect in acute anterior myocardial infarction. Am J Cardiol 2000;86(8):830–4.

[43] Birnbaum Y, Fishbein MC, Blanche C, et al. Ventricular septal rupture after acute myocardial infarction. N Engl J Med 2002;347(18):1426–32.

[44] Bursi F, Enriquez-Sarano M, Jacobsen SJ, et al. Mitral regurgitation after myocardial infarction: a review. Am J Med 2006;119:103–12.

[45] Cheitlin M, Armstrong WF, Aurigemma GP, et al. ACC/AHA/ASE2003 guideline update for the clinical application of echocardiography: summary article. A report of the American College of Cardiology/American Heart Association Task Force of Practice Guidelines (ACC/AHA/ASE committee to update the 1997 guidelines for the Clinical Application of echocardiography). J Am Coll Cardiol 2003;42:954–70.

[46] Gurm HS, Bates ER. Cardiogenic shock complicating myocardial infarction. Crit Care Clin 2007;23:759–77.

[47] Ohman EM, Nanas J, Stomel RJ, et al. Thrombolysis and counterpulsation to improve survival in myocardial infarction complicated by hypotension and suspected cardiogenic shock or heart failure: results of the TACTICS Trial. Thrombolysis 2005;19:33–9.

[48] Antman EM, Anbe DT, Armstrong PW, et al. ACC/AHA guidelines for the management of patients with ST elevation myocardial infarction: a report of the American College of Cardiology/American Heart Association Task Force on Practice Guidelines. Committee to revise the 1999 guidelines for the management of patients with acute myocardial infarction. Circulation 2004;110:e82–292.

[49] Wilcox RG, von der Lippe G, Olsson CG, et al. Trial of tissue plasminogen activator for mortality reduction in acute myocardial infarction. Anglo-Scandinavian Study of Early Thrombolysis (ASSET). Lancet 1988;8585:525–30.

[50] Long-term effects of intravenous anistreplase in acute myocardial infarction: final report of the AIMS study. AIMS Trial Study Group. Lancet 1990;224:427–31.

[51] Bates ER, Topol EJ. Limitations of thrombolytic therapy for acute myocardial infarction complicated by congestive heart failure and cardiogenic shock. J Am Coll Cardiol 1991;18:1077–84.

[52] Becker RC. Hemodynamic, mechanical and metabolic determinants of thrombolytic efficacy: a theoretic framework for assessing the limitations of thrombolysis in patients with cardiogenic shock [Editorial]. Am Heart J 1993;125:919–29.

[53] Grines CL, Browne KF, Marco J, et al. A comparison of immediate angioplasty with thrombolytic therapy for acute myocardial infarction: The Primary Angioplasty in Myocardial Infarction Study Group. N Engl J Med 1993;328:673–9.

[54] Califf RM, Topol EJ, George BS, et al. Hemorrhagic complications associated with the use of intravenous tissue plasminogen activator in treatment of acute myocardial infarction. Am J Med 1988;85(3):353–9.

[55] Rao AK, Pratt C, Berke A, et al. Thrombolysis in Myocardial Infarction (TIMI) Trail— phase I: hemorrhagic manifestations and changes in plasma fibrinogen and the fibrinolytic system in patients treated with recombinant tissue plasminogen activator and streptokinase. J Am Coll Cardiol 1998;11:1–11.

[56] Berkowitz SD, Granger CB, Pieper KS, et al. Incidence and predictors of bleeding after contemporary thrombolytic therapy for myocardial infarction. Circulation 1997;95:2508–16.

[57] Moscucci M, Fox KAA, Cannon CP, et al. Predictors of major bleeding in acute coronary syndromes: the Global Registry of Acute Coronary Events (GRACE). Eur Heart J 2003;24: 1815–23.

[58] Kandzari DE, Granger CB, Simoons ML, et al. Risk factors for intracranial hemorrhage and nonhemorrhagic stroke after fibrinolytic therapy (from the GUSTO-I trial). Am J Cardiol 2004;93:458–61.

[59] Huynh T, Cox JL, Massel D, et al. Predictors of intracranial hemorrhage with fibrinolytic therapy in unselected community patients: a report from the FASTRAK II project. Am Heart J 2004;148:86–91.

[60] Gurwitz JH, Gore JM, Goldberg RJ, et al. Risk for intracranial hemorrhage after tissue plasminogen activator treatment for acute myocardial infarction. Participants in the National Registry of Myocardial Infarction 2. Ann Intern Med 1998;129(8):597–604.

[61] Brass LM, Lichtman JH, Wang Y, et al. Intracranial hemorrhage associated with thrombolytic therapy for elderly patients with acute myocardial infarction. Results for the Cooperative Cardiovascular Project. Stroke 2000;31:1802–11.

[62] Estess JM, Topol EJ. Fibrinolytic treatment for elderly patients with acute myocardial infarction. Heart 2002;87:308–11.

[63] Pollack CV Jr, Diercks DB, Roe MT, et al. 2004 American College of Cardiology/American Heart Association guidelines for the management of patients with ST-elevation myocardial infarction: implications for emergency department practice. Ann Emerg Med 2005;45:363–76.

[64] Ellis SG, Ribeiro da Silva E, Heyndrick GR, et al. Randomized comparison of rescue angioplasty with conservative management of patients with early failure of thrombolysis for acute anterior myocardial infarction. Circulation 1994;90:2280–4.

[65] Sutton AG, Campbell PG, Graham R, et al. A randomized trial of rescue angioplasty versus a conservative approach for failed fibrinolysis in ST-segment elevation myocardial infarction: the Middlesbrough Early Revascularization to Limit Infarction (MERLIN) trial. J Am Coll Cardiol 2004;44:287–96.

[66] Schomig A, Ndrepepe J, Mehilli J, et al. A randomized trial of coronary stenting versus balloon angioplasty as a rescue intervention after failed thrombolysis in patients with acute myocardial infarction. J Am Coll Cardiol 2004;44:2073–9.

[67] Gershlick AH, Stephens-Lloyd A, Hughes S, et al. Rescue angioplasty after failed thrombolytic therapy for acute myocardial infarction. N Engl J Med 2005;353:2758–68.

[68] Patel TN, Bavry AA, Kumbhani DJ, et al. A meta-analysis of randomized trials of rescue percutaneous coronary intervention after failed fibrinolysis. Am J Cardiol 2006;97(12): 1685–90.

[69] Wijeysundera HC, Vijayaraghavan R, Nallamothu BK, et al. Rescue angioplasty or repeat fibrinolysis after failed fibrinolytic therapy for ST-segment myocardial infarction: a meta-analysis of randomized trial. J Am Coll Cardiol 2007;49:422–30.

[70] Collet JP, Montalescot G, Le MM, et al. Percutaneous coronary intervention after fibrinolysis: a multiple meta-analyses approach according to the type of strategy. J Am Coll Cardiol 2006;48:1326–35.

[71] Deepa S, Mishra P. Risk factors for reperfusion failure following fibrinolytic therapy for ST segment elevation myocardial infarction (STEMI). American Journal of Clinical Medicine 2005;2:11–4.

[72] Bigger JT Jr, Dresdale FJ, Heissenbuttel RH, et al. Ventricular arrhythmias in ischemic heart disease: mechanism, prevalence, significance, and management. Prog Cardiovasc Dis 1977; 19:255–300.

[73] Rotman M, Wagner GS, Wallace AG. Bradyarrhythmias in acute myocardial infarction. Circulation 1972;45:703–22.

[74] Crimm A, Severance HW Jr, Coffey K, et al. Prognostic significance of isolated sinus tachycardia during first three days of acute myocardial infarction. Am J Med 1984;76(6):983–8.

[75] Pizzetti F, Turazza FM, Franzosi MG, et al. Incidence and prognostic significance of atrial fibrillation in acute myocardial infarction: the GISSI-3 data. Heart 2001;86(5):527–32.

[76] Schwartz PJ, Zipes DP. Autonomic modulation of cardiac arrhythmias. In: Zipes DP, Jalife J, editors. Cardiac electrophysiology: from cell to bedside. 3rd edition. Philadelphia: WB Saunders; 1999. p. 300–14.

[77] Downar E, Janse MJ, Durrer D. The effect of acute coronary artery occlusion on subepicardial transmembrane potentials in the intact porcine heart. Circulation 1977;56(2):217–24.

[78] Sobel BE, Corr PB, Robison AK, et al. Accumulation of lysophosphoglycerides with arrhythmogenic properties in ischemic myocardium. J Clin Invest 1978;62(3):546–53.

[79] Cinca J, Blanch P, Carreno A, et al. J Acute ischemic ventricular arrhythmias in pigs with healed myocardial infarction: comparative effects of ischemia at a distance and ischemia at the infarct zone. Circulation 1997;96(2):653–8.

[80] Feigl D, Ashkenazy J, Kishon Y. Early and late atrioventricular block in acute inferior myocardial infarction. J Am Coll Cardiol 1984;4(1):35–8.

[81] Rubart M, Zipes DP. Genesis of cardiac arrhythmias: electrophysiological considerations. In: Libby P, Bonow RO, Mann DL, et al, editors. Braunwald's heart disease: a textbook of cardiovascular medicine. Philadelphia: Saunders Elsevier; 2007. p. 727–61.

[82] Antman EM, Hand M, Armstrong PW, et al. 2007 focused update of the ACC/AHA 2004 guidelines for the management of patients with ST-elevation myocardial infarction: a report of the American College of Cardiology/American Heart Association Task Force on Practice Guidelines (Writing Group to Review New Evidence and Update the ACC/AHA 2004 guidelines for the management of patients with ST-elevation myocardial infarction). J Am Coll Cardiol 2008;51:210–47.

[83] Brady WJ, Perron AD. Administration of atropine in the setting of acute myocardial infarction: potentiation of the ischemic process? Am J Emerg Med 2001;19(1):81–3.

[84] Crenshaw BS, Ward SR, Granger CB, et al. Atrial fibrillation in the setting of acute myocardial infarction: the GUSTO-I experience. J Am Coll Cardiol 1997;30(2):406–13.

[85] Wong CK, White HD, Wilcox RG, et al. New atrial fibrillation after acute myocardial infarction independently predicts death: the GUSTO-III experience. Am Heart J 2000; 140(6):878–85.

[86] Pedersen OD, Bagger H, Kober L, et al. The occurrence and prognostic significance of atrial fibrillation/-flutter following acute myocardial infarction. TRACE Study group. Eur Heart J 1999;20(10):748–54.

[87] Al-Khatib SM, Pieper KS, Lee KL, et al. Atrial fibrillation and mortality among patients with acute coronary syndromes without ST-segment elevation: results from the PURSUIT trial. Am J Cardiol 2001;88:76–9.

[88] Echt DS, Liebson PR, Mitchell LB, et al. Mortality and morbidity in patients receiving encainide, flecainide, or placebo. The Cardiac Arrhythmia Suppression Trial. N Engl J Med 1991;324(12):781–8.

[89] Matsumura K, Jeremy RW, Schaper J, et al. Progression of myocardial necrosis during reperfusion of ischemic myocardium. Circulation 1998;97(8):795–804.

[90] Wehrens XH, Doevendans PA, Ophuis TJ, et al. A comparison of electrocardiographic changes during reperfusion of acute myocardial infarction by thrombolysis or percutaneous transluminal coronary angioplasty. Am Heart J 2000;139(3):430–6.

[91] Gressin V, Louvard Y, Pezzano M, et al. Holter recording of ventricular arrhythmias during intravenous thrombolysis for acute myocardial infarction. Am J Cardiol 1992;69(3):152–9.

ELSEVIER
SAUNDERS

Emerg Med Clin N Am
26 (2008) 703–713

EMERGENCY
MEDICINE
CLINICS OF
NORTH AMERICA

# Ensuring Emergency Medicine Performance Standards for Stroke and Transient Ischemic Attack Care

## Marian P. LaMonte, MD, MSN[a,b,]*

[a]*Neurological Services, St. Agnes Hospital, 900 Caton Avenue, 2nd Floor,
Baltimore, MD 21229, USA*
[b]*Stroke Center, St. Agnes Hospital, 900 Caton Avenue, 2nd Floor, Baltimore, MD 21229, USA*

In 2000, the Brain Attack Coalition published its "Recommendations for the Establishment of Primary Stroke Centers" [1]. These recommendations were adopted by the Joint Commission on Accreditation of Hospitals Organization (JCAHO) in an effort to provide standards for hospitals wishing to improve care of cerebrovascular event (CE) patients. The commission's Primary Stroke Center Certification program was developed in collaboration with the American Stroke Association and is based on the Brain Attack Coalition's recommendations [2]. Since that time, hospitals across the country have devoted resources to improving aspects of care for CE patients that conform to standards addressed by organizations leading quality improvement efforts for these patients. Position papers, review articles, and manuscripts reviewing emergency medicine care of stroke and TIA patients are widely available in general medical, neurologic, and emergency medicine literature [1–8]. This article reviews emergency medicine evaluation and management for cerebrovascular event patients and provides a practical process for ensuring high quality care. Areas of practice that most frequently generate questions and controversy are highlighted. The term "cerebrovascular event" or CE is used throughout the text when both stroke and transient ischemic attack (TIA) are under discussion. Recommendations are based on literature review and the author's experience with the successful certification of multiple primary stroke centers and appointments in neurology, emergency medicine, and nursing specialties.

* Corresponding author. Division of Neurology, St. Agnes Hospital, 900 Caton Avenue, 2nd Floor, Baltimore, MD 21229.
   *E-mail address:* mlamonte@stagnes.org

0733-8627/08/$ - see front matter
doi:10.1016/j.emc.2008.05.002

## Standards for emergency medicine evaluation and management of cerebrovascular events

A distillation of the standards for emergency medicine evaluation and management of CE patients includes: 1) establishing the historical and physical findings supporting a definite, probable or possible diagnosis of CE; 2) establishing an exact time that the patient was in a baseline neurologic state; 3) performing laboratory and radiological testing to support or refute the diagnosis and; 4) to identify metabolic, medical and infectious comorbidities; 5) initiating correction of metabolic, medical and infectious comorbidities that worsen neurologic function; 6) evaluating for the benefit and risk of administering intravenous (IV) tissue plasminogen activator (tPA); 7) determining the benefit and risk of administering antithrombotic; 8) assessing swallowing function; 9) establishing fluid and nutritional support; 10) producing parameters for vital signs and neurologic assessments that are effective in identifying changes from baseline; and 11) providing specific nursing intervention orders.

## Practical processes for ensuring quality care for cerebrovascular event patients

### The clinical pathway for cerebrovascular event patients

A clinical pathway (also known as a clinical practice guideline) is a hospital designated process that is structured to ensure every CE patient entering the emergency department (or who has a CE while hospitalized) receives certain standards of care during their stay. These standards are health provider and patient care behaviors that can be directly linked through research to better patient outcomes. Those that are specific to the prehospital (emergency department) phase of care are outlined in the previous section of this article. These behaviors are translated into practical actions that are taken by emergency department personnel and start with the first health professional encountered by the patient. Application of the clinical pathway to the set of all CE patients allows for data collection that can be used for quality improvements. The data collected for CE patients from institutions with JCAHO stroke center certification is tested for adherence to performance measures. The current set of performance measures are seen in Box 1.

### When and for whom to initiate the clinical pathway

A main concern of emergency medicine staff is establishing the accurate diagnosis of CE among patients who present with a myriad of symptoms that may mimic the condition. During the course of emergency department evaluation to establish the diagnosis, an opportunity exists to begin care for neurologic complaints and deficits. The decision of when and for whom to initiate the specific behaviors required for the best CE care remains difficult for

**Box 1. JCAHO Stroke Center Certification performance measures**

For patients with diagnosis of ischemic or hemorrhagic stroke defined as:
- ICD-9-CM principal diagnosis code
- Age 18 years or older
- Treated at a Primary Stroke Center that is a certified Disease Specific Care Program

Performance measure: 1

Thrombolytic therapy administered

Population:

Acute ischemic stroke patients who arrive at the hospital within 120 minutes (2 hours) of time last known well and for whom IV tPA was initiated at this hospital within 180 minutes (3 hours) of time last known well

Excluded populations:
- Patients admitted for the performance of elective carotid endarterectomy
- Time last known well to arrival in the emergency department greater than (>) 2 hours or unknown

Performance measure: 2

Dysphagia screening performed

Population:

Patients with ischemic or hemorrhagic stroke who undergo screening for dysphagia with a simple valid bedside testing protocol before being given any food, fluids, or medication by mouth

Excluded populations:
- Patients admitted for the performance of elective carotid endarterectomy
- Patients who are NPO throughout the hospital stay

Performance measure: 3

Antithrombotic therapy initiated by end of hospital day 2

Population:

Patients with ischemic stroke who receive antithrombotic therapy by the end of hospital day 2

Excluded Populations:
- Patients discharged before the end of hospital day 2

Performance measure: 4

Deep vein thrombosis (DVT) prophylaxis initiated

Population:

Nonambulatory ischemic or hemorrhagic stroke patients should start receiving DVT prophylaxis by end of hospital day 2

Excluded populations:
- Patients who are discharged before end of hospital day 2:
- Patients receiving comfort measures only by end of hospital day 2
- Patients admitted for the performance of elective carotid endarterectomy
- Patients ambulating by end of hospital day 2

Performance measure: 5

Discharged on antithrombotic therapy

Population:

Patients with an ischemic stroke prescribed antithrombotic therapy at discharge

Excluded populations:
- Patients discharged/transferred to another short-term general hospital for inpatient care
- Patients who expired
- Patients who expired from a medical facility
- Patients who left against medical advice
- Patients discharged to hospice (home or facility)
- Patients receiving comfort measures only
- Patients for whom discharge destination cannot be determined or missing
- Patients admitted for the performance of elective carotid endarterectomy

Performance measure: 6

Patients with atrial fibrillation receiving anticoagulation therapy

Population:

Patients with an ischemic stroke with atrial fibrillation discharged on anticoagulation therapy

Excluded populations:
- Patients discharged/transferred to another short-term general hospital for inpatient care
- Patients who expire
- Patients who left against medical advice
- Patients discharged to hospice
- Patients receiving comfort measures only
- Patients admitted for the performance of elective carotid endarterectomy

Performance measure: 7

Discharged on cholesterol-reducing medication

Population:

Ischemic stroke patients with LDL >100, or LDL not measured, or on cholesterol-reducer before admission, who are discharged on cholesterol reducing drugs.

Excluded populations:

- Patients discharged/transferred to another short-term general hospital for inpatient care
- Patients who expired
- Patients who left against medical advice
- Patients discharged to hospice
- Patients receiving comfort measures only
- Patients admitted for the performance of elective carotid endarterectomy

Performance measure: 8

Stroke education provided

Population:

Patients with ischemic or hemorrhagic stroke or their caregivers who were given education or educational materials during the hospital stay addressing all of the following: personal risk factors for stroke, warning signs for stroke, activation of emergency medical system, need for follow-up after discharge, and medications prescribed.

Excluded populations:

- Patients who expired
- Patients discharged against medical advice
- Patients discharged/transferred to another short-term hospital for inpatient care
- Patients discharged to hospice
- Patients receiving comfort measures only
- Patients admitted for the performance of elective carotid endarterectomy

Performance measure: 9

Smoking cessation/advice/counseling

Population:

Patients with ischemic or hemorrhagic stroke with a history of smoking cigarettes, who are, or whose caregivers are, given smoking cessation advice or counseling during hospital stay. For the purposes of this measure, a smoker is defined as someone who has smoked cigarettes anytime during the year before hospital arrival

Excluded populations:

- Patients discharged/transferred to another short-term hospital for inpatient care
- Patients who expired
- Patients who left against medical advice
- Patients discharged to hospice
- Patients receiving comfort measures only

- Patients admitted for the performance of elective carotid endarterectomy

Performance measure: 10

Assessed for rehabilitation

Population:

Patients with an ischemic stroke or hemorrhagic stroke who were assessed for rehabilitation services

Excluded populations:

- Patients discharged/transferred to another short-term hospital for inpatient care
- Patients who expired
- Patients who left against medical advice
- Patients discharged to hospice
- Patients receiving comfort measures only
- Patients admitted for the performance of elective carotid endarterectomy

---

*Data from* The Joint Commission Certification Disease-Specific Care. Stroke performance measurement implementation guide. Available at: http://www.jointcommission.org.

a portion of patients because a final definitive diagnosis of stroke or TIA can only be established after hospital admission. This proves challenging because the performance measures that apply to stroke centers are based on final diagnosis of stroke. A practical approach to this problem would be to establish an "if–then" model for initiating stroke care behaviors. In such a model, patients who have an unequivocal diagnosis of stroke would begin the clinical pathway immediately upon arrival. Those who have another specific diagnosis as the condition inciting neurologic dysfunction or CE-like symptoms, ie, hypoglycemia, are not required to engage in a stroke pathway. For all other patients with CE (stroke or TIA) as a probable or possible diagnosis, the clinical pathway is initiated as soon as the diagnosis is entertained. The model would indicate the following: 1) If definite stroke, then initiate stroke pathway immediately upon arrival; 2) If probable or possible CE, then initiate stroke pathway as soon as the diagnosis is entertained; 3) If not stroke (another diagnosis is established as the condition inciting neurologic dysfunction), then stroke pathway is not required. A diagram of this model is visualized in Box 2.

In summary, the pathway is applied to all patients who have definite, probable, or possible diagnosis of CE as determined at the first point of care (emergency department, or the location of the patient with CE while hospitalized).

For those patients arriving by ambulance, the first health professional encountered by the patient will likely be emergency department personnel proper; for those arriving by non-EMS transport, it is likely the greeting

---

**Box 2. Model for initiating clinical pathway for CE**

Definite CE: Initiate clinical pathway upon arrival; all patients
in this category who arrive at the hospital within 120 minutes
(2 hours) of time last known in baseline state must have
documentation of IV tissue plasmogen activator (tPA)
evaluation and determination

Probable/possible CE: Initiate clinical pathway as soon as
diagnosis is entertained

Not CE: Another diagnosis is established as the condition inciting
neurologic deficits; clinical pathway not required

---

room attendant (or registrar). Because the possibility of providing therapeutics with IV tPA exists for every patient with stroke, the immediate recognition of stroke as a cause of patient's complaint must be a priority for training of these personnel. For hospitals with an accredited stroke program, greeting staff (registrars), triage nurses, and emergency department personnel proper are required to have training in stroke annually [8]. Prompting signs that clearly state stroke symptoms and signs can also be posted so that personnel who encounter these patients less frequently can be reminded of the need for immediate action. An example of a sign used by St. Agnes Hospital's greeting staff is seen in Box 3.

### Special considerations for IV tPA administration

The benchmark for ultra fast workup for possible IV tPA administration is that acute stroke patients (those who arrive within two hours of time last known to be at neurologic baseline) have completed diagnostic workup within one hour of arrival, or in a time period that would ensure IV tPA

---

**Box 3. Registrar's quick triage for stroke**

Hospital Emergency Department, Brain Pain–Stroke Quick Triage
for Registrars

Does the patient complain of any of the following symptoms?
- Sudden loss of speech
- Sudden loss of strength in an arm, leg, or both
- Sudden loss of vision
- Sudden loss of balance
- A sudden, severe headache unlike a previous headache

If yes, to any above: immediately triage to RN

---

administration is commenced within three hours from time last known to be at neurologic baseline. When time last known to be at neurologic baseline requires further investigation, it is wise to perform the workup as if the patient could receive tPA until the actual time is confirmed.

All CE patients must have time last at neurologic baseline documented. Because the older term "time of symptom onset" is fraught with misunderstanding and easily misinterpreted by patients and health providers, the newer terms of "time last at neurologic baseline" or "time last normal" are often used. This is the time the patient or a witness knows for a fact that the patient was last talking and walking normally. Determining this time can easily be categorized into an "A" or "B," that is to say, "either/or" diagram based on the patient's capability to communicate. Either "A," the patient is not aphasic and can pinpoint the time when last walking and talking normally, or "B," a witness can pinpoint the time visually observing the patient walking and talking normally. When "B" is required, the emergency department staff must personally confirm the time last normal with the witness.

Documentation of time of administration of IV tPA (for those receiving therapy) and for the reason that IV tPA was not administered (for those not receiving therapy) is required for all definite stroke patients arriving within 2 hours from the time last known to be at neurologic baseline. Documentation can be provided in the form of a checklist, numbering system, or as

---

**Box 4. Contraindications to IV tPA for stroke patients**

1. Evidence of intracranial hemorrhage on pretreatment evaluation
2. Suspicion of subarachnoid hemorrhage
3. Recent intracranial surgery or serious head trauma or recent previous stroke
4. History of intracranial hemorrhage
5. Uncontrolled hypertension at time of treatment (eg, >185 mm Hg systolic or >110 mm Hg diastolic)
6. Seizure at the onset of stroke
7. Active internal bleeding
8. Intracranial neoplasm, arteriovenous malformation, or aneurysm
9. Known bleeding diathesis including but not limited to:
   a. Current use of oral anticoagulants (eg, warfarin sodium) with prothrombin time (PT) >15 seconds
   b. Administration of heparin within 48 hours preceding the onset of stroke and have an elevated activated partial thromboplastin time (aPTT) at presentation
   i. Platelet count <100,000/mm$^3$

narrative by the physician managing the patient. Box 4 for IV tPA indications and contraindications.

Clarification of which physician can order and administer IV tPA is provided by the JCAHO on the organization's Web site as [2]:

A Board Certified emergency department physician can order and administer IV tPA using the clinical practice guidelines and clinical protocols without consulting a neurologist or the stroke team. Therefore, when a stroke team approved clinical pathway for stroke exists, the emergency medicine physician, as part of the stroke team, orders and administers IV tPA even in the event that a stroke team neurologist is not contacted.

IV tPA is indicated in adult stroke patients who, at the time of assessment, have a neurologic deficit. Therefore a standardized neurologic assessment tool is required for communication and documentation of the patient's deficit. Because the interrater reliability and validity of the National Institutes of Health Stroke Scale (NIHSS) has been established, and because it can be performed quickly, it is an ideal assessment tool used to determine the neurologic status of a CE patient. By definition, a patient with an NIHSS score of zero has no neurologic deficit, and therefore, no indication for IV tPA. Patients with scores of one or more would be considered for tPA therapy. There is no definitive lowest score cut off for which it is known that the risk outweighs the benefit. Likewise, although the highest scores in very elderly patients with large strokes may result in greater risk of hemorrhagic conversion, these patients are also seen to have greater odds of benefit.

NIHSS scoring is required for all CE patients, not only those for whom IV tPA is considered. When NIHSS scoring is performed serially, it can establish changes from the initial baseline deficits. Serial scoring is particularly useful when the patient has a change in physician and nursing providers such as when the patient is admitted and relocated from the emergency department to a hospital bed. Neurologic worsening, as indicated by any standard assessment tool, requires immediate investigation and treatment of neurologic and medical complications or comorbidities impacting recovery.

### Best practice aids for emergency medicine providers

Ensuring documentation for all aspects of diagnostics, IV tPA evaluation, swallowing assessment, and neurologic and medical status support can be challenging. Several national organizations have developed tool sets to assist in ensuring that standards of emergency medicine evaluation and management of CE patients are met. The National Institute of Neurologic Disorders and Stroke, the American Academy of Neurology, the American Stroke Association, the National Stroke Association, and others provide information online or via order that can be used fundamentally or incorporated into the clinical pathway for CE patients at any emergency department. Aids include prompts for emergency department personnel so that every CE patient has uniform evaluation and management, and communication is by documentation in the medical record and never inferred. Prompts may be forms, charts, tables, checklists, diagrams, posters, or other creative avenues to ensure performance of best practice for CE care. Multiple documentation requirements can be satisfied by template order sets and assessment tools. Our facility uses template forms for the NIH stroke scale scoring and dysphagia screening. Specific documentation requirements related to IV tPA, including time that the patient was last at neurologic baseline, total NIHSS score, and reason tPA not given, are written directly into the emergency department order sets. Templates should be used judiciously for stroke care, not purely for data collection purposes. All data collection must be handled in accordance with Health Information Protection and Portability Act regulations.

## Quality improvement processes

Data collected from clinical pathways offers an excellent opportunity to determine strengths and weaknesses of the care process. Because data can be collected in nearly real-time (while the patient is still hospitalized), feedback on the need for changes can be communicated back to providers and acted upon during a period of time still pertinent to ongoing care. When data is reviewed in regular time periods, need for improvement in specific performance measures can be addressed by usual process improvement steps. All emergency medicine departments should have designated periodic review time for identified problem areas and for special patient case reviews. Having a regularly designated time for improvement meetings and case reviews promotes collegiality among the many disciplines involved in stroke care. This avoids a sense of professional alienation of any one specialty in caring for this complex disorder whose care needs stretch across the spectrum from 911 call takers to emergency department care to hospitalization, rehabilitation, and family or out-of-home long-term care.

## Summary

Emergency department personnel are the largest and most influential group of health providers for patients in the early phase of CE. Evaluation and management performance standards are based on measures that are known to promote improved outcome for CE. Challenges in diagnosis, time constraints in workup, and documentation of the multiple facets of evaluation and management can be overcome by initiating a clinical pathway for CE patients and making use of available tools and aids for improving the process of care. Multidisciplinary conferences to review patient cases and clinical pathway data should be held regularly to ensure timely process improvements and strengthen teamwork.

# References

[1] Alberts MJ, Hademenos G, Latchaw RE, et al. Recommendations for the establishment of primary stroke centers. Brain attack coalition. JAMA 2000;283(23):3102–9.

[2] Available at: http://www.jointcommission.org.

[3] Ralph L Sacco, Robert Adams, Greg Albers, et al. Guidelines for prevention of stroke in patients with ischemic stroke or transient ischemic attack: a statement for healthcare professionals from the American Heart Association/American Stroke Association Council on Stroke: co-sponsored by the Council on Cardiovascular Radiology and Intervention. Stroke 2006;37:577–617.

[4] Harold Adams, Robert Adams, Gregory Del Zoppo, et al. American Heart Association/ American Stroke Association guidelines update a scientific statement from the stroke council of the guidelines for the early management of patients with ischemic stroke: 2005. Stroke 2005;36:916–23.

[5] Scott PA, Starkman S, Choi JY, et al. Provider support systems for acute stroke, in improving the chain of recovery for acute stroke in your community. National Institutes of Health, National Institute of Neurological Disorders and Stroke. September 2003, NIH Publication No. 03-5384.

[6] LaMonte MP, Medlin T, Gaasch W. Intravenous thrombolytic therapy for stroke: a review of recent studies and controversies. Ann Emerg Med 1999;34(2):244–55.

[7] LaMonte MP, Bahouth MN, Magder LS, et al. A regional system of stroke care provides thrombolytic outcomes comparable with the NINDS Stroke Trial. Ann Emerg Med 2008, in press.

[8] LaMonte MP. Evaluation and management of transient ischemic attacks. Clin Geriatr Med 2007;23(2):401–12.

ELSEVIER
SAUNDERS

Emerg Med Clin N Am
26 (2008) 715–739

EMERGENCY
MEDICINE
CLINICS OF
NORTH AMERICA

# Critical Care Toxicology

## Christopher P. Holstege, MD[a,b,c,]*,
## Stephen G. Dobmeier, BSN[c], Laura K. Bechtel, PhD[a]

[a]Division of Medical Toxicology, Department of Emergency Medicine, University of
Virginia School of Medicine, PO Box 800774, 1222 Jefferson Park Avenue,
4th Floor, Charlottesville, VA 22908–0774, USA
[b]Department of Pediatrics, University of Virginia School of Medicine, PO Box 800774,
Charlottesville, VA 22908–0774, USA
[c]Blue Ridge Poison Center, University of Virginia Health System, Room 4601,
1222 Jefferson Park Avenue, Charlottesville, VA 22903, USA

Critically poisoned patients are commonly encountered in emergency medicine. Exposure to potential toxins can occur by either accident (ie, occupational incidents or medication interactions) or intentionally (ie, substance abuse or intentional overdose). The outcome following a poisoning depends on numerous factors, such as the type of substance, the dose, the time from exposure to presentation to a health care facility, and the pre-existing health status of the patient. If a poisoning is recognized early and appropriate supportive care is initiated quickly, most patient outcomes are favorable. In modern hospitals with access to life support equipment the case fatality rate for self-poisonings is approximately 0.5%, but this can be as high as 10% to 20% in the developing world lacking critical care resources [1].

This article introduces the basic concepts for the initial approach to the critically poisoned patient and the steps required for stabilization. It introduces some key concepts in diagnosing the poisoning, using clinical clues and ancillary testing (ie, laboratory, ECG, and radiology). Finally, specific management issues are discussed.

## Clinical evaluation

When evaluating a patient who has presented with a potential toxicologic emergency, the health care practitioner should not limit the differential diagnosis. A comatose patient who smells of ethanol may be harboring an

* Corresponding author. PO Box 800774, Charlottesville, VA 22908–0774.
E-mail address: ch2xf@virginia.edu (C.P. Holstege).

intracranial hemorrhage; an agitated patient who seems anticholinergic may actually be encephalopathic from an infectious etiology. Patients must be thoroughly assessed and appropriately stabilized. Rarely is there a specific antidote for a poisoned patient; supportive care is the most important intervention.

All patients presenting with toxicity should be aggressively managed. Poisoned patients may seem to be in extremis (ie, brain dead), but most fully recover. The patient's airway should be patent and adequate ventilation ensured. If necessary, endotracheal intubation should be performed. Too often physicians are lulled into a false sense of security when a patient's oxygen saturations are adequate on high-flow oxygen. If the patient has either inadequate ventilation or poor airway protective reflexes, then the patient may be at risk for subsequent $CO_2$ narcosis with risk for worsening acidosis and the potential for aspiration. The initial treatment of hypotension for all poisonings consists of intravenous fluids. Close monitoring of the patient's pulmonary status should be performed to ensure that pulmonary edema does not develop as fluids are infused. The health care providers should place the patient on continuous cardiac monitoring with pulse oximetry and make frequent neurologic checks. Glucose should be checked at bedside in all patients with altered mental status. Poisoned patients should receive a large-bore peripheral intravenous line and all symptomatic patients should have a second line placed in either the peripheral or central venous system.

Many toxins can potentially cause seizures. In general, toxin-induced seizures are treated in a similar fashion to other seizures. Clinicians should ensure the patient maintains a patent airway and the blood glucose should be measured. Most toxin-induced seizures are self-limiting. For seizures requiring treatment, the first-line agent should be parenteral benzodiazepines. If benzodiazepines are not effective at controlling seizures, a second-line agent, such as phenobarbital, should be used. In rare poisoning cases (ie, isoniazid) pyridoxine should be administered. In cases of toxin-induced seizures, phenytoin is generally not recommended. It is usually ineffective and may add to the underlying toxicity of some agents, such as cyclic antidepressants, theophylline, cocaine, and lidocaine [2]. If a poisoned patient requires intubation, it is important to avoid the use of long-acting paralytic agents because these agents may mask seizures if they develop.

Rapid recognition of a toxidrome, if present, can help determine whether a poison is involved in a patient's condition and can help determine the class of toxin involved. Toxidromes are the constellation of signs and symptoms associated with a class of poisons. Table 1 lists selected toxidromes and their characteristics. Patients may not present with every component of a toxidrome and toxidromes can be clouded in mixed ingestions. Certain aspects of a toxidrome can have great significance. For example, noting dry axilla may be the only way of differentiating an anticholinergic patient from a sympathomimetic patient, and miosis may distinguish opioid toxicity from a benzodiazepine overdose. There are several notable exceptions to the

Table 1
Toxidromes

| Toxidrome | Clinical effects |
| --- | --- |
| Opioid | Sedation, miosis, decreased bowel sounds, decreased respirations |
| Anticholinergic | Mydriasis, dry skin, dry mucous membranes, decreased bowel sounds, sedation, altered mental status, hallucinations, tachycardia, urinary retention |
| Sympathomimetic | Agitation, mydriasis, tachycardia, hypertension, hyperthermia, diaphoresis |
| Cholinergic | Miosis, lacrimation, diaphoresis, bronchospasm, bronchorrhea, vomiting, diarrhea, bradycardia |
| Serotonin syndrome | Altered mental status, tachycardia, hypertension, hyperreflexia, clonus, hyperthermia |

recognized toxidromes. For example, several opioid agents do not cause miosis (ie, meperidine and tramadol). In most cases, a toxidrome does not indicate a specific poison, but rather a class of poisons.

## Testing in the critically poisoned patient

When evaluating the critically ill poisoned patient, there is no substitute for a thorough history and physical examination. Numerous television medical shows depict a universal toxicology screen that automatically determines the agent causing a patient's symptoms. Unfortunately, samples cannot be simply "sent to the laboratory" with the correct diagnosis to a clinical mystery returning on a computer printout. Clues from a patient's physical examination are generally more likely to be helpful than a "shotgun" laboratory approach that involves indiscriminate testing of blood or urine for multiple agents [3].

When used appropriately, diagnostic tests may be of help in the management of the intoxicated patient. When a specific toxin or even class of toxins is suspected, requesting qualitative or quantitative levels may be appropriate [4]. In the suicidal patient whose history is generally unreliable or in the unresponsive patient where no history is available, the clinician may gain further clues as to the etiology of a poisoning by responsible diagnostic testing. In the intentionally poisoned patient, an acetaminophen level should be obtained to rule out coexisting toxicity.

### Anion gap

A basic metabolic panel should be obtained in all suicidal poisoned patients. When low serum bicarbonate is discovered on a metabolic panel, the clinician should determine if an elevated anion gap exists. The formula most commonly used for the anion gap calculation is [5]

$$[\text{Na}^+] - [\text{Cl}^- + \text{HCO}_3]$$

   This equation allows one to determine if serum electroneutrality is being maintained. The primary cation (sodium) and anions (chloride and bicarbonate) are represented in the equation [6]. There are other contributors to this equation that are unmeasured [7]. Other serum cations are not commonly included in this calculation, because either their concentrations are relatively low (ie, potassium) or assigning a number to represent their respective contribution is difficult (ie, magnesium, calcium) [7]. Similarly, there is also a multitude of other serum anions (ie, sulfate, phosphate, organic anions) that are also difficult to measure and quantify in an equation [6,7]. These unmeasured ions represent the anion gap calculated using the previously mentioned equation. The normal range for this anion gap is accepted to be 8 to 16 mEq/L [7], but some have recently suggested that because of changes in the technique for measuring chloride, the range should be lowered to 6 to 14 mEq/L [6]. An increase in the anion gap beyond an accepted normal range, accompanied by a metabolic acidosis, represents an increase in unmeasured endogenous (ie, lactate) or exogenous (ie, salicylates) anions [5]. A list of the more common causes of this phenomenon is organized in the classic MUDILES pneumonic as shown (the "P" has been removed from the older acronym of MUDPILES, because paraldehyde is no longer available):

   Methanol
   Uremia
   Diabetic ketoacidosis
   Iron, inhalants (ie, carbon monoxide, cyanide, toluene), isoniazid, ibuprofen
   Lactic acidosis
   Ethylene glycol, ethanol ketoacidosis
   Salicylates, starvation ketoacidosis, sympathomimetics

   It is imperative that clinicians who evaluate poisoned patients initially presenting with an increased anion gap metabolic acidosis investigate the etiology of that acidosis. Symptomatic poisoned patients may have an initial mild metabolic acidosis on presentation because of an elevation of serum lactate that can be caused by a number of processes before stabilization (ie, agitation, hypoxia, hypotension). With adequate supportive care including hydration and oxygenation, the anion gap acidosis should begin to resolve. If, despite adequate supportive care, an anion gap metabolic acidosis worsens in a poisoned patient, the clinician should consider toxins that form acidic metabolites (ie, ethylene glycol, methanol) [8]; toxins that themselves can worsen the acidosis as absorption increases (ie, ibuprofen) [9]; or toxins that cause lactic acidosis by interfering with aerobic energy production (ie, cyanide or iron) [10].

*Osmole gap*

   The serum osmole gap is a common laboratory test that may be useful when evaluating poisoned patients. This test is most often discussed in the context of evaluating the patient suspected of toxic alcohol (ie, ethylene glycol, methanol, and isopropanol) intoxication. Although this test may have use in such situations, it has many pitfalls and limitations to its effectiveness.

Osmotic concentrations are themselves expressed in both terms of osmolality (milliosmoles per kilogram of solution) and osmolarity (milliosmoles per liter of solution) [11,12]. This concentration can be measured by use of an osmometer, a tool that most often uses the technique of freezing point depression and is expressed in osmolality ($Osm_M$) [13]. A calculated serum osmolarity ($Osm_C$) may be obtained by any of a number of equations [14], involving the patient's glucose, sodium, and urea that contribute to almost all of the normally measured osmolality [15]. One of the most commonly used of these calculations is expressed below:

$$Osm_C = 2[Na^+] + [BUN]/2.8 + [glucose]/18$$

The correction factors in the equation are based on the relative osmotic activity of the substance in question [11]. Assuming serum neutrality, sodium as the predominant serum cation is doubled to account for the corresponding anions. Finding the osmolarity contribution of any other osmotically active substances that is reported in milligrams per deciliter (like blood, urea, nitrogen [BUN] and glucose) is accomplished by dividing by one tenth its molecular weight in daltons [11]. For BUN this conversion factor is 2.8 and for glucose it is 18. Similar conversion factors may be added to this equation to account for ethanol and the various toxic alcohols as shown below:

$$Osm_C = 2[Na^+] + [BUN]/2.8 + [glucose]/18 + [ethanol]/4.6$$
$$+ [methanol]/3.2 + [ethylene\ glycol]/6.2 + [isopropanol]/6.0$$

The difference between the measured ($Osm_M$) and calculated ($Osm_C$) is the osmole gap (OG) and is depicted by the equation below [11]:

$$OG = Osm_M - Osm_C$$

If a significant osmole gap is discovered, the difference in the two values may represent presence of foreign substances in the blood [13]. Possible causes of an elevated osmole gap are listed as follows:

Acetone
Ethanol
Ethylene glycol
Isopropanol
Methanol
Propylene glycol

Unfortunately, what constitutes a normal osmole gap is widely debated. Traditionally, a normal gap has been defined as less than or equal to 10 mOsm/kg. The original source of this value is an article from Smithline and Gardner [16] that declares this number as pure convention. Further clinical study has not shown this assumption to be correct. Glasser and colleagues [17] studied 56 healthy adults and reported that they found the normal osmole gap to range from −9 to 5+ mOsm/kg. A study examining a pediatric emergency department population (N = 192) found a range from −13.5 to 8.9 [18]. Another study by Aabakken and colleagues [19] looked at the osmole gaps of 177 patients admitted to their emergency department and reported their range to be from −10 to 20 mOsm/kg. A vital point brought forth by the authors of this study is that the day-to-day co-efficient of variance for their laboratory in regards to sodium was 1%. They believed this variance translated to a calculated analytic standard deviation of 9.1 mOsm in regards to osmole gap. This analytic variance alone may account for the variation found in patient's osmole gaps. This concern that even small errors in the measurement of sodium can result in large variations of the osmole gap has been voiced by other researchers [18,20]. Overall, the clinician should recognize that there is likely a wide range of variability in a patient's baseline osmole gap.

There are several concerns in regard to using the osmole gap as a screening tool in the evaluation of the potentially toxic-alcohol poisoned patient. The lack of a well-established normal range is particularly problematic. For example, a patient may present with an osmole gap of 9 mOsm, a value considered normal by the traditionally accepted normal maximum gap value of 10 mOsm. If this patient had an osmole gap of −5 just before ingestion of a toxic alcohol, the patient's osmole gap must have been increased by 14 mOsm to reach the new gap of 9 mOsm. If this increase was caused by ethylene glycol, it corresponds to a toxic level of 86.8 mg/dL [21]. In addition, if a patient's ingestion of a toxic alcohol occurred at a time distant from the actual blood sampling, the osmotically active parent compound has been metabolized to the acidic metabolites. The subsequent metabolites have no osmotic activity of their own and hence no osmole gap is detected [14,22]. It is possible that a patient may present at a point after ingestion with only a moderate rise in their osmole gap and anion gap. Steinhart [23] reported a patient with ethylene glycol toxicity who presented with an osmole gap of 7.2 mOsm caused by delay in presentation. Darchy and colleagues [20] presented two other cases of significant ethylene glycol toxicity with osmole gaps of 4 and 7, respectively. The lack of an abnormal osmole gap in these cases was speculated either to be caused by metabolism of the parent alcohol or a low baseline osmole gap that masked the toxin's presence.

The osmole gap should be used with caution as an adjunct to clinical decision making and not as a primary determinant to rule out toxic alcohol ingestion. If the osmole gap obtained is particularly large, it suggests an agent from the previous list may be present. A normal osmole should be interpreted with caution; a negative study may not rule out the presence of such an ingestion; and the test result must be interpreted within the context of the clinical presentation. If such a poisoning is suspected, appropriate therapy should be initiated presumptively (ie, ethanol infusion, 4-methyl-pyrazole, hemodialysis, and so forth) while confirmation from serum levels of the suspected toxin are pending.

## Urine drug screening

Many clinicians regularly obtain urine drug screening on altered patients or on those suspected of ingestion. Such routine urine drug testing is of questionable benefit. Kellermann and colleagues [24] found little impact of urine drug screening on patient management in an urban emergency setting, and Mahoney and colleagues [25] similarly conclude that toxic screening added little to treatment or disposition of overdose patients in their emergency department. In a study of over 200 overdose patients, Brett [26] showed that although unsuspected drugs were routinely detected, the results rarely led to changes in management and likely never affected outcome. In a similar large study of trauma patients, Bast and colleagues [27] noted that a positive drug screen had minimal impact on patient treatment.

Some authors do argue in favor of routine testing. Fabbri and colleagues [28] countered that comprehensive screening may aid decisions on patient disposition, resulting in fewer admissions to the hospital and less demand on critical care units. The screen used in their retrospective study tested for over 900 drugs and is not available to most clinicians. Milzman and colleagues [29] argued in favor of screening trauma victims, stating that the prognosis of intoxicated patients is unduly poor secondary to low Glasgow Coma Scores, although patient treatment and disposition did not seem to be affected [29].

The effect of such routine screening on patient management is low because most of the therapy is supportive and directed at the clinical scenario (ie, mental status, cardiovascular function, respiratory condition). Interpretation of the results can be difficult even when the objective for ordering a comprehensive urine screen is adequately defined. Most assays rely on the antibody identification of drug metabolites, with some drugs remaining positive days after use, and may not be related to the patient's current clinical picture. The positive identification of drug metabolites is likewise influenced by chronicity of ingestion, fat solubility, and coingestions. In one such example, Perrone and colleagues [30] showed a cocaine retention time of 72 hours following its use. Conversely, many drugs of abuse are not detected on most urine drug screens, including gamma hydroxybutyrate, fentanyl, and ketamine.

Interpretation is further confounded by false-positive and false-negative results. George and Braithwaite [31] evaluated five popular rapid urine screening kits and found all lacked significant sensitivity and specificity. The monoclonal antibodies used in these immunoassays may detect epitopes from multiple drug classes. For example, a relatively new antidepressant, venlafaxine, produced false-positive results by cross-reactivity with the antiphencyclidine antibodies used in a urine test device [32]. False-positive benzodiazepine results were found in patients receiving the nonsteroidal anti-inflammatory drug oxaprozin who were screened using urine immuno-assays [33]. Conversely, antibodies used in the immunoassays may not detect all drugs classified within a specific drug class. For example, one urine immunoassay does not detect physiologic doses of methadone. This assay detects codeine and its metabolites: morphine and morphine-3-glucuronide. Additionally, cross-reactivity of both prescription and over-the-counter medications used in therapeutic amounts for true illness may elicit positive screens. Diphenhydramine has been documented to interfere with one urine immunoassay for propoxyphene [34].

The use of ordering urine drug screens is fraught with significant testing limitations, including false-positive and false-negative results. Many authors have shown that the test results rarely affect management decisions. Routine drug screening of those with altered mental status, abnormal vital signs, or suspected ingestion is not warranted and rarely guides patient treatment or disposition.

*Radiographic studies*

The role of radiologic testing specifically in the diagnosis and manage-ment of the critically poisoned patient is limited. Radiologic testing is com-monly used to diagnose complications associated with poisonings, such as aspiration pneumonitis and anoxic brain injury.

In some circumstances, plain radiography can assist in the diagnosis and management of poisonings if the substance in question is radiopaque. The primary use of radiography in the critically ill poisoned patient is in the detection and management of iron poisoning (Fig. 1) [35–37]. Attempts to use the presence or absence of radiopacities consistently to predict severe iron toxicity have not been successful [38,39]. Not all iron products are equally radiopaque; whereas ferrous sulfate and ferrous fumarate are typically radiopaque, other preparations may not be radiopaque [40]. For example, chewable iron supplements are unlikely to be seen on abdominal radiographs [37] secondary to both the low elemental content in these chew-able products and as a result of their quick dissolution in the gastrointestinal tract [37]. In using abdominal radiographs in diagnosing iron poisonings, time from ingestion is important; as time passes visualization becomes more difficult [35].

Another situation where plain radiography may prove useful is with body packers. These couriers, also known as "mules," swallow multiple packages of illicit drugs for the purposes of transporting without detection. The con-tainer of choice is often condoms, latex, or cellophane formed into balls or ovals that are 2 to 4 cm in size [41]. Besides the illegal nature of this occupa-tion, there is a serious health risk to these patients who may suffer from

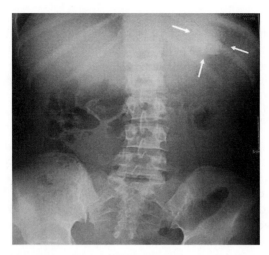

Fig. 1. A radiograph demonstrating a grouping of iron tablets in the stomach (*arrows*) following a suicidal ingestion of ferrous fumarate.

intestinal obstruction or from the direct effects of the illicit drugs themselves if the packages leak [42]. One study by Karhunen and colleagues [43] in Finland looked at a total of 82 patients admitted for abdominal radiographs because of suspected body packing. Twelve of these were read as positive, and nine of these proved to be true positives (75%). The three false-positives (3.6%) were thought secondary to constipation involving compact feces with increased radiodensity mimicking narcotic packages. There were 70 films that were read as negative with only one false-negative (1.2%) that was attributed to the inexperience of the radiologist. In a recent review of the literature, plain abdominal radiography was identified as the radiologic method of choice for finding these packets, as opposed to ultrasound and CT [41]. The authors based this decision on ease of use, availability, patient tolerance, and the relatively high sensitivity and specificity shown by the Karhunen study.

Besides these established examples, plain radiography of the abdomen has also been studied to identify other pills that may be radiopaque in acute overdose. Multiple studies regarding the radiopacity of ingested pharmaceuticals have not consistently supported the use of radiography in management of these patients. O'Brien and colleagues [44] studied the detect ability of 459 different tablets and capsules using plain radiography. The investigators used a ferrous sulfate tablet as a control grading the other tablets' radiopacity. These pills were then placed in the middle of a plastic container that contained 20 cm of water to simulate the human body density. Overall, of the wide variety of pills tested, only 29 drugs (6.3%) were graded as having the same or greater radiopacity as ferrous sulfate; 136 pills (29.6%) were regarded as having at least moderate opacity; and the largest remaining portion of pills, 294 (64%), were regarded as no more than min-imally detectable. The authors concluded that indiscriminate use of plain abdominal radiographs was not justified and that a negative film could not be relied on to rule out potential toxic pill ingestions, especially if there is time to allow the pills to dissolve.

*Electrocardiogram*

The interpretation of ECG in the poisoned patient can challenge even the most experienced clinician. There are numerous drugs that can cause ECG changes. The incidence of ECG changes in the poisoned patient is unclear and the significance of various changes may be difficult to define. Despite the fact that drugs have widely varying indications for therapeutic use, many unrelated drugs share common cardiac electrocardiographic effects if taken in overdose. Potential toxins can be placed into broad classes based on their cardiac effects. Two such classes, agents that block the cardiac potassium efflux channels and agents that block cardiac fast sodium chan-nels, can lead to characteristic changes in cardiac indices consisting of QRS prolongation and QT prolongation, respectively. The recognition of specific ECG changes associated with other clinical data (toxidromes) can be potentially life saving [45].

Studies suggest that approximately 3% of all noncardiac prescriptions are associated with the potential for QT prolongation [46]. Myocardial re-polarization is driven predominantly by outward movement of potassium ions [47]. Blockade of the outward potassium currents by drugs prolongs the action potential, resulting in QT interval prolongation and the poten-tial emergence of T- or U-wave abnormalities on the ECG [48,49]. The prolongation of repolarization causes the myocardial cell to have less charge difference across its membrane, which may result in the activation of the inward depolarization current (early afterdepolarization) and pro-mote triggered activity. These changes may lead to reentry and subsequent polymorphic ventricular tachycardia, most often as the torsades de pointes variant of polymorphic ventricular tachycardia [50]. The QT interval is simply measured from the beginning of the QRS complex to the end of the T wave. Within any ECG tracing, there is lead-to-lead variation of the QT interval. In general, the longest measurable QT interval on an ECG is regarded as determining the overall QT interval for a given tracing [51]. The QT interval is influenced by the patient's heart rate. Several for-mulas have been developed to correct the QT interval for the effect of heart rate (QTc) using the RR interval (RR), with Bazett's formula ($QTc = QT/RR^{1/2}$) being the most commonly used. QT prolongation is considered to occur when the QTc interval is greater than 440 milliseconds in men and 460 milliseconds in women, with arrhythmias most commonly associated with values greater than 500 milliseconds (Fig. 2). The potential for an arrhythmia for a given QT interval varies from drug to drug and

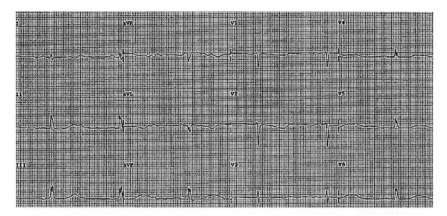

Fig. 2. ECG demonstrating sinus bradycardia with marked QT prolongation (660 ms) following an overdose of sotalol.

patient to patient [47]. Drugs associated with QT prolongation are listed in Box 1 [52].

Other etiologies involved in possible prolongation of the QT interval include congenital long QT syndrome, mitral valve prolapse, hypokalemia, hypocalcemia, hypomagnesemia, hypothermia, myocardial ischemia, neurologic catastrophes, and hypothyroidism [53].

The ability of drugs to induce cardiac $Na^+$ channel blockade and prolong the QRS complex has been well described in numerous literature reports (Fig. 3) [54]. This $Na^+$ channel blockade activity has been described as a membrane stabilizing effect, a local anesthetic effect, or a quinidine-like effect. Cardiac voltage-gated sodium channels reside in the cell membrane and open in conjunction with cell depolarization. Sodium channel blockers bind to the transmembrane $Na^+$ channels and decrease the number available for depolarization. This creates a delay of $Na^+$ entry into the cardiac myocyte during phase 0 of depolarization. As a result, the upslope of depolarization is slowed and the QRS complex widens [55]. In some cases, the QRS complex may take the pattern of recognized bundle branch blocks [56,57]. In the most severe cases, the QRS prolongation becomes so profound that it is difficult to distinguish between ventricular and supraventricular rhythms [58,59]. Continued prolongation of the QRS may result in a sine wave pattern and eventual asystole (Fig. 4). It has been theorized that the $Na^+$ channel blockers can cause slowed intraventricular conduction, unidirectional block, the development of a reentrant circuit, and a resulting ventricular tachycardia [60]. This can then degenerate into ventricular fibrillation. Differentiating a prolongation of the QRS complex because of $Na^+$ channel blockade in the poisoned patient versus other nontoxic etiologies can be difficult. Rightward axis deviation of the terminal 40 milliseconds of the QRS axis has been associated with tricyclic antidepressant poisoning [61,62]. The occurrence of this finding in other $Na^+$ channel blocking agents is unknown.

**Box 1. K⁺ efflux channel blocking drugs**

Antihistamines
  Astemizole
  Clarithromycin
  Diphenhydramine
  Loratidine
  Terfenadine
Antipsychotics
  Chlorpromazine
  Droperidol
  Haloperidol
  Mesoridazine
  Pimozide
  Quetiapine
  Risperidone
  Thioridazine
  Ziprasidone
Arsenic trioxide
Bepridil
Chloroquine
Cisapride
Citalopram
Clarithromycin
Class IA antiarrhythmics
  Disopyramide
  Quinidine
  Procainamide
Class IC antiarrhythmics
  Encainide
  Flecainide
  Moricizine
  Propafenone
Class III antiarrhythmics
  Amiodarone
  Dofetilide
  Ibutilide
  Sotalol
Cyclic antidepressants
  Amitriptyline
  Amoxapine
  Desipramine
  Doxepin

Imipramine
Nortriptyline
Maprotiline
Erythromycin
Fluoroquinolones
  Ciprofloxacin
  Gatifloxacin
  Levofloxacin
  Moxifloxacin
  Sparfloxacin
Hydroxychloroquine
Levomethadyl
Methadone
Pentamidine
Quinine
Tacrolimus
Venlafaxine

Myocardial $Na^+$ channel blocking drugs comprise a diverse group of pharmaceutical agents (Box 2).

Patients poisoned with these agents have a variety of clinical presentations. For example, sodium channel blocking medications, such as diphenhydramine, propoxyphene, and cocaine, may also develop anticholinergic, opioid, and sympathomimetic syndromes, respectively [63–65]. In addition, specific drugs may affect not only the myocardial $Na^+$ channels, but also calcium influx and potassium efflux channels [66,67]. This may result in ECG changes and rhythm disturbances not related entirely to the drug's $Na^+$ channel blocking activity. All the agents listed in Box 2 are similar in that they may induce myocardial $Na^+$ channel blockade and may respond to therapy with hypertonic saline or sodium bicarbonate [59,64,65]. It is

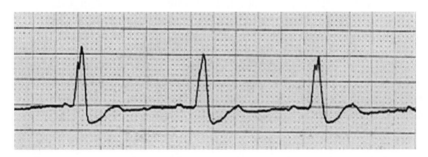

Fig. 3. A rhythm strip demonstrating marked QRS prolongation following a propoxyphene overdose.

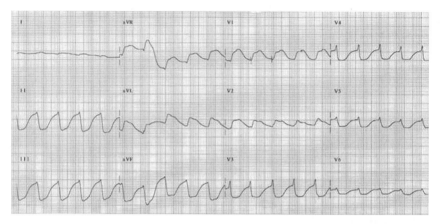

Fig. 4. An ECG demonstrating a sinusoidal wave pattern secondary to the sodium channel blockade induced by an acute overdose of hydroxychloroquine.

reasonable to treat poisoned patients with a prolonged QRS interval, particularly those with hemodynamic instability, empirically with 1 to 2 mEq/kg of sodium bicarbonate. A shortening of the QRS can confirm the presence of a sodium channel blocking agent. It can also improve inotropy and help prevent arrhythmias [54].

There are multiple agents that can result in cardiotoxicity and subsequent ECG changes from the changes noted previously to other alterations, such as bradycardia and tachycardia. Physicians managing patients who have taken overdoses on medications should be aware of the various electrocardiographic changes that can potentially occur in the overdose setting.

## Management

After initial evaluation and stabilization of the critically poisoned patient as described previously, the physician can consider whether there is a need for the administration of specific therapies. Decontamination should be considered. Several poisons have specific antidotes that if used in a timely and appropriate manner can be of great benefit. Finally, the safe disposition of the patient must be determined (ie, monitored floor bed or ICU).

Approximately 80% of all poisonings occur by ingestion and the most common type of decontamination performed is gastrointestinal decontamination using a variety of techniques including emesis, gastric lavage, activated charcoal, cathartics, and whole-bowel irrigation. Poisonings may also occur by dermal and ocular routes, which necessitate external decontamination. Significant controversy exists concerning the need for routine gastric emptying in the poisoned patient. Current available evidence dissuades from the routine use of gastric decontamination. Gastric decontamination may be considered in select cases and specific scenarios. Before

---

**Box 2. Na$^+$ channel blocking drugs**

Amantadine
Carbamazepine
Chloroquine
Class IA antiarrhythmics
   Disopyramide
   Quinidine
   Procainamide
Class IC antiarrhythmics
   Encainide
   Flecainide
   Propafenone
Citalopram
Cocaine
Cyclic antidepressants
Diltiazem
Diphenhydramine
Hydroxychloroquine
Loxapine
Orphenadrine
Phenothiazines
   Medoridazine
   Thioridazine
Propranolol
Propoxyphene
Quinine
Verapamil

---

performing gastrointestinal decontamination techniques, the clinician responsible for the care of the poisoned patient must clearly understand whether the benefit of decontamination outweighs any potential harm.

The number of pharmacologic antagonists or antidotes available to treat the critically poisoned patient is quite limited (Table 2). There are few antidotes that rapidly reverse toxic effects and restore a patient to a previously healthy baseline state. Administering some pharmacologic antagonists may worsen patient outcome compared with simply optimizing basic supportive care. Antidotes should be used cautiously, with a clear understanding of indications and contraindications.

*Atropine*

Atropine is the initial drug of choice in symptomatic patients poisoned with organophosphates or carbamates. Atropine acts as a muscarinic

Table 2
Antidotes

| Agent or clinical finding | Antidote |
| --- | --- |
| Acetaminophen | N-acetylcysteine |
| Benzodiazepines | Flumazenil |
| β-blockers | Glucagon |
| Cardiac glycosides | Digoxin immune Fab |
| Crotalid envenomation | Crotalidae polyvalent immune Fab |
| Cyanide | Hydroxocobalamin |
| Ethylene glycol | Fomepizole |
| Iron | Deferoxamine |
| Isoniazid | Pyridoxine |
| Methanol | Fomepizole |
| Methemoglobinemia | Methylene blue |
| Opioids | Naloxone |
| Organophosphates | Atropine |
|  | Pralidoxime |
| Sulfonylureas | Octreotide |

receptor antagonist and blocks neuroeffector sites on smooth muscle, cardiac muscle, secretory gland cells, and the central nervous system. Atropine is useful in alleviating bronchoconstriction, bronchorrhea, tenesmus, abdominal cramps, nausea, vomiting, bradydysrythmias, and seizure activity. Atropine can be administered by the intravenous, intraosseous, intramuscular, or endotracheal route. The dose varies with the type of exposure, requiring a few milligrams in mild cases and hundreds of milligrams in extreme cases [68]. For the mildly and moderately symptomatic patient, 2 mg for adults and 0.02 mg/kg for children (minimum of 0.1 mg) is administered every 5 minutes. In the severely poisoned patient, dosages may need to be increased and given more rapidly [69]. Tachycardia is not a contraindication to atropine administration in these patients. Drying of the respiratory secretions and resolution of bronchoconstriction are the therapeutic end points used to determine the appropriate dose of atropine. This is clinically apparent as the patient's work of breathing improves [68]. Atropine has no effect on the nicotinic receptors and has no effect on autonomic ganglia and neuromuscular junction [69]. Muscle weakness, fasciculations, tremors, and paralysis are not indications for further atropine dosing. It does have a partial effect on the central nervous system and is helpful in resolving or preventing seizures [70]. It is most effective in preventing seizures if given within 5 minutes of organophosphate exposure [71]. After 5 to 10 minutes anticholinergic treatment alone is not effective at terminating seizures and benzodiazepines must be added to treat seizures effectively [71,72].

*Deferoxamine*

Deferoxamine is an effective chelator of iron. Deferoxamine chelates iron and converts it to a water-soluble complex, ferrioxamine, which is eliminated readily by the urine. Indications for deferoxamine infusion include significant clinical signs of iron toxicity, metabolic acidosis, shock, profound lethargy, coma, serum iron levels greater than 500 µg/dL, or a radiograph positive for multiple pills [73]. Deferoxamine should be infused intravenously at a starting rate of 15 mg/kg/h, not to exceed 1 g/h, over a total of 6 hours, followed by re-evaluation. Deferoxamine-induced hypotension may occur at fast rates, and adequate hydration should be ensured before infusion initiation [73]. As iron is chelated and excreted, urine may develop a characteristic rusty-red (vine rose) appearance.

## Crotalidae antivenin

Use of antivenin in the appropriate doses can control local swelling and serious systemic effects (ie, coagulopathy) that occur in patients who have been envenomated [74]. Antivenin should not be used prophylactically because a significant number of snake bites are dry bites. There are numerous dosage regimens that vary with the degree of systemic toxicity and regional treatment preferences. Consultation with a poison center or a clinical toxicologist is advised for the most contemporary treatment recommendations.

## Digoxin immune Fab

Digoxin-specific Fab fragments are antibody fragments produced by enzymatic cleavage of sheep IgG antibodies to digoxin. Fab fragments can reverse digitalis-induced dysrhythmias, conduction disturbances, myocardial depression, and hyperkalemia in severely poisoned patients [75]. Patients can have reversal of ventricular arrhythmia within 2 minutes and most patients have settling of toxic dysrhythmias within 30 minutes of Fab administration [76]. Within 6 hours 90% of patients have complete or partial response [75]. Animal studies and case reports have demonstrated the efficacy of Fab fragments to the cardiac glycoside contained in plants [77–79]. Digoxin-specific Fab fragment therapy should be administered in a digoxin poisoned patient for the following indications: (1) potassium greater than 5 mEq/L following acute ingestion, (2) hemodynamic instability, and (3) patients with potentially life-threatening dysrhythmias [76].

Although serum digoxin levels should not be the sole factor in determining the need to administer Fab, dosage calculations for Fab are based on the serum digoxin level, or estimated body load of digoxin. It is assumed that equimolar doses of antibody fragments are required to achieve neutralization. Forty milligrams of Fab (one vial) bind 0.6 mg of digoxin. When presented with a severely poisoned patient in whom the quantity ingested acutely is unknown, an empiric dose of 5 to 10 vials at a time should be given and the clinical response observed. If cardiac arrest is imminent or has occurred, the dose can be given as a bolus, but it should be infused over 30 minutes in stable patients. For patients with chronic therapeutic overdoses the digoxin levels are often only mildly elevated and one to two vials of Fab may be sufficient [75]. The recommended dose for a given patient can be determined using the tables in the package insert or by contacting a regional poison center or toxicology consultant.

## Flumazenil

Benzodiazepines are involved in many intentional overdoses. Although these overdoses are rarely fatal when a benzodiazepine is the sole ingestant, they often complicate overdoses with other central nervous system depressants (eg, ethanol, opioids, and other sedatives) because of their synergistic activity. Flumazenil finds its greatest use in the reversal of benzodiazepine-induced sedation from minor surgical procedures. The initial flumazenil dose is 0.2 mg and should be administered intravenously over 30 seconds. If no response occurs after an additional 30 seconds, a second dose is recommended. Additional incremental doses of 0.5 mg may be administered at 1-minute intervals until the desired response is noted or until a total of 3 mg has been administered. It is important to note that resedation may occur [80], and patients should be observed with close monitoring after requiring reversal. Flumazenil should not be administered as a nonspecific coma-reversal drug and should be used with extreme caution after intentional benzodiazepine overdose because it has the potential to precipitate withdrawal in benzodiazepine-dependent individuals or induce seizures in those at risk [80].

## Fomepizole

Fomepizole (4-methyl-pyrazole) is an alcohol dehydrogenase inhibitor. It is administered in cases of suspected or confirmed ingestion and intoxication with ethylene glycol or methanol [81]. Fomepizole should be administered intravenously as a loading dose of 15 mg/kg, followed by doses of 10 mg/kg every 12 hours for four doses (48 hours) then 15 mg/kg every 12 hours thereafter [8,82]; all doses should be administered as a slow intravenous infusion over 30 minutes. During hemodialysis, the frequency of dosing should be increased to every 4 hours. Therapy should be continued until ethylene glycol or methanol concentrations are less than 20 mg/dL and the patient is asymptomatic.

## Hydroxocobalamin

Hydroxocobalamin is a safe and effective treatment of cyanide toxicity that has recently been approved in the United States. The reaction of hydroxocobalamin with cyanide results in the displacement of a hydroxyl group by a cyano group to form cyanocobalamin (vitamin $B_{12}$), which is then excreted in the urine [83]. The usual adult dose of hydroxocobalamin is 5 g, which may be repeated in cases of massive cyanide poisoning [84,85]. The pediatric dose is 70 mg/kg up to 5 g [86]. Virtually every patient receiving this antidote develops orange-red discoloration of the skin, mucous membranes, and urine. This resolves within 24 to 48 hours [87].

## N-Acetylcysteine

Significant acetaminophen overdoses may need to be treated with N-acetylcysteine if the patient has a toxic serum acetaminophen concentration or has indicators of hepatocellular damage [88]. N-acetylcysteine increases glutathione levels and serves as a glutathione surrogate. An acetaminophen overdose may deplete glutathione, permitting the toxic metabolite to destroy hepatocytes. N-acetylcysteine is most effective if administered within 8 hours of the acetaminophen ingestion; however, it can still be effective days after the ingestion when patients are already in hepatic failure and acetaminophen levels are no longer detectable [88].

N-acetylcysteine can be given by both oral and intravenous administration [88]. Oral is 140 mg/kg loading dose followed by 70 mg/kg every 4 hours for 17 doses. Intravenous is 150 mg/kg loading dose followed by 50 mg/kg over 4 hours followed by 100 mg/kg infused over 16 hours.

Parenteral administration of N-acetylcysteine eliminates compliance problems associated with oral therapy (adverse taste and odor caused by the sulfhydryl groups) and circumvents the problems associated with acetaminophen-induced vomiting.

## Naloxone

Opioid poisoning from the abuse of morphine derivatives or synthetic narcotic agents may be reversed with the opioid antagonist naloxone [89]. Naloxone is commonly used in comatose patients as a therapeutic and diagnostic agent. The standard dosage regimen is to administer from 0.4 to 2 mg slowly, preferably intravenously. The intravenous dose should be readministered at 5-minute intervals until the desired end point is achieved: restoration of respiratory function, ability to protect the airway, and an improved level of consciousness [90]. If the intravenous route of administration is not viable, alternative routes include intramuscular and intraosseous [90]. A patient may not respond to naloxone administration for a variety of reasons: insufficient dose of naloxone, the absence of an opioid exposure, a mixed overdose with other central nervous and respiratory system depressants, or medical or traumatic reasons.

Naloxone can precipitate profound withdrawal symptoms in opioid-dependant patients. Symptoms of withdrawal include agitation, vomiting, diarrhea, piloerection, diaphoresis, and yawning [90]. Care should be taken to administer this agent as necessary only to restore adequate respiration and airway protection. Naloxone's clinical efficacy can last for as little as 45 minutes [89]. Patients are at risk for recurrence of narcotic effect. This is particularly true for patients exposed to methadone or sustained-release opioid products. In addition, renal insufficiency increases naloxone's elimination half-life, placing the patient at risk for resedation hours after the initial dose. Patients should be observed in a monitored setting for resedation for at least 4 hours after reversal with naloxone. If a patient does resedate, it is reasonable to administer naloxone as an infusion. An infusion of two thirds the effective initial bolus per hour is usually effective [90].

*Pralidoxime chloride*

Pralidoxime chloride reactivates acetylcholinesterase by exerting a nucleophilic attack on the phosphorus resulting in an oxime-phosphate bond that splits from the acetylcholinesterase leaving the regenerated enzyme. This reactivation is clinically most apparent at skeletal neuromuscular junctions, with less activity at muscarinic sites [91]. Pralidoxime must be administered concurrently with adequate atropine doses. The process of aging prevents pralidoxime from regenerating the acetylcholinesterase-active site, and is ineffective after aging has occurred. The sooner pralidoxime is administered, the greater the clinical effect. The recommended dose of pralidoxime is 1 to 2 g for adults or 20 to 50 mg/kg for children by intravenous route. Slow administration over 15 to 30 minutes has been advocated to minimize side effects [68,92]. These side effects include hypertension, headache, blurred vision, epigastric discomfort, nausea, and vomiting. Rapid administration can result in laryngospasm, muscle rigidity, and transient impairment of respiration [91].

Pralidoxime is rapidly excreted by the kidney with a half-life of approximately 90 minutes [93]. A continuous infusion is often recommended after the loading dose to maintain therapeutic levels [94–97]. Currently, the World Health Organization recommends a bolus of greater than 30 mg/kg followed by an infusion of greater than 8 mg/kg/h [98].

*Pyridoxine*

Isoniazid, hydrazine, and the *Gyrometria* species of mushrooms can decrease the brain concentrations of γ-aminobutyric acid by inhibiting pyridoxal-5-phosphate activity, resulting in the development of severe seizure activity [99,100]. The administration of pyridoxine (vitamin $B_6$) can prevent or actively treat the central nervous system toxicity associated with these toxins [101]. Pyridoxine is administered on a gram-for-gram basis with isoniazid (ie, the amount of pyridoxine should equal the amount of isoniazid). If the ingested amount of agent is unknown, the dose of pyridoxine should be 5 g administered intravenously [101]. This dose can be repeated.

**Summary**

The emergency physician often is required to care for critically poisoned patients. Prompt action must be taken for patients who present with serious toxic effects or after potentially fatal ingestions. Because many poisons have no true antidote and the poison involved may initially be unknown, the first step is simply focused on supportive care. Identifying the causative poison, through a detailed history, recognizing a toxidrome, or laboratory analysis may help direct care. There are several antidotes available that can be life saving, and the clinician should promptly identify those patients who may benefit from these agents.

# References

[1] Eddleston M, Haggalla S, Reginald K, et al. The hazards of gastric lavage for intentional self-poisoning in a resource poor location. Clin Toxicol 2007;45(2):136–43.

[2] Wills B, Erickson T. Drug- and toxin-associated seizures. Med Clin North Am 2005;89(6): 1297–321.

[3] Brett AS. Implications of discordance between clinical impression and toxicology analysis in drug overdose. Arch Intern Med 1988;148(2):437–41.

[4] Wu AH, McKay C, Broussard LA, et al. National Academy of Clinical Biochemistry laboratory medicine practice guidelines: recommendations for the use of laboratory tests to support poisoned patients who present to the emergency department. Clin Chem 2003;49(3):357–79.

[5] Chabali R. Diagnostic use of anion and osmoleal gaps in pediatric emergency medicine. Pediatr Emerg Care 1997;13(3):204–10.

[6] Ishihara K, Szerlip HM. Anion gap acidosis. Semin Nephrol 1998;18(1):83–97.

[7] Gabow PA. Disorders associated with an altered anion gap. Kidney Int 1985;27(2):472–83.

[8] Mégarbane B, Borron SW, Baud FJ. Current recommendations for treatment of severe toxic alcohol poisonings. Intensive Care Med 2005;31(2):189–95.

[9] Marciniak K, Thomas I, Brogan T, et al. Massive ibuprofen overdose requiring extracorporeal membrane oxygenation for cardiovascular support. Pediatr Crit Care Med 2007; 8(2):180–2 [Report].

[10] Judge BS. Metabolic acidosis: differentiating the causes in the poisoned patient. Med Clin North Am 2005;89(6):1107–24.

[11] Suchard JR. Osmoleal gap. In: Dart RC, editor. Medical toxicology. 3rd edition. Philadelphia: Lippincott Williams & Wilkins; 2004. p. 106–9.

[12] Kruse JA, Cadnapaphornchai P. The serum osmol gap. J Crit Care 1994;9(3):185–97.

[13] Erstad BL. Osmoleality and osmolearity: narrowing the terminology gap. Pharmacotherapy 2003;23(9):1085–6.

[14] Glaser DS. Utility of the serum osmole gap in the diagnosis of methanol or ethylene glycol ingestion. Ann Emerg Med 1996;27(3):343–6.

[15] Worthley LI, Guerin M, Pain RW. For calculating osmoleality, the simplest formula is the best. Anaesth Intensive Care 1987;15(2):199–202.

[16] Smithline N, Gardner KD Jr. Gaps–anionic and osmoleal. JAMA 1976;236(14):1594–7.

[17] Glasser L, Sternglanz PD, Combie J, et al. Serum osmoleality and its applicability to drug overdose. Am J Clin Pathol 1973;60(5):695–9.

[18] McQuillen KK, Anderson AC. Osmole gaps in the pediatric population. Acad Emerg Med 1999;6(1):27–30.

[19] Aabakken L, Johansen KS, Rydningen EB, et al. Osmolal and anion gaps in patients admitted to an emergency medical department. Hum Exp Toxicol 1994;13(2):131–4.

[20] Darchy B, Abruzzese L, Pitiot O, et al. Delayed admission for ethylene glycol poisoning: lack of elevated serum osmole gap. Intensive Care Med 1999;25(8):859–61.

[21] Hoffman RS, Smilkstein MJ, Howland MA, et al. Osmole gaps revisited: normal values and limitations. J Toxicol Clin Toxicol 1993;31(1):81–93.

[22] Eder AF, McGrath CM, Dowdy YG, et al. Ethylene glycol poisoning: toxicokinetic and analytical factors affecting laboratory diagnosis. Clin Chem 1998;44(1):168–77.

[23] Steinhart B. Case report: severe ethylene glycol intoxication with normal osmoleal gap– a chilling thought. J Emerg Med 1990;8(5):583–5.

[24] Kellermann AL, Fihn SD, LoGerfo JP, et al. Impact of drug screening in suspected overdose. Ann Emerg Med 1987;16(11):1206–16.

[25] Mahoney JD, Gross PL, Stern TA, et al. Quantitative serum toxic screening in the management of suspected drug overdose. Am J Emerg Med 1990;8(1):16–22.

[26] Brett A. Toxicologic analysis in patients with drug overdose. Arch Intern Med 1988;148(9): 2077.

[27] Bast RP, Helmer SD, Henson SR, et al. Limited utility of routine drug screening in trauma patients. South Med J 2000;93(4):397–9.

[28] Fabbri A, Marchesini G, Morselli-Labate AM, et al. Comprehensive drug screening in decision making of patients attending the emergency department for suspected drug overdose. Emerg Med J 2003;20(1):25–8.

[29] Milzman DP, Boulanger BR, Rodriguez A, et al. Pre-existing disease in trauma patients: a predictor of fate independent of age and injury severity score. J Trauma 1992;32(2): 236–43.

[30] Perrone J, De Roos F, Jayaraman S, et al. Drug screening versus history in detection of substance use in ED psychiatric patients. Am J Emerg Med 2001;19(1):49–51.

[31] George S, Braithwaite RA. A preliminary evaluation of five rapid detection kits for on site drugs of abuse screening. Addiction 1995;90(2):227–32.

[32] Sena SF, Kazimi S, Wu AH. False-positive phencyclidine immunoassay results caused by venlafaxine and O-desmethylvenlafaxine. Clin Chem 2002;48(4):676–7.

[33] Camara PD, Audette L, Velletri K, et al. False-positive immunoassay results for urine benzodiazepine in patients receiving oxaprozin (Daypro). Clin Chem 1995;41(1): 115–6.

[34] Schneider S, Wennig R. Interference of diphenhydramine with the EMIT II immunoassay for propoxyphene. J Anal Toxicol 1999;23(7):637–8.

[35] Ng RC, Perry K, Martin DJ. Iron poisoning: assessment of radiography in diagnosis and management. Clin Pediatr (Phila) 1979;18(10):614–6.

[36] Kaczorowski JM, Wax PM. Five days of whole-bowel irrigation in a case of pediatric iron ingestion. Ann Emerg Med 1996;27(2):258–63.

[37] Everson GW, Oudjhane K, Young LW, et al. Effectiveness of abdominal radiographs in visualizing chewable iron supplements following overdose. Am J Emerg Med 1989;7(5): 459–63.

[38] Chyka PA, Butler AY. Assessment of acute iron poisoning by laboratory and clinical observations. Am J Emerg Med 1993;11(2):99–103.

[39] Palatnick W, Tenenbein M. Leukocytosis, hyperglycemia, vomiting, and positive X-rays are not indicators of severity of iron overdose in adults. Am J Emerg Med 1996;14(5): 454–5.

[40] Savitt DL, Hawkins HH, Roberts JR. The radiopacity of ingested medications. Ann Emerg Med 1987;16(3):331–9.

[41] Hergan K, Kofler K, Oser W. Drug smuggling by body packing: what radiologists should know about it. Eur Radiol 2004;14(4):736–42.

[42] McCleave NR. Drug smuggling by body packers: detection and removal of internally concealed drugs. Med J Aust 1993;159(11–12):750–4.

[43] Karhunen PJ, Suoranta H, Penttila A, et al. Pitfalls in the diagnosis of drug smuggler's abdomen. J Forensic Sci 1991;36(2):397–402.

[44] O'Brien RP, McGeehan PA, Helmczi AW, et al. Detectability of drug tablets and capsules by plain radiography. Am J Emerg Med 1986;4(4):302–12.

[45] Holstege C, Baer A, Brady WJ. The electrocardiographic toxidrome: the ECG presentation of hydrofluoric acid ingestion. Am J Emerg Med 2005;23(2):171–6.

[46] De Ponti F, Poluzzi E, Montanaro N. QT-interval prolongation by non-cardiac drugs: lessons to be learned from recent experience. Eur J Clin Pharmacol 2000;56(1):1–18.

[47] Yap YG, Camm AJ. Drug induced QT prolongation and torsades de pointes. Heart 2003; 89(11):1363–72.

[48] Anderson ME, Al-Khatib SM, Roden DM, et al. Cardiac repolarization: current knowledge, critical gaps, and new approaches to drug development and patient management. Am Heart J 2002;144(5):769–81.

[49] Sides GD. QT interval prolongation as a biomarker for torsades de pointes and sudden death in drug development. Dis Markers 2002;18(2):57–62.

[50] Nelson LS. Toxicologic myocardial sensitization. J Toxicol Clin Toxicol 2002;40(7): 867–79.

[51] Chan T, Brady W, Harrigan R, et al, editors. ECG in emergency medicine and acute care. Philadelphia: Elsevier-Mosby; 2005.

[52] De Ponti F, Poluzzi E, Cavalli A, et al. Safety of non-antiarrhythmic drugs that prolong the QT interval or induce torsades de pointes: an overview. Drug Saf 2002;25(4):263–86.

[53] Priori SG, Cantu F, Schwartz PJ. The long QT syndrome: new diagnostic and therapeutic approach in the era of molecular biology. Schweiz Med Wochenschr 1996;126(41):1727–31.

[54] Kolecki PF, Curry SC. Poisoning by sodium channel blocking agents. Crit Care Clin 1997; 13(4):829–48.

[55] Harrigan RA, Brady WJ. ECG abnormalities in tricyclic antidepressant ingestion. Am J Emerg Med 1999;17(4):387–93.

[56] Heaney RM. Left bundle branch block associated with propoxyphene hydrochloride poisoning. Ann Emerg Med 1983;12(12):780–2.

[57] Fernandez-Quero L, Riesgo MJ, Agusti S, et al. Left anterior hemiblock, complete right bundle branch block and sinus tachycardia in maprotiline poisoning. Intensive Care Med 1985;11(4):220–2.

[58] Brady WJ, Skiles J. Wide QRS complex tachycardia: ECG differential diagnosis. Am J Emerg Med 1999;17(4):376–81.

[59] Clark RF, Vance MV. Massive diphenhydramine poisoning resulting in a wide-complex tachycardia: successful treatment with sodium bicarbonate. Ann Emerg Med 1992;21(3): 318–21.

[60] Joshi AK, Sljapic T, Borghei H, et al. Case of polymorphic ventricular tachycardia in diphenhydramine poisoning. J Cardiovasc Electrophysiol 2004;15(5):591–3.

[61] Wolfe TR, Caravati EM, Rollins DE. Terminal 40-ms frontal plane QRS axis as a marker for tricyclic antidepressant overdose. Ann Emerg Med 1989;18(4):348–51.

[62] Berkovitch M, Matsui D, Fogelman R, et al. Assessment of the terminal 40-millisecond QRS vector in children with a history of tricyclic antidepressant ingestion. Pediatr Emerg Care 1995;11(2):75–7.

[63] Zareba W, Moss AJ, Rosero SZ, et al. Electrocardiographic findings in patients with diphenhydramine overdose. Am J Cardiol 1997;80(9):1168–73.

[64] Stork CM, Redd JT, Fine K, et al. Propoxyphene-induced wide QRS complex dysrhythmia responsive to sodium bicarbonate–a case report. J Toxicol Clin Toxicol 1995; 33(2):179–83.

[65] Kerns W II, Garvey L, Owens J. Cocaine-induced wide complex dysrhythmia. J Emerg Med 1997;15(3):321–9.

[66] Bania TC, Blaufeux B, Hughes S, et al. Calcium and digoxin vs. calcium alone for severe verapamil toxicity. Acad Emerg Med 2000;7(10):1089–96.

[67] Dorsey ST, Biblo LA. Prolonged QT interval and torsades de pointes caused by the combination of fluconazole and amitriptyline. Am J Emerg Med 2000;18(2):227–9.

[68] Newmark J. Nerve agents. Neurologist 2007;13(1):20–32.

[69] Eddleston M, Dawson A, Karalliedde L, et al. Early management after self-poisoning with an organophosphorus or carbamate pesticide: a treatment protocol for junior doctors. Crit Care 2004;8(6):R391–7.

[70] Shih TM, Rowland TC, McDonough JH. Anticonvulsants for nerve agent-induced seizures: the influence of the therapeutic dose of atropine. J Pharmacol Exp Ther 2007; 320(1):154–61.

[71] McDonough JH, Shih T-M. Neuropharmacological mechanisms of nerve agent-induced seizure and neuropathology. Neurosci Biobehav Rev 1997;21(5):559–79.

[72] Myhrer T, Enger S, Aas P. Pharmacological therapies against soman-induced seizures in rats 30 min following onset and anticonvulsant impact. Eur J Pharmacol 2006;548(1–3): 83–9.

[73] Madiwale T, Liebelt E. Iron: not a benign therapeutic drug. Curr Opin Pediatr 2006;18(2): 174–9.

[74] Singletary EM, Rochman AS, Bodmer JC, et al. Envenomations. Med Clin North Am 2005;89(6):1195–224.

[75] Kirk M, Judge B. Digitalis poisoning. In: Irwin J, editor. Intensive care medicine. 5th edition. Baltimore (MD): Lippincott Williams & Wilkins; 2003. p. 1551–5.

[76] Flanagan RJ, Jones AL. Fab antibody fragments: some applications in clinical toxicology. Drug Saf 2004;27(14):1115–33.

[77] Shumaik GM, Wu AW, Ping AC. Oleander poisoning: treatment with digoxin-specific Fab antibody fragments. Ann Emerg Med 1988;17(7):732–5.

[78] Camphausen C, Haas N, Mattke A. Successful treatment of oleander intoxication (cardiac glycosides) with digoxin-specific Fab antibody fragments in a 7-year-old child. Z Kardiol 2005;94(12):817–23.

[79] Clark RF, Selden BS, Curry SC. Digoxin-specific Fab fragments in the treatment of oleander toxicity in a canine model. Ann Emerg Med 1991;20(10):1073–7.

[80] Seger DL. Flumazenil–treatment or toxin. J Toxicol Clin Toxicol 2004;42(2):209–16.

[81] Brent J, McMartin K, Phillips S, et al, The Methylpyrazole for Toxic Alcohols Study Group. Fomepizole for the treatment of methanol poisoning. N Engl J Med 2001;344(6):424–9.

[82] Lushine KA, Harris CR, Holger JS. Methanol ingestion: prevention of toxic sequelae after massive ingestion. J Emerg Med 2003;24(4):433–6.

[83] Hall AH, Dart R, Bogdan G. Sodium thiosulfate or hydroxocobalamin for the empiric treatment of cyanide poisoning? Ann Emerg Med 2007;49(6):806–13.

[84] Borron SW, Baud FJ, Barriot P, et al. Prospective study of hydroxocobalamin for acute cyanide poisoning in smoke inhalation. Ann Emerg Med 2007;49(6):794–801, e2.

[85] Megarbane B, Delahaye A, Goldgran-Toledano D, et al. Antidotal treatment of cyanide poisoning. J Chin Med Assoc 2003;66(4):193–203.

[86] Geller RJ, Barthold C, Saiers JA, et al. Pediatric cyanide poisoning: causes, manifestations, management, and unmet needs. Pediatrics 2006;118(5):2146–58.

[87] DesLauriers CA, Burda AM, Wahl M. Hydroxocobalamin as a cyanide antidote. Am J Ther 2006;13(2):161–5.

[88] Rowden AK, Norvell J, Eldridge DL, et al. Updates on acetaminophen toxicity. Med Clin North Am 2005;89(6):1145–59.

[89] Chamberlain JM, Klein BL. A comprehensive review of naloxone for the emergency physician. Am J Emerg Med 1994;i2(6):650–60.

[90] Clarke SF, Dargan PI, Jones AL. Naloxone in opioid poisoning: walking the tightrope. Emerg Med J 2005;22(9):612–6.

[91] Eyer P. The role of oximes in the management of organophosphorus pesticide poisoning. Toxicol Rev 2003;22(3):165–90.

[92] Rotenberg JS, Newmark J. Nerve agent attacks on children: diagnosis and management. Pediatrics 2003;112(3):648–58.

[93] Sidell F. Nerve agents. In: Sidell FR, Franz DR, editors. Medical aspects of chemical and biological warfare. Washington, DC: Office of the Surgeon General at TMM publications; 1997. p. 129–80.

[94] Tush GM, Anstead MI. Pralidoxime continuous infusion in the treatment of organophosphate poisoning. Ann Pharmacother 1997;31(4):441–4.

[95] Pawar KS, Bhoite RR, Pillay CP, et al. Continuous pralidoxime infusion versus repeated bolus injection to treat organophosphorus pesticide poisoning: a randomised controlled trial. Lancet 2006;368(9553):2136–41.

[96] Farrar HC, Wells TG, Kearns GL. Use of continuous infusion of pralidoxime for treatment of organophosphate poisoning in children. J Pediatr 1990;116(4):658–61.

[97] Holstege CP, Kirk M, Sidell FR. Chemical warfare: nerve agent poisoning. Crit Care Clin 1997;13(4):923–42.

[98] Bawaskar HS, Joshi SR. Organophosphorus poisoning in agricultural India: status in 2005 [comment]. J Assoc Physicians India 2005;53:422–4.

[99] Karlson-Stiber C, Persson H. Cytotoxic fungi: an overview. Toxicon 2003;42(4):339–49.

[100] Knapp JF, Johnson T, Alander S. Seizures in a 13-year-old girl. Pediatr Emerg Care 2003; 19(1):38–40.

[101] Lheureux P, Penaloza A, Gris M. Pyridoxine in clinical toxicology: a review. Eur J Emerg Med 2005;12(2):78–85 [Review].

ELSEVIER
SAUNDERS

Emerg Med Clin N Am
26 (2008) 741–757

EMERGENCY
MEDICINE
CLINICS OF
NORTH AMERICA

# Monitoring the Critically Ill Emergency Department Patient

Michael E. Winters, MD, FAAEM, FACEP[a,b,c,d,*],
Michael T. McCurdy, MD[a,d], Jeff Zilberstein, MD[a,d]

[a]Department of Emergency Medicine, University of Maryland School of Medicine,
110 South Paca Street, 6th Floor, Suite 200, Baltimore, MD 21201, USA
[b]Department of Medicine, University of Maryland School of Medicine, 110 South Paca Street,
6th Floor, Suite 200, Baltimore, MD 21201, USA
[c]Combined Emergency Medicine/Internal Medicine Program, University of Maryland School
of Medicine, 110 South Paca Street, 6th Floor, Suite 200, Baltimore, MD 21201, USA
[d]Combined Emergency Medicine/Internal Medicine/Critical Care Program,
University of Maryland School of Medicine, 110 South Paca Street,
6th Floor, Suite 200, Baltimore, MD 21201, USA

Emergency physicians (EPs) diagnose and manage critically ill patients on a daily basis. With the persistent problems of hospital overcrowding and emergency department (ED) boarding, EPs now are managing critically ill patients long after initial resuscitative efforts. Continued care of the critically ill ED patient is challenging, because delays in diagnosis or therapy may lead to rapid cardiovascular collapse and death. Fundamental to the care of the critically ill ED patient is the use of various noninvasive and invasive monitoring modalities. Because these monitoring modalities are used to detect hemodynamic compromise, initiate treatment, and monitor the response to therapies, it is imperative that the EP understand the utility and limitations of current monitoring methods. This article discusses the methods commonly used to monitor the critically ill ED patient. Armed with this information, the EP can provide effective and efficient care of the critically ill patient.

## The cardiovascular system

A goal of the cardiovascular system is to deliver sufficient amounts of oxygen to the tissues to maintain normal cellular function. Tissue oxygen

* Corresponding author. Department of Emergency Medicine, University of Maryland School of Medicine, 110 South Paca Street, 6th Floor, Suite 200, Baltimore, MD 21201.
  E-mail address: mwint001@umaryland.edu (M.E. Winters).

delivery depends primarily on cardiac output and on the oxygen content of arterial blood. Cardiac output, in turn, depends on the interaction of pre-load, contractility, and afterload. Any disturbance in one or several of these components leads to tissue hypoperfusion and impaired oxygen delivery. Impaired tissue oxygen delivery, regardless of the cause, leads to progressive cellular dysfunction, organ injury, and death.

A primary objective of monitoring the critically ill patient in the ED is to assess the cardiovascular system and ensure adequate tissue perfusion and oxygen delivery. Currently, a number of monitoring techniques are used to evaluate the essential factors that affect tissue oxygen delivery, namely, oxygenation, ventilation, arterial perfusion pressure, intravascular volume, and cardiac output. In addition, there now are several new monitoring methods that directly evaluate tissue perfusion. Although each monitoring modality is discussed separately in this article, no technique used in isolation is sufficient to assess the circulatory system. Rather, the collective information provided by these monitoring tools provides the most useful assessment of the circulatory system and, ultimately, of oxygen delivery.

## Monitoring oxygenation by pulse oximetry

Pulse oximetry is regarded by many as one of the most important advances in monitoring critically ill patients. In the ED, pulse oximetry provides the EP with a continuous, noninvasive method to assess arterial oxygen saturation. Displayed readings are determined primarily by two components: the different absorption spectra of oxyhemoglobin and deoxyhemoglobin at different wavelengths of light, and the characteristics of pulsatile arterial blood [1,2]. The monitoring device uses a probe (finger, ear, or forehead) that contains two light-emitting diodes that emit light at 660 nm and 940 nm. A photoreceptor located on the opposite side of the diodes receives the transmitted light, and a signal processor compares the ratio of absorption of the two wavelengths, removes the nonpulsatile component, and provides the EP with the arterial oxygen saturation reading ($S_pO_2$) [1]. Despite its routine use, pulse oximetry has several limitations that must be recognized when monitoring critically ill ED patients.

In general, pulse oximeters have been shown to be accurate in critically ill patients [3]. The accuracy of the device, however, depends on the initial calibration data [3]. These data are obtained by the manufacturer using healthy volunteers who are subjected to various hypoxic environments. Most manufacturers report accuracies of $S_pO_2$ within 2% for arterial oxygen saturations above 70% [3–5]. In the critically ill patient, however, pulse oximetry readings become less accurate when arterial oxygen saturations fall below 90% [6]. Inaccuracies in the critically ill patient are caused primarily by hypotension, hypothermia, low cardiac output, vasoconstriction, and/or therapy with vasoactive medications [1,3,7,8]. These conditions result in a decrease in the pulsatile component of blood flow, thereby reducing signal strength and quality. Additional inaccuracies are caused by the presence of dyshemoglobinemias (carboxyhemoglobin, methemoglobin), methylene blue, indocyanine green, and sickling red cells [1,9]. Hyperbilirubinemia and anemia do not affect the accuracy of pulse oximetry [1,10].

In addition to inaccuracies, pulse oximeters may have a delayed response time to an hypoxic event in the critically ill patient. $S_pO_2$ readings depend on signal averaging time, blood flow, and the site of the oximeter probe [3]. Hypotension, hypothermia, and vasoactive medications can delay significantly the response time of the pulse oximeter to a decrease in actual arterial oxygen saturation. Patients may have arterial oxygen saturations below 80% despite a normal reading on the pulse oximeter. This delay in response time occurs more often with finger probes [11].

Perhaps the greatest limitation to the use of pulse oximetry in the critically ill patient is that it provides no measure of ventilation or acid base status [4]. $S_pO_2$ simply provides an estimate of arterial oxygen saturation. It cannot be used to estimate arterial oxygen tension ($P_aO_2$), arterial carbon dioxide tension ($P_aCO_2$), or pH [1,3]. Depending on where a patient is on the oxygen dissociation curve, large fluctuations in $P_aO_2$ may occur with minimal change in the $S_pO_2$ [3]. Similarly, significant increases in $P_aCO_2$ can occur with normal readings for $S_pO_2$. EPs must not rely on pulse oximetry to provide information about ventilatory or acid-base status.

## Monitoring ventilation using end-tidal carbon dioxide

Although pulse oximetry tells nothing about ventilatory status, end-tidal carbon dioxide ($P_{et}CO_2$) monitoring can provide useful information regarding alveolar ventilation. $P_{et}CO_2$ is the concentration of carbon dioxide at end expiration and is determined by tissue carbon dioxide production, pulmonary perfusion, and alveolar ventilation. It can be measured in both mechanically ventilated and spontaneously breathing patients. $P_{et}CO_2$ is displayed as either a numerical value (capnometry) or as a graphic waveform plotted against time (capnography). In healthy patients who have stable cardiopulmonary function, $P_{et}CO_2$ often is used to estimate $P_aCO_2$ [2]. In general, $P_{et}CO_2$ underestimates $P_aCO_2$ by 2 to 5 mm Hg because of the influence of dead space ventilation [3]. Importantly, the gradient between $P_{et}CO_2$ and $P_aCO_2$ remains constant (2–5 mm Hg) as long as patients are hemodynamically stable, have a normal capnogram, and have no significant pulmonary pathology [3].

Unfortunately, the relationship between $P_{et}CO_2$ and $P_aCO_2$ is unreliable in critically ill patients. Frequent alterations in tidal volumes, variable changes in physiologic dead space, increases in venous shunt, and hemodynamic instability can have unpredictable effects on the normal gradient between $P_{et}CO_2$ and $P_aCO_2$. As a result, $P_{et}CO_2$ should not be used as a reliable surrogate for $P_aCO_2$ in the critically ill ED patient.

Despite the limitation of $P_{et}CO_2$ as an estimate of $P_aCO_2$, capnography has several useful applications in the critically ill patient. Confirming endotracheal tube placement, detecting endotracheal tube dislodgment, detecting ventilator malfunction, diagnosing pulmonary embolism, assessing the success of cardiopulmonary resuscitation, evaluation of weaning from mechanical ventilation, and determining the optimal level of positive end-expiratory pressure are uses of capnography in the critically ill patient. Many of these applications are suitable primarily for the ICU. Perhaps the most useful application of capnography for critically ill patients in the ED is in the detection of airway accidents and ventilator dysfunction. After initial resuscitation, many critically ill patients undergo a series of radiology and diagnostic procedures that place them at risk for endotracheal tube accidents. The sudden loss of the capnogram waveform indicates endotracheal tube obstruction (mucus plug, kinked ventilator tubing), extubation, ventilator malfunction, or cardiac arrest [12]. A sudden drop of the waveform to a low but non-zero value signals partial obstruction of the endotracheal tube, an airway leak, or the development of hypotension [12].

In addition to monitoring for endotracheal tube dislodgement or ventilator malfunction, capnography can be used to monitor patients in whom hypercarbia may be detrimental [13]. As discussed previously, $P_{et}CO_2$ is not a reliable estimate of $P_aCO_2$ in the critically ill patient. Nevertheless, because $P_{et}CO_2$ typically underestimates $P_aCO_2$, the gradient $(P_aCO_2 - P_{et}CO_2)$ nearly always is positive. $P_{et}CO_2$ values greater than 40 mm Hg nearly always correlate with at least an equal or higher value of $P_aCO_2$ [14]. Elevated $P_{et}CO_2$ values in patients at risk of the effects of hypercarbia (elevated intracranial pressure, status asthmaticus, exacerbations of chronic obstructive pulmonary disease) indicate the need for alterations in management.

## Monitoring arterial pressure

Maintaining adequate organ perfusion is crucial for patient survival. Organ perfusion depends on the organ metabolic demand and on perfusion pressure, which in turn are determined by local vasomotor tone and cardiac output [15]. Under normal circumstances, tissue perfusion is maintained through alterations in the alpha-adrenergic tone of afferent vessels, termed "autoregulation" [16]. Although autoregulatory thresholds are different for each organ, organ perfusion remains fairly constant over a wide range of perfusion pressures. Unfortunately, both the cerebral and coronary vessels have very few, if any, alpha-adrenergic receptors. As a result, organ perfusion to these vital organs depends directly on perfusion pressure. As Polcano and Pinsky [15] note, "The body will protect perfusion pressure above everything else in its autonomic hierarchy."

Unfortunately, organ perfusion pressure cannot be measured directly at the bedside [17]. As a surrogate for tissue perfusion pressure, clinicians measure arterial blood pressure. Arterial blood pressure is the input pressure for organ perfusion [15]. As long as venous pressure and vascular resistance remain constant, arterial blood pressure provides a reasonable estimate of the adequacy of organ perfusion [16,17].

## Noninvasive measurements of arterial pressure

The most common method of determining arterial pressure is through the use of a noninvasive sphygmomanometer cuff applied to the upper arm. The arterial pressure can be determined either manually through the auscultation of Korotkoff sounds (auscultatory method) or by an automated device (oscillometric method). In general, oscillometric devices are more accurate than the traditional auscultatory method [14]. Oscillometric devices, however, determine the mean arterial pressure (MAP) and then, using a variety of extrapolations and calculations, provide readings for systolic and diastolic blood pressures. In the critically ill patient, noninvasive measurements of arterial pressure, regardless of the method used, must be interpreted with caution. Oscillometric devices have been shown to underestimate systolic blood pressure by as much as 6% to 19% and to overestimate diastolic blood pressure by as much as 5% to 27% [18–20]. Furthermore, noninvasive measurements of arterial pressure become less reliable in patients who have marked hypovolemia and/or abnormal cardiac function [21–23]. Oscillometric measurements also are limited by the cycling delay of the device. For these reasons, noninvasive measurements of arterial pressure must be used with great caution when monitoring hemodynamically unstable, critically ill patients.

## Invasive monitoring of arterial pressure

Currently, there is no evidence to support the routine placement of an arterial catheter in every critically ill patient [15]. Nevertheless, relative indications for continuous intra-arterial pressure monitoring include hemodynamic instability, titration of vasopressor or vasodilator medications, cardiac output monitoring, and the need for frequent arterial blood sampling [15]. The two most common sites of arterial cannulation are the radial and femoral arteries. Except in states of marked peripheral vasoconstriction, in which radial measurements may underestimate central pressure [24], radial and femoral artery readings are clinically interchangeable. Additional sites include the brachial, axillary, and dorsalis pedis arteries. Because of the lack of collateral circulation and the risk of thrombosis and permanent ischemia, the brachial and dorsalis pedis sites are rarely used.

Placement of an indwelling arterial catheter is not without risks. In perhaps the largest study of complications of arterial cannulation, a recent review found the most common complications to be temporary occlusion and hematoma formation [25]. Reviewing more than 19,000 radial artery cannulations, the authors found that temporary occlusion occurred in 19.7% of cases, and hematomas formed in 14.4% [25]. Serious ischemic damage, sepsis, and pseudoaneurysm formation occurred in less than 1% of patients who had a radial catheter [25]. Similarly, a review of 3900 cases of femoral artery cannulations found that temporary occlusion occurred in less than 2% of cases, hematomas formed in 6%, and permanent ischemic damage occurred in less than 0.02% [25]. Although catheter-related blood stream infections occur more often with femoral artery catheters, the overall incidence remains low [26].

When measuring arterial pressure with invasive catheters, correct set-up and maintenance of tubing is critical to avoid errors in measurements. One of the most common sources of error in invasive arterial pressure monitoring is the presence of air bubbles in the tubing system [27]. Air bubbles alter the mechanical signal interpreted by the transducer, thereby providing inaccurate readings. Leveling or placement of the transducer is less important clinically in measuring arterial pressure than in measuring central venous pressure (CVP).

*The importance of mean arterial pressure*

MAP is the mean organ perfusion pressure throughout the cardiac cycle. In contrast to systolic and diastolic blood pressures, MAP remains relatively constant throughout the arterial circulation [27,28]. MAP is less affected by wave reflection, characteristics of the hemodynamic monitoring system, and small-vessel vasoconstriction than is systolic blood pressure. Furthermore, it is more accurate in patients who have low-flow states [21]. Given the variability in measurements of systolic and diastolic blood pressures, MAP more closely approximates organ perfusion pressure in the critically ill patient.

MAP forms the basis of autoregulation. The normal autoregulatory range for most tissues is a MAP from 65 to 120 mm Hg. Below a MAP of 60 mm Hg, autoregulation fails, and tissue perfusion becomes directly dependent on perfusion pressure. Although a normal arterial pressure does not necessarily reflect hemodynamic stability, a MAP below 60 mm Hg always should be considered pathologic [29]. Thus, a primary goal of monitoring and managing a critically ill patient in the ED is to maintain a MAP higher than 65 mm Hg. Currently, there is no literature to support increasing the MAP to values higher than 65 mm Hg [24]. In fact, limited data indicate increased mortality when higher target values of MAP are obtained using vasopressor agents [30].

**Assessing and monitoring intravascular volume**

Fundamental to the treatment of critically ill patients is the administration of intravenous fluids. Intravenous fluids are given to augment cardiac output and restore arterial pressure so that an adequate amount of oxygen is delivered to vital organs. Importantly, 50% of critically ill patients respond to intravenous fluid administration alone [31–33]. In other words, half of critically ill patients will augment cardiac output, and thus oxygen delivery, when given an appropriate fluid challenge. Additionally, the cardiac index has been shown to improve by 35% to 40% after appropriate fluid resuscitation [34]. To date, clinicians have relied on static measurements of volume status to guide resuscitation and continued therapy. More recent literature has focused on dynamic measurements of volume to guide decisions regarding fluid therapy.

## Static measurements of intravascular volume

The two most common static measurements used by clinicians to determine intravascular volume status are CVP and pulmonary artery occlusion pressure. Because the pulmonary artery catheter is not a monitoring tool used in the emergency department, the following discussion focuses on the limitations of using CVP as a measure of intravascular volume status.

CVP is the pressure in the great thoracic veins proximal to the right atrium [15]. It is measured at end expiration, preferably from a central venous catheter placed in either the subclavian or internal jugular vein, and is determined relative to atmospheric pressure. It traditionally is believed that CVP represents right atrial pressure, from which estimates of right ventricular end-diastolic pressure and, ultimately, right ventricular end-diastolic volume (preload) can be made. The normal range for CVP is 4 to 6 mm Hg. It commonly is taught that low values of CVP correspond to hypovolemia, whereas values higher than 10 mm Hg indicate adequate volume status and preload.

Unfortunately, CVP monitoring has many limitations that affect its clinical usefulness in determining volume status and preload. First, numerous physiologic and anatomic factors affect CVP measurements adversely. These factors include tricuspid valve disease, pericardial disease, abnormal right ventricular function, dysrhythmias, myocardial disease, pulmonary vascular disease, and changes in intrathoracic pressure produced by positive-pressure ventilation [15]. Another important limitation is the reference level chosen to take measurements. The reference level chosen by the clinician for zeroing the monitoring device can have significant impact on CVP values. Furthermore, clinicians measure CVP relative to atmospheric pressure, when the true pressure that determines CVP and preload is the transmural pressure surrounding the heart [35].

The usefulness of static measurements of CVP as predictors of changes in cardiac output with fluid administration, termed "fluid responsiveness," is limited. The relationship between intravascular volume and changes in cardiac output is defined by the Starling curve. Unfortunately, a static CVP measurement provides no information about the location of an individual patient on the Starling curve. A patient may have a high CVP but still increase cardiac output with additional intravenous fluids. Conversely, a patient may have a low CVP with an expanded volume and not respond to further fluid administration. As a result, isolated measurements of CVP are not reliable in predicting fluid responsiveness [36,37].

Regardless of the tool used, static measurements are limited in their ability to reflect dynamic intravascular change. Despite its limitations, however, CVP may be the most clinically pertinent of the options available in the ED, especially when treating patients who also will require vasopressor therapy.

*Dynamic measurements of intravascular volume*

Because of the limitations of static measurements, recent literature has focused on dynamic measurements of intravascular volume in an effort to improve accuracy [38]. Dynamic measurements evaluated thus far include systolic pressure variation (SPV), pulse pressure variation (PPV), and stroke volume variation (SVV). Studies using these markers of intravascular volume have been limited primarily to sedated, mechanically ventilated patients in sinus rhythm. Nevertheless, each has been shown to be superior to static measures of filling pressures in determining overall volume status and predicting fluid responsiveness [33].

SPV (the difference between the maximum systolic blood pressure during inspiration and the minimum systolic blood pressure during expiration), PPV (the difference between the maximum pulse pressure during inspiration and the minimum pulse pressure during expiration), and SVV use the effects of changes in pleural pressure during positive-pressure ventilation on right ventricular function. During a positive-pressure breath, blood is "squeezed" out of the lungs, thereby augmenting left ventricular return and temporarily increasing left ventricular cardiac output. Simultaneously, the positive-pressure breath decreases venous return to the right heart so that left ventricular output decreases a few beats later secondary to the temporary decrease in venous return. This response is exaggerated in hypovolemic patients. The differences in maximum and minimum values for systolic blood pressure, pulse pressure, and stroke volume define SPV, PPV, and SVV. An SPV, PPV, or SVV greater than 13% has been shown to be highly sensitive and specific in identifying hypovolemic patients who are fluid responsive [29,39]. Unfortunately, these dynamic markers lose accuracy in patients who have variations in tidal volumes or dysrhythmias [40].

The use of dynamic measurements of volume status and fluid responsiveness is more challenging in the spontaneously breathing patient, because pleural pressures vary in the opposite direction when compared with positive-pressure ventilation. Thus far, the literature addressing the use of dynamic measurements to evaluate spontaneously breathing patients is limited. In one study evaluating the use of dynamic CVP measurements in spontaneously breathing patients [41], the investigators found that an inspiratory decrease in CVP of at least 1 mm Hg accurately predicted patients who were fluid responsive. Further studies are needed to confirm this finding, however.

Finally, bedside echocardiography is gaining popularity as a dynamic measure of volume status and fluid responsiveness [42]. Several studies have evaluated the behavior of the inferior vena cava during mechanical ventilation as a predictor of fluid responsiveness [43]. Inferior vena cava collapsibility of more than 12% has been shown to be highly sensitive and specific for predicting patients who will augment cardiac output with fluid administration [44]. Although additional studies are required to determine appropriate cut-off levels, it is likely that with the increasing popularity of ultrasound, emergency echocardiography will play an increasing role in the evaluation of volume status in patients in the ED.

## Monitoring tissue perfusion

Despite optimization of oxygenation, ventilation, MAP, and intravascular volume status, tissue hypoperfusion and impaired oxygen delivery still may be present. Recent literature has focused on evaluating the microcirculation by measuring both global and regional markers of tissue hypoxia. Global markers of tissue hypoxia, such as serum lactate and central venous oxygen saturation ($S_{cv}O_2$), provide information regarding anaerobic metabolism. Unfortunately, these markers do not identify which vascular bed is underperfused. In contrast, regional markers of tissue hypoxia monitor specific vascular beds, namely the cutaneous and splanchnic circulation, to identify local tissue hypoperfusion. Although they remain primarily investigational, promising methods of monitoring regional impaired oxygen delivery include sublingual capnometry, orthogonal polarization spectroscopy (OPS), near-infrared spectroscopy (NIRS), and transcutaneous oxygen tension.

### Global markers of tissue perfusion

### Lactate

Lactate is the byproduct of anaerobic metabolism, resulting from the inability of pyruvate to enter the Krebs cycle. Although an elevated lactate level can result from other causes (increased pyruvate production [45], inhibition of pyruvate dehydrogenase [46], impaired hepatic clearance), it often is considered a marker of tissue hypoxia. The normal serum value for lactate is less than 2 mmol/L. It is well documented that lactate levels above 4 mmol/L are strongly associated with worse patient outcome. Perhaps more important than single values is the time to normalization of lactate levels, termed "lactate clearance time." Multiple studies have documented the usefulness of lactate clearance time as a predictor of patient mortality [47–50]. Patients who have a prolonged lactate clearance time ($>$ 48 hours) have significantly higher rates of infection, organ dysfunction, and death [47,51]. The best chance of survival seems to correlate with a lactate clearance time of less than 24 hours [51]. For the purposes of following serial levels, there is good correlation between arterial and venous samples of lactate [52]. Based on the available evidence, EPs should monitor serial venous or arterial lactate levels when managing critically ill patients.

## Central venous oxygen saturation

Mixed venous oxygen saturation ($S_vO_2$) is used in the assessment of oxygen delivery as a measure of tissue hypoxia. $S_vO_2$ is obtained using a pulmonary artery catheter and reflects the pooled venous oxygen saturation returning to the pulmonary artery from the body [15]. $S_vO_2$ is influenced by arterial oxygen saturation, hemoglobin concentration, cardiac output, and tissue oxygen consumption. Normal values for $S_vO_2$ range from 70% to 75%. $S_vO_2$ values below 60% indicate cellular oxidative impairment, whereas values below 50% are consistently associated with anaerobic metabolism [15]. Although $S_vO_2$ is a useful monitor of global tissue hypoxia, pulmonary artery catheters are not placed routinely, if ever, in the ED setting. As such, recent literature has focused on the use of $S_{cv}O_2$ as a surrogate for $S_vO_2$.

$S_{cv}O_2$ is the venous oxygen saturation near the junction of the superior vena cava and right atrium. $S_{cv}O_2$ can be measured intermittently or continuously and is obtained from either a subclavian or internal jugular central venous catheter. Because $S_{cv}O_2$ neglects venous return from the lower body, values for $S_{cv}O_2$ typically are 3% to 5% less than $S_vO_2$ in healthy patients (the lower half of the body extracts less oxygen than the upper body) [53]. Despite the discrepancy, $S_{cv}O_2$ and $S_vO_2$ generally change in parallel with impaired tissue oxygen delivery. $S_{cv}O_2$ values lower than 65% indicate ongoing oxidative impairment. In critically ill patients, $S_{cv}O_2$ values higher than 80% are common because of cellular dysfunction with impaired oxygen consumption. Typically, such values are seen in late stages of shock and cardiovascular dysfunction. $S_{cv}O_2$ values above 80% should not be interpreted mistakenly as indicating adequate tissue oxygen delivery. As with most of the monitoring methods previously discussed, $S_{cv}O_2$ readings should be used in context with other markers of tissue perfusion (eg, lactate).

## Regional markers of tissue perfusion

### Sublingual capnometry

In states of hypoperfusion and impaired oxygen delivery, the body preferentially redistributes blood flow to vital organs. Often, this redistribution shunts blood away from the splanchnic and cutaneous circulations. As oxygen delivery is restored to normal values, these vascular beds typically are the last to regain normal perfusion. Therefore research has focused on monitoring these vascular beds as a marker of the success of resuscitation.

Early research regarding the splanchnic circulation focused on the use of gastric tonometry. Gastric tonometry uses the premise that decreased blood flow to an organ results in the accumulation of carbon dioxide. The monitoring device uses a special nasogastric tube to measure the partial pressure of carbon dioxide in the gastric mucosa. Given the limitations of the device and the controversies regarding interpretation of the data, gastric tonometry has remained a tool used in primarily research laboratories.

Newer studies evaluating the perfusion of the splanchnic circulation have used sublingual capnometry. Sublingual capnometry is performed using a sensor placed under the tongue that measures the partial pressure of carbon dioxide in the sublingual tissue ($P_{sl}CO_2$). Although studies are limited, available data indicate that $P_{sl}CO2$ can be used as a predictor of patient outcome. Normal values for $P_{sl}CO2$ are reported to range from 43 to 47 mmHg [54]. A $P_{sl}CO_2$ higher than 70 mm Hg has been shown to correlate with elevated arterial lactate levels and is predictive of decreased hospital survival [54]. Perhaps more important than the actual value for $P_{sl}CO_2$ is the difference between $P_{sl}CO_2$ and $P_aCO_2$, termed the "$P_{sl}CO_2$ gap." A $P_{sl}CO_2$ gap of more than 25 mm Hg is reported to identify patients at a high risk of mortality [55,56]. Further studies are required to define optimal values for $P_{sl}CO_2$ and the $P_{sl}CO_2$ gap; however, because it is a noninvasive and inexpensive method of monitoring, sublingual capnometry is likely to be used more widely by EPs to monitor the critically ill patient.

## Orthogonal polarization spectroscopy

OPS uses polarized light to visualize the microcirculation directly. Direct visualization is possible because hemoglobin absorbs polarized light, allowing real-time images to be reflected to a videomicroscope [21]. From these images, investigators can measure functional capillary density. Functional capillary density has been shown to be a sensitive marker of tissue perfusion and an indirect measurement of oxygen delivery [57]. Tissues evaluated thus far using OPS include the oral mucosa, sublingual mucosa, rectal mucosa, and vaginal mucosa. Unfortunately, OPS is limited by movement artifacts, the presence of saliva, and observer related bias [57]. As a result, this monitoring method remains primarily investigational.

## Near-infrared spectroscopy

NIRS measures the concentrations of hemoglobin, oxygen saturation, and cytochrome aa3 using the principle of light transmission [57]. Cytochrome aa3 is the final receptor in the electron transport chain and is responsible for approximately 90% of cellular oxygen consumption. When tissue hypoxia exists, cytochrome aa3 remains in a reduced state that can be measured using NIRS. NIRS has been used primarily to evaluate the perfusion of skeletal muscle. Although promising, the use of NIRS to measure the reduced state of cytochrome aa3 remains controversial because of signal contamination by light scatter, variable interpretations of the data, and the lack of a reference standard for comparison [57].

## Transcutaneous oxygen tension

Monitors to measure either transcutaneous oxygen or carbon dioxide use heated probes placed on the skin. Like the splanchnic circulation, the skeletal muscle and cutaneous circulations receive less blood flow during states of shock. Direct measurements of oxygen or carbon dioxide tension in these tissues are thought to be markers of regional tissue hypoperfusion. Several studies have demonstrated increased mortality in patients who have either low concentrations of transcutaneous oxygen or high concentrations of carbon dioxide [58]. Transcutaneous monitoring is limited by tissue trauma from probe insertion, thermal injury if probes are not moved every 4 hours, and the lack of established critical values to guide resuscitation.

## Monitoring cardiac output

Cardiac output is a primary determinant of oxygen delivery. As discussed previously, cardiac output is determined by the interaction of preload, contractility, and afterload. In patients who do not respond to initial resuscitative treatment, knowledge of cardiac output may be helpful in guiding further therapy. Unfortunately, vital signs and the bedside physical examination are not sufficiently precise to estimate cardiac output [38]. As a result, a number of monitoring modalities have been developed to measure cardiac output. All these devices have limitations that affect their overall clinical usefulness. At present, no data indicate that knowing, or targeting, cardiac output improves outcome. Furthermore, there is no normal value for cardiac output: it is either sufficient or insufficient to meet the body's metabolic demands. The following sections provide a brief discussion of the modalities currently used to monitor cardiac output.

### Pulmonary artery catheter

Developed in the 1940s and later refined by Swan and Ganz in 1970, the pulmonary artery catheter (PAC) became the standard hemodynamic monitoring tool used in the ICU. The PAC can provide a number of measurements including preload, pulmonary artery pressure, $S_VO_2$, and cardiac output. The PAC measures cardiac output using the thermodilution technique. Newer methods to monitor cardiac output typically are compared with the PAC thermodilution technique.

Most EPs are familiar with the controversies surrounding the PAC. A number of studies have demonstrated increased patient risk with the use of the device [59–61]. Furthermore, many of these studies have failed to demonstrate that use of the PAC improves patient morbidity or mortality [62–65]. Explanations for the lack of patient improvement have been debated in the literature for years. Nevertheless, given the controversies and risk associated with the PAC, this monitoring modality should not be used routinely in the ED.

### Pulse contour analysis

Pulse contour analysis permits the continuous monitoring of cardiac output by estimating stroke volume. Taking diastolic blood pressure as the baseline, the arterial pulse pressure waveform is a function of stroke volume and arterial compliance. Stroke volume is estimated by taking the area under the pulse pressure curve from end diastole to end systole. Arterial compliance then is calculated using either a series of assumptions based on patient age, height, weight, heart rate, and MAP or is estimated using another form of cardiac output monitoring. From the calculated arterial compliance and the measured stroke volume, the device determines cardiac output.

Several commercial devices that use pulse contour analysis to display cardiac output are available. Each device has limitations. Most require frequent recalibration because of the changing hemodynamic status in the critically ill patient. In addition, each is limited by the assumptions used in determining arterial compliance. Importantly, pulse contour analysis of cardiac output has not been validated in patients who have rapidly changing arterial tone, a common clinical scenario in the critically ill patient.

## Transthoracic electrical bioimpedance

Transthoracic electrical bioimpedance (TEB) determines cardiac output by applying a low-voltage electrical current from the neck to the thorax and measuring changes in impedance, which reflect changes in thoracic blood volume. The device uses an arrangement of skin electrodes placed on the thorax and is timed with the ECG to determine the correlation between electrical and mechanical cardiac events. Using a serious of assumptions and equations, TEB devices determine blood flow in the aorta, from which values for cardiac output are determined.

Although current studies report reasonable correlation with thermodilution techniques, TEB has several technical limitations. TEB is very sensitive to the arrangement and placement of skin electrodes [15]. Any improper placement or altered contact of skin electrodes affects the results. Furthermore, any process that increases intrathoracic blood volume adversely affects cardiac output measurements. Disease processes common in critically ill patients that increase intrathoracic blood volume include pulmonary edema, pleural effusions, pulmonary contusion, acute respiratory distress syndrome, and chest wall edema. Last, the accuracy of TEB is decreased in the presence of cardiac dysrhythmias.

## Esophageal Doppler monitoring

Esophageal Doppler monitoring (EDM) determines cardiac output by measuring the change in frequency of an ultrasound beam reflected from red blood cells as they pass through the descending aorta. Essentially, the device measures stroke volume by multiplying the cross-sectional area of the aorta by the time-integrated velocity of blood flow [66]. The cross-sectional area of the descending aorta is measured using M-mode ultrasonography or is calculated using a proprietary algorithm using the patient's age and body mass index. Once the stroke volume is determined, it is multiplied by the heart rate to yield the cardiac output. In addition to heart rate, EDM can provide estimates on preload and cardiac contractility.

EDM has several limitations. The device is placed similar to a nasogastric tube. Successful placement and direction of the probe is operator dependent and is an acquired skill. Because of the frequent movement of the patient, the device must be repositioned frequently to ensure proper signal. In addition to these technical issues, several key assumptions made in cardiac output readings may not be true in the critically ill patient. Most important, the device assumes that the aorta is cylindrical. In reality, the aorta is dynamic, and the cross-sectional area is dependent on pulse pressure and compliance. In addition, EDM assumes a stable blood flow in the descending aorta. Diseases that produce tachycardia, anemia, or aortic valve disease affect blood velocity measurements [66]. Notwithstanding these limitations, studies to date have demonstrated good correlation with thermodilution techniques [67]. Further evidence demonstrating the value of EDM in critically ill patients is needed before the device can be recommended for routine use.

*Transthoracic echocardiography*

With EPs' increasing use of and familiarity with ultrasonography, transthoracic echocardiography is being used more frequently in the assessment of the critically ill patient. Volume-based or Doppler-based methods can be used to measure cardiac output using transthoracic echocardiography. Because of their dependence on quality resolution, volume-based measurements of cardiac output correlate poorly with absolute measurements obtained using thermodilution [68]. Doppler-based measurements have demonstrated very good agreement with thermodilution when images are obtained at the level of the aortic valve [69]. Although precise measurements of stroke volume and cross-sectional area are difficult in untrained hands, estimates of global function can help guide resuscitation.

**Summary**

It is clear that EPs are managing an increasing proportion of critically ill patients. With the problem of ED boarding, many of these critically ill patients remain in the ED for extended periods of time. During these prolonged ED stays, potential delays in diagnosis and/or therapy may increase patient morbidity and mortality. All EPs use monitoring modalities in critically ill patients. The goal of that monitoring is to detect early cardiovascular compromise and impaired oxygen delivery before disastrous collapse occurs. With the pearls and pitfalls discussed in this article regarding the monitoring of oxygenation, ventilation, arterial perfusion pressure, intravascular volume, markers of tissue hypoxia, and cardiac output, the EP can continue to provide optimal care for this complicated patient population.

## Acknowledgments

The authors thank Linda Kesselring for assisting in the preparation of this article.

## References

[1] McMorrow RC, Mythen MG. Pulse oximetry. Curr Opin Crit Care 2006;12(3):269–71.
[2] Caples SM, Hubmayr RD. Respiratory monitoring tools in the intensive care unit. Curr Opin Crit Care 2003;9(3):230–5.
[3] Soubani AO. Noninvasive monitoring of oxygen and carbon dioxide. Am J Emerg Med 2001;19(2):141–6.
[4] Keogh BF. When pulse oximetry monitoring of the critically ill is not enough. Anesth Analg 2002;94(Suppl 1):S96–9.
[5] Jubran A. Pulse oximetry. In: Tobin MJ, editor. Principles and practice of intensive care monitoring. New York: McGraw Hill; 1998. p. 261–302.
[6] Kallet RH, Tang JF. Bedside monitoring of pulmonary function. In: Fink MP, editor. Textbook of critical care. 5th edition. Philadelphia: Elsevier; 2005. p. 445–61.
[7] Clayton DG, Webb RK, Ralston AC, et al. A comparison of the performance of 20 pulse oximeters under conditions of poor perfusion. Anaesthesia 1991;46(1):3–10.
[8] Ibanez J, Velasco J, Raurich JM. The accuracy of the Biox 3700 pulse oximeter in patients receiving vasoactive therapy. Intensive Care Med 1991;17(8):484–6.
[9] Scheller MS, Unger RJ, Kelner MJ. Effects of intravenously administered dyes on pulse oximetry readings. Anesthesiology 1986;65(5):550–2.
[10] Jay GD, Hughes L, Renzi FP. Pulse oximetry is accurate in acute anemia from hemorrhage. Ann Emerg Med 1994;24(1):32–5.
[11] Jubran A, Tobin MJ. Monitoring during mechanical ventilation. Clin Chest Med 1996;17(3): 453–73.
[12] Zwerneman K. End-tidal carbon dioxide monitoring: a VITAL sign worth watching. Crit Care Nurs Clin North Am 2006;18(2):217–25, xi.
[13] Anderson CT, Breen PH. Carbon dioxide kinetics and capnography during critical care. Crit Care 2000;4(4):207–15.
[14] Myers C. Critical care monitoring in the emergency department. Emergency Medicine Practice 2007;9(7).
[15] Polanco PM, Pinsky MR. Practical issues of hemodynamic monitoring at the bedside. Surg Clin North Am 2006;86(6):1431–56.
[16] Stucchi R, Poli G, Fumagalli R. Hemodynamic monitoring in ICU. Minerva Anestesiol 2006;72(6):483–7.
[17] Bigatello LM, George E. Hemodynamic monitoring. Minerva Anestesiol 2002;68(4): 219–25.
[18] Umana E, Ahmed W, Fraley MA, et al. Comparison of oscillometric and intraarterial systolic and diastolic blood pressures in lean, overweight, and obese patients. Angiology 2006; 57(1):41–5.
[19] Araghi A, Bander JJ, Guzman JA. Arterial blood pressure monitoring in overweight critically ill patients: invasive or noninvasive? Crit Care 2006;10(2):R64.
[20] Bur A, Hirschl MM, Herkner H, et al. Accuracy of oscillometric blood pressure measurement according to the relation between cuff size and upper-arm circumference in critically ill patients. Crit Care Med 2000;28(2):371–6.
[21] Wilson M, Davis DP, Coimbra R. Diagnosis and monitoring of hemorrhagic shock during the initial resuscitation of multiple trauma patients: a review. J Emerg Med 2003;24(4): 413–22.
[22] Gardner RM. Direct blood pressure measurement—dynamic response requirements. Anesthesiology 1981;54(3):227–36.

[23] Ellestad MH. Reliability of blood pressure recordings. Am J Cardiol 1989;63(13):983–5.

[24] Pinsky MR. Hemodynamic monitoring in the intensive care unit. Clin Chest Med 2003;24(4): 549–60.

[25] Scheer B, Perel A, Pfeiffer UJ. Clinical review: complications and risk factors of peripheral arterial catheters used for haemodynamic monitoring in anaesthesia and intensive care medicine. Crit Care 2002;6(3):199–204.

[26] Cousins TR, O'Donnell JM. Arterial cannulation: a critical review. AANA J 2004;72(4): 267–71.

[27] McGhee BH, Bridges EJ. Monitoring arterial blood pressure: what you may not know. Crit Care Nurse 2002;22(2):60–4, 66–70 [73 passim].

[28] Darovic GO. Hemodynamic monitoring: invasive and noninvasive clinical application. 2nd edition. Philadelphia: Saunders; 1995.

[29] Pinsky MR, Payen D. Functional hemodynamic monitoring. Crit Care 2005;9(6):566–72.

[30] Hayes MA, Timmins AC, Yau EH, et al. Elevation of systemic oxygen delivery in the treatment of critically ill patients. N Engl J Med 1994;330(24):1717–22.

[31] Pinsky MR. At the threshold of noninvasive functional hemodynamic monitoring. Anesthesiology 2007;106(6):1084–5.

[32] Michard F, Teboul JL. Predicting fluid responsiveness in ICU patients: a critical analysis of the evidence. Chest 2002;121(6):2000–8.

[33] Perel A. The value of functional hemodynamic parameters in hemodynamic monitoring of ventilated patients. Anaesthesist 2003;52(11):1003–4.

[34] Hollenberg SM, Ahrens TS, Annane D, et al. Practice parameters for hemodynamic support of sepsis in adult patients: 2004 update. Crit Care Med 2004;32:1928–48.

[35] Magder S. Central venous pressure: a useful but not so simple measurement. Crit Care Med 2006;34(8):2224–7.

[36] Vincent JL, Weil MH. Fluid challenge revisited. Crit Care Med 2006;34(5):1333–7.

[37] Bellomo R, Uchino S. Cardiovascular monitoring tools: use and misuse. Curr Opin Crit Care 2003;9(3):225–9.

[38] Antonelli M, Levy M, Andrews PJ, et al. Hemodynamic monitoring in shock and implications for management. International Consensus Conference, Paris, France, 27–28 April 2006. Intensive Care Med 2007;33(4):575–90.

[39] Michard F, Boussat S, Chemla D, et al. Relation between respiratory changes in arterial pulse pressure and fluid responsiveness in septic patients with acute circulatory failure. Am J Respir Crit Care Med 2000;162(1):134–8.

[40] Pinsky MR. Hemodynamic evaluation and monitoring in the ICU. Chest 2007;132(6): 2020–9.

[41] Magder S, Lagonidis D, Erice F. The use of respiratory variations in right atrial pressure to predict the cardiac output response to PEEP. J Crit Care 2001;16(3):108–14.

[42] Beaulieu Y. Bedside echocardiography in the assessment of the critically ill. Crit Care Med 2007;35(Suppl 5):S235–249.

[43] Andrews P, Azoulay E, Antonelli M, et al. Year in review in intensive care medicine, 2004. II. Brain injury, hemodynamic monitoring and treatment, pulmonary embolism, gastrointestinal tract, and renal failure. Intensive Care Med 2005;31(2):177–88.

[44] Feissel M, Michard F, Faller JP, et al. The respiratory variation in inferior vena cava diameter as a guide to fluid therapy. Intensive Care Med 2004;30(9):1834–7.

[45] Gore DC, Jahoor F, Hibbert JM, et al. Lactic acidosis during sepsis is related to increased pyruvate production, not deficits in tissue oxygen availability. Ann Surg 1996;224(1):97–102.

[46] Vary TC, Siegel JH, Nakatani T, et al. Effect of sepsis on activity of pyruvate dehydrogenase complex in skeletal muscle and liver. Am J Physiol 1986;250(6 Pt 1):E634–40.

[47] McNelis J, Marini CP, Jurkiewicz A, et al. Prolonged lactate clearance is associated with increased mortality in the surgical intensive care unit. Am J Surg 2001;182(5):481–5.

[48] Abramson D, Scalea TM, Hitchcock R, et al. Lactate clearance and survival following injury. J Trauma 1993;35(4):584–8 [discussion: 588–9].

[49] Manikis P, Jankowski S, Zhang H, et al. Correlation of serial blood lactate levels to organ failure and mortality after trauma. Am J Emerg Med 1995;13(6):619–22.

[50] Jeng JC, Jablonski K, Bridgeman A, et al. Serum lactate, not base deficit, rapidly predicts survival after major burns. Burns 2002;28(2):161–6.

[51] Husain FA, Martin MJ, Mullenix PS, et al. Serum lactate and base deficit as predictors of mortality and morbidity. Am J Surg 2003;185(5):485–91.

[52] Middleton P, Kelly AM, Brown J, et al. Agreement between arterial and central venous values for pH, bicarbonate, base excess, and lactate. Emerg Med J 2006;23(8):622–4.

[53] Marx G, Reinhart K. Venous oximetry. Curr Opin Crit Care 2006;12(3):263–8.

[54] Weil MH, Nakagawa Y, Tang W, et al. Sublingual capnometry: a new noninvasive measurement for diagnosis and quantitation of severity of circulatory shock. Crit Care Med 1999; 27(7):1225–9.

[55] Marik PE, Bankov A. Sublingual capnometry versus traditional markers of tissue oxygenation in critically ill patients. Crit Care Med 2003;31(3):818–22.

[56] Marik PE. Sublingual capnography: a clinical validation study. Chest 2001;120(3):923–7.

[57] Lima A, Bakker J. Noninvasive monitoring of peripheral perfusion. Intensive Care Med 2005;31(10):1316–26.

[58] Tatevossian RG, Wo CC, Velmahos GC, et al. Transcutaneous oxygen and CO2 as early warning of tissue hypoxia and hemodynamic shock in critically ill emergency patients. Crit Care Med 2000;28(7):2248–53.

[59] Harvey S, Harrison DA, Singer M, et al. Assessment of the clinical effectiveness of pulmonary artery catheters in management of patients in intensive care (PAC-Man): a randomised controlled trial. Lancet 2005;366(9484):472–7.

[60] Binanay C, Califf RM, Hasselblad V, et al. Evaluation study of congestive heart failure and pulmonary artery catheterization effectiveness: the ESCAPE trial. JAMA 2005;294(13): 1625–33.

[61] Polanczyk CA, Rohde LE, Goldman L, et al. Right heart catheterization and cardiac complications in patients undergoing noncardiac surgery: an observational study. JAMA 2001; 286(3):309–14.

[62] Sandham JD, Hull RD, Brant RF, et al. A randomized, controlled trial of the use of pulmonary-artery catheters in high-risk surgical patients. N Engl J Med 2003;348(1):5–14.

[63] Richard C, Warszawski J, Anguel N, et al. Early use of the pulmonary artery catheter and outcomes in patients with shock and acute respiratory distress syndrome: a randomized controlled trial. JAMA 2003;290(20):2713–20.

[64] Connors AF Jr, Speroff T, Dawson NV, et al. The effectiveness of right heart catheterization in the initial care of critically ill patients. SUPPORT Investigators. JAMA 1996;276(11): 889–97.

[65] Shah MR, Hasselblad V, Stevenson LW, et al. Impact of the pulmonary artery catheter in critically ill patients: meta-analysis of randomized clinical trials. JAMA 2005;294(13): 1664–70.

[66] Chaney JC, Derdak S. Minimally invasive hemodynamic monitoring for the intensivist: current and emerging technology. Crit Care Med 2002;30(10):2338–45.

[67] Dark PM, Singer M. The validity of trans-esophageal doppler ultrasonography as a measure of cardiac output in critically ill adults. Intensive Care Med 2004;30(11):2060–6.

[68] Brown JM. Use of echocardiography for hemodynamic monitoring. Crit Care Med 2002; 30(6):1361–4.

[69] Huttemann E. Transoesophageal echocardiography in critical care. Minerva Anestesiol 2006;72(11):891–913.

ELSEVIER
SAUNDERS

Emerg Med Clin N Am
26 (2008) 759–786

EMERGENCY
MEDICINE
CLINICS OF
NORTH AMERICA

# The Use of Vasopressors and Inotropes in the Emergency Medical Treatment of Shock

Timothy J. Ellender, MD[a,b,*], Joseph C. Skinner, MD[a,b]

[a]Department of Emergency Medicine, Indiana University Hospital, Emergency Medical
Group Inc., 1701 North Senate Boulevard EMTC-AG001, Indianapolis, IN 46202, USA
[b]Multidisciplinary Critical Care Fellowship, Methodist Hospital/Clarian Health,
1701 North Senate Boulevard, Indianapolis, IN 46202, USA

Shock is a final common pathway associated with regularly encountered emergencies including myocardial infarction, microbial sepsis, pulmonary embolism, significant trauma, and anaphylaxis. Shock results in impaired tissue perfusion, cellular hypoxia, and metabolic derangements that cause cellular injury. Although this early injury is often reversible, persistent hypoperfusion leads to irreversible tissue damage, progressive organ dysfunction, and can progress to death [1].

Cardiovascular collapse (shock) is a common life-threatening condition that requires prompt stabilization and correction. Lambe and coworkers [2] reported a 59% increase in critically ill patients between 1990 and 1999. National estimates report an increase in potential shock with an estimated 1.1 Americans presenting to emergency departments nationally with potential shock (requiring emergent resuscitation within 15 minutes). This marks an estimated increase in emergent resuscitation requirements from 17% (1998) to 22% (2002) [3]. Depending on the etiology, mortality figures vary from 23% to 75% for some causes [3–11]. The clinical manifestations and prognosis of shock are largely dependent on the etiology and duration of insult. It is important that emergency physicians, familiar with the broad differential diagnosis of shock, be prepared to rapidly recognize, resuscitate, and target appropriate therapies aimed at correcting the underlying process. This article focuses on the basic pathophysiology of shock states and reviews

---

* Corresponding author. Department of Emergency Medicine, Indiana University, Emergency Medical Group Inc., 1701 North Senate Boulevard EMTC-AG001, Indianapolis, IN 46202.

E-mail address: tellende@iupui.edu (T.J. Ellender).

0733-8627/08/$ - see front matter © 2008 Elsevier Inc. All rights reserved.
doi:10.1016/j.emc.2008.04.001　　　　　　　　　　　　　　　*emed.theclinics.com*

the rationale regarding vasoactive drug therapy for cardiovascular support of shock within an emergency environment.

Vasoactive drugs have been used to treat the hemodynamic changes associated with shock for over 40 years [12]. In the emergency medical management of patients, vasoactive drug therapy is used to manipulate the relative distribution of blood flow and restore tissue perfusion. These agents are classically subdivided, based on their predominant pathway of activity, into two separate class types: vasopressors and inotropes. Vasopressors modulate vasoconstriction and thereby increase blood pressure, whereas inotropes increase cardiac performance and thereby improve cardiac output (CO). Vasopressor and inotropic agents function primarily through stimulation of adrenergic receptors or through the induction of intracellular processes that mimic sympathetic end points (increased cAMP). Many of the drugs in use have varied effects because of their mixed receptor activity. Most of these act directly or indirectly on the sympathetic nervous system with effects that vary according to the strength of sympathetic receptor stimulus and affinity. Direct-acting drugs operate by stimulating the sympathetic nervous system receptor, whereas indirect-acting drugs cause the release of norepinephrine, which produces the effect.

The composite treatment of shock largely depends on correctly identifying the aberrant mechanisms, eliminating the causative agents, and supporting recovery. Vasoactive drugs are used largely to right cardiovascular imbalances, and the proper selection of one or more agents greatly depends on a basic understanding of the physiologic mechanisms driving a particular shock state [12,13].

Shock is a physiologic state characterized by a systemic reduction in tissue perfusion necessary to meet the metabolic needs of the tissues. Hypoperfusion results in oxygen debt, occurring as oxygen delivery becomes unable to meet metabolic requirements [14–16]. This state of oxygen debt is derived from disruption within the oxygen delivery pathway.

Hypoperfusion and resulting oxygen debt leads to tissue ischemia, general cellular hypoxia, and derangements of critical biochemical processes [4,17] further propagating autonomic dysregulation and organ failure. These effects may be reversible if the shock state is promptly recognized and corrected. Recognized hypoperfusion is a time-dependent emergency. This concept is already established in hemorrhagic-traumatic [18–21], cardiovascular [22–25], septic [26–29], and general critical shock presenting to the emergency department [30–32]. Efforts to correct shock are largely aimed at restoring balance to one or all of three main systems: (1) the pump (CO); (2) the transport system (peripheral circulation); and (3) the transport medium (blood volume) (Table 1) [4].

Shock may be caused by a primary decrease in CO (cardiogenic-obstructive shock); vasodilatation (distributive shock); or low circulating blood volume (hypovolemic shock) (Table 2) [1]. Cardiogenic shock can be further defined by intrinsic dysfunction caused by myopathies, infarction, acute

Table 1
Categories of shock and primary treatment strategies

| 1° Therapy | Causes of inadequate blood or plasma volume | |
| --- | --- | --- |
| Volume infusion | Hemorrhagic shock | Traumatic |
| | | Gastrointestinal |
| | | Cavitary hemorrhage |
| | Hypovolemic shock | Dehydration |
| | | Gastrointestinal loss (vomitus, diarrhea) |
| | | Third-spacing caused by inflammation (burns, pancreatitis) |

| 1° Therapy | Causes of cardiogenic (pump) dysfunction and decreased cardiac output | |
| --- | --- | --- |
| Chemical support with inotropic agents | Myocardial ischemia | Coronary thrombosis |
| | | Hypotension with global hypoxia/ischemia |
| | Cardiomyopathy | Myocarditis |
| | | Chronic myopathies (ischemic, diabetic, infiltrative, congenital) |
| | Late hypodynamic septic shock[a] | |
| | Structural cardiac damage | Ventricular rupture |
| | | Acute valvular or papillary muscle dysfunction |
| | Toxic drug overdose[a] | Calcium channel blocker overdose |
| | | β-blocker overdose |
| Require correction of underlying process or relief of obstructive processes | Pulmonary embolism[a] | |
| | Cardiac tamponade | |
| | Tension pneumothorax | |
| | Cardiac arrhythmia | Atrial fibrillation with rapid ventricular response |
| | | Supraventicular tachycardia |
| | | Ventricular tachycardia |

| 1° Therapy | Causes of abnormal vasomotor tone and vasodilation | |
| --- | --- | --- |
| Early volume infusion and chemical support with vasopressor agents | Early hyperdynamic septic shock[a] | |
| | Anaphylactic shock | |
| | Central neurogenic shock | |
| | Toxic drug overdose | Tricyclic antidepressants |
| | | Opiates |
| | | Alpha antagonists |

[a] Denotes mixed physiologic processes that often necessitate mixed chemical support (inotropes/vasopressors).

*Data from* Jones AE, Kline JA. Shock. In: Marx, editor. Rosen's emergency medicine: concepts and clinical practice. 6th edition, vol 1. Philadelphia: Mosby; 2006. p. 42.

Table 2
Classification of shock and hemodynamic variables

| Shock type | Heart rate | Stroke volume | Cardiac output | Systemic vascular resistance |
|---|---|---|---|---|
| Cardiogenic | Increased | Decreased | Decreased | Increased |
| Hypovolemic | Increased | No change or decreased | No change or decreased | Increased |
| Distributive (spinal[a]) | Increased (normal or decreased[a]) | Increased (no change[a]) | Increased | Decreased |

[a] Denotes physiologic variation in spinal shock caused by a predominant decrease in sympathetic input.

valvular dysfunction, and arrhythmias or by extrinsic dysfunction caused by obstructive disorders, such as pulmonary embolism, constrictive pericarditis, pericardial tamponade, or tension pneumothorax [33,34]. Hypovolemic shock, caused by a relative or absolute decreased circulating blood volume, results in a decreased preload that alters stroke volume and leads to a decreased CO. Hypovolemic shock can be caused by hemorrhage from trauma, aneurysm rupture, or gastrointestinal bleeding, or from basic fluid loss caused by diarrhea, burns, or "third spacing." Distributive or vasodilatory shock results from vascular changes that lead to a decrease in vasomotor tone and a loss of peripheral vascular resistance. There are multiple subcauses of distributive shock including sepsis, anaphylaxis, toxic shock syndrome, and central neurologic injury. It is also important to note that vasodilatory shock is the final common pathway of prolonged and severe shock of any cause [35].

Pathologic maldistribution of blood flow is hard to measure [7,36] and shock is hard to define using hemodynamic criteria alone [4,7,14,27, 37–39]. Any set mean arterial pressure (MAP) or cardiac index might define dysfunction in one individual, yet it might also represent normal physiology in another [33,36,40]. The identification and treatment of shock is grossly dependent on surrogate markers and estimations of tissue blood flow [32,40–42]. Assessment of the major features of shock (eg, hypotension, decreased capillary blood flow, oliguria, mental status changes, and acidosis) should be done in any patient with a critical illness, or who is at risk of developing shock. Markers of regional perfusion, urine output, and mentation have not been shown to be superior to markers of global perfusion, such as blood lactate levels and measures of arterial base excess [4,7,13]. A current approach to the diagnosis of shock and monitoring of the response to therapy must integrate physical examination findings (eg, confusion, delayed capillary refill, oliguria); hemodynamic variables (eg, MAP, shock index, pulse pressure); and global metabolic parameters (eg, lactate, arterial base excess, mixed venous oxygen saturations) [4,13,32,37–50]. A composite picture of patient parameters is best used to correct or assess the adequacy of perfusion.

Global tissue perfusion and oxygen delivery is determined by blood oxygenation and MAP. Oxygen delivery ($DO_2$) is a function of arterial oxygen content ($Cao_2$) and CO [$DO_2 = Cao_2 \times CO \times 10$]. Arterial oxygen content is the sum of bound arterial oxygen ($Hb \times Sao_2 \times 1.38$) and dissolved arterial oxygen ($0.0031 \times Pao_2$). $Pao_2$ is usually disregarded because the number is diminutive. How much oxygen is delivered to the tissues through the microvasculature depends on how many oxygen-carrying units are present, how many of those hemoglobin units are effectively carrying oxygen, and how effectively the heart is working to transport the oxygenated units [15,16]. CO is the product of heart rate and stroke volume; in turn, stroke volume depends on preload, myocardial contractility, and afterload (Table 3).

MAP is derived from the product of systemic vascular resistance (SVR) and CO. SVR is governed by blood viscosity, vessel length, and the inverse of vessel diameter. SVR and CO are important clinical concepts that distinguish the different forms of shock. Consequently, any basic approach to hypotension should begin with an assessment of the patient's volume status and CO. Low CO states are clinically linked to a narrowed pulse pressure, a rising shock index, and a delayed capillary refill with cool peripheral extremities [33,34]. Widened pulse pressures with low diastolic pressures, bounding pulses, warm extremities, and normal capillary refill can be seen with increased CO states [4,32,42].

In patients with evidence of hypoperfusion and increased CO, a decreased SVR or a decreased relative volume should be suspected. Conditions that cause high output and low resistance are classically linked to inflammatory states. The prototypical high output–low resistance condition is septic shock, although severe pancreatitis, anaphylaxis, burns, and liver failure share similar physiologic alterations. Perfusion deficits observed in hyperdynamic shock are derived from a complex interaction of humoral and microcirculatory processes that result in uneven local regional blood flow and a derangement of cellular metabolic processes [49]. In patients with suspected hypoperfusion and clinical evidence of low CO, an assessment of cardiac volumes and global intravascular volume must be reassessed. Historical and physical features often easily differentiate the hypovolemic state whether caused by hemorrhage (trauma) or volume loss (diarrhea, vomiting). Clinical features, such as elevated jugular venous pulses, peripheral edema, a cardiac gallop, or pulmonary rales, help to distinguish the hypotensive patient with low CO and high intravascular volumes [7,33,34]. These patients tend to be cold and clammy because of their increased SVR and usually have historical features and clinical signs (EKG changes) that help further differentiate the cardiac origins of shock.

## Principles of management

The management of shock first focuses on identifying the underlying cause and applying some combination of fluid resuscitation, vasoconstrictors,

Table 3
Hemodynamic measurements and physiologic variables

| Measurement | Determining parameters | Formulas/ measurements | Normal values |
|---|---|---|---|
| MAP | SVR<br>CO<br>SBP<br>DBP | MAP = SVR × CO<br>MAP = (SBP + DBP)/2 | Normal MAP should be 65 mmHg or greater |
| SVR | Blood vessel diameter<br>Blood vessel length<br>Blood viscosity | | In a 70-kg person, the resting SVR is 900–1200 $dyn \cdot s/cm^5$ (90–120 $MPa \cdot s/m^3$) |
| CO | HR<br>SV | CO = HR × SV | In a 70-kg person, a normal resting CO is approximately 4900 mL/min |
| SV | Preload/EDV<br>Afterload<br>ESV<br>Contractility<br>EF | SV = EDV − ESV | In a 70-kg person, the given SV is approximately 70 mL at rest |
| EF | SV<br>EDV | EF = (SV/EDV) × 100% | In a healthy 70-kg person, the SV is approximately 70 mL and the left ventricular EDV is 120 mL, giving an ejection fraction of 70/120, or 58% |
| Preload | Left ventricular stretch<br>Relates to EDV<br>LVEDP<br>LVEDR | (LVEDP × LVEDR)/2 × ventricular thickness | |
| Afterload | LVESP<br>MAP<br>SVR | | |
| PP | SBP<br>DBP | PP = SBP − DBP | In a 70-kg person, the resting PP is 40 mm Hg |
| SI | HR<br>DBP | SI = HR/SBP | In a 70-kg person, a normal SI is <0.5 |

*Abbreviations:* CO, cardiac output; DBP, diastolic blood pressure; EDV, end diastolic volume; EF, ejection fraction; ESV, end systolic volume; HR, heart rate; LVEDP, left ventricular end diastolic pressure; LVEDR, left ventricular end diastolic radius; MAP, mean arterial pressure; PP, pulse pressure; SBP, systolic blood pressure; SI, shock index; SV, stroke volume; SVR, systemic vascular resistance.

inotropic agents, and potentially vasodilators in a coordinated attempt to right physiologic irregularity, correct perfusion deficits, and maintain oxygen delivery (Table 4). Clinically, this is achieved by improving blood pressure and CO through the optimization of preload, augmentation of SVR, and the increase of cardiac contractility. To achieve these goals,

Table 4
Pharmacologic agents used to support cardiac output and blood pressure

| Vasoactive agent | α1 | α2 | β1 | β2 | Dopamine | Other | Clinical effect |
|---|---|---|---|---|---|---|---|
| Epinephrine | ++++ | ++(+) | +++ | 0(+) | 0 | | ▲ in SVR predominates, vasodilator in low dose; ▲CO by ▲inotrope and ▲HR |
| Ephedrine | ++ | 0 | ++(+) | ++ | 0 | | ▲ in SVR predominates; Mild ▲CO by ▲inotrope |
| Norepinephrine | ++++ | +++ | +++ | 0(+) | 0 | | ▲ in SVR predominates because of alpha effects; ▼CO s/t ▲ in SVR offset by inotrope; ▲HR at higher doses may limit clinical effectiveness |
| Phenylepherine | +++ | 0 | 0 | 0 | 0 | | ▲▲ in SVR predominates; CO neutral at low doses s/t ▲venous return offsets the ▲SVR effect on CO; At high doses, ▲ in SVR predominates with ▼CO |
| Dopamine | | | | | | Dopamine | |
| 0.5–2 µg/kg/min | 0 | (+) | + | + | ++ | | Dose 1-▲CO by ▲inotrope |
| 3.0–10 µg/kg/min | + | (+) | ++ | + | ++ | | Dose 2-▲SVR and ▲CO by ▲inotrope and ▲HR |
| 10–20 µg/kg/min | +(++) | (+) | ++(++) | +(+) | ++ | | Dose 3-▲ in SVR predominates |
| Dobutamine | 0(+) | 0(+) | ++++ | +++ | 0 | | ▲HR at higher doses may limit clinical effectiveness; ▼▲SVR; ▲CO by ▲inotrope; Minimal stimulation to HR |
| Isoproterenol | 0 | 0 | ++++ | ++++ | 0 | | ▼SVR; ▲CO by ▲inotrope and ▲HR |
| Vasopressin | 0 | 0 | 0 | 0 | 0 | V1 receptor | SVR often limits utility in shock; ▲▲ in SVR predominates |
| Amrinone/milrinone | 0 | 0 | 0 | 0 | 0 | PDE inhibition | ▼SVR; ▲CO by phosphodiesterase inhibition |

0, no effect; +, minimal receptor stimulation; ++, mild; +++, moderate; ++++, strong receptor stimulation; -, debated activity; 0, variable effects; ▲, increase; ▼, decrease.
Abbreviations: CO, cardiac output; HR, heart rate; PDE, phosphodiesterase; SVR, systemic vascular resistance.

the physician can use a number of vasoactive agents. Vasopressor agents largely improve perfusion pressure and preserve regional distribution of CO through an increase in MAP above autoregulatory thresholds [12,51]. Vasopressor agents may also improve cardiac preload and increase CO by decreasing venous compliance and augmenting venous return [7,12]. Inotropes improve oxygen delivery and CO through an increase in rate and contractility [13,29,40,52,53].

## Receptor physiology

Vasopressors and inotropes are broadly divided into adrenergic agonists and nonadrenergic agonists. The main categories of adrenergic receptors relevant to vasoactive therapy are the $\alpha_1$-, $\alpha_2$-, $\beta_1$-, and $\beta_2$-adrenergic receptors, and the dopamine receptors. Discussion of nonadrenergic mechanisms typically revolves around activation of vasopressin-specific receptors, in particular $V_1$, and the modulation of internal cellular phosphodiesterase activity.

### Alpha-adrenergic receptors

Alpha receptors share a number of general functions including some vasoconstriction of the veins and coronary arteries [12,51]. $\alpha_1$ Receptor stimulation exerts a primary effect on smooth muscle with resultant constriction. In the smooth muscle of blood vessels, the principal effect is vasoconstriction. $\alpha_1$ activity has been linked to metabolic alterations and potentially to increased cardiac contractility, although the exact mechanisms of these activities are unclear [54–56]. Stimulation of postsynaptic $\alpha_2$ receptors causes vasodilatation by endothelial nitric oxide production [51,57]. It is thought that this mixed constrictive-dilatory alpha activity helps maintain perfusion balance, particularly within the coronary arteries [58].

### Beta-adrenergic receptors

$\beta_1$ Receptor stimulation primarily affects the heart. $\beta_1$ Agonism produces increases in heart rate and contractility, leading to improved cardiac performance and output. Heart rate increases are enacted by increased sinoatrial nodal conduction (chronotropic effect); increased automaticity and conduction of the ventricular cardiac muscle; and increased atrioventricular nodal conduction (dromotrophic effect) [59]. Stroke volumes increase as a result of cardiac muscle contractility (inotropic effect). $\beta_2$ Receptor stimulation causes relaxation of smooth muscle. In smooth muscle beds of small coronary arteries, arteries of visceral organs, and arteries of skeletal muscle $\beta_2$ activation results in vasodilation. Additionally, $\beta_2$ stimulation results in mild chronotropic and inotropic improvement, although these effects are minimal [59].

## Dopaminergic receptors

There are over seven subtypes of dopamine receptor [60,61]. $D_4$ receptors have been identified in human hearts. Through dopamine receptors, dopamine increases CO by improving myocardial contractility, and at certain doses increasing heart rate [60]. In the kidney, dopamine acts by $D_1$ and $D_2$ receptors to stimulate diuresis and naturesis [61]. In the human pulmonary artery $D_1$, $D_2$, $D_4$, and $D_5$ receptor subtypes may account for vasorelaxive effects of dopamine [62].

## Vasopressin receptors

Vasopressin is a peptide hormone whose primary role is to regulate the body's retention of water. Vasopressin, or antidiuretic hormone, is released when the body is dehydrated, causing the kidneys to conserve water (but not salt), concentrating the urine and reducing urine volume. It also raises blood pressure by inducing moderate vasoconstriction through its stimulation of $V_1$ receptors present throughout the vasculature, but most predominantly within the smooth muscle of peripheral arterioles [63–65]. High-level activation greatly increases vascular resistance and is a dominant compensatory mechanism for restoring blood pressure in hypovolemic shock [65]. Under normal physiologic conditions, $V_1$ stimulated vasoconstriction results in no net change in blood pressure because of baroreflex activation [64,65]. Vasopressin has also been linked to paradoxical vasodilation that is largely dependent on the vascular bed type and on the degree of receptor activation [64–66].

## Therapeutic considerations

There are several important concepts to consider when selecting individual agent-receptor pathways. Many of the agents used to treat shock act on multiple different receptors and can cause mixed effects, some of which can be undesirable. Secondly, many of these agents have specific dose-response curves for which different receptor subtypes are activated at varying dose-dependent levels. This is particularly challenging when titrating or mixing these agents. Lastly, the human body uses many autoregulatory functions. Many of the desired responses (eg, vasoconstriction) can stimulate feedback responses that might counter the intended effect (increased perfusion). In this example, stimulated vasoconstriction leads to an increase in SVR and a resultant increase in MAP. Elevated MAPs can trigger reflexive bradycardia causing a decrease in CO (decreased perfusion). Additionally, increases in SVR (afterload) can also negatively impact CO, particularly in patients with weakened or ischemic myocardium. Common complications associated with vasopressors and inotropic agents include dysrhythmias, myocardial ischemia, hyperglycemia, and hypoperfusion. With all of these factors in mind, the choice of agent should be selective and titrated to the minimal effective dose to achieve target end points (MAP, urine output, and mentation).

## Specific agents

Epinephrine is a circulating catecholamine hormone that is synthesized from norepinephrine primarily in the adrenal medulla. It has a full range of alpha and beta agonistic properties with a host of effects that ultimately limit the ease of clinical use [67]. Epinephrine's main limitations are its potential provocation of dysrhythmias [67,68], potential for myocardial ischemia, and more profound splanchnic vasoconstriction than other agents that may cause abdominal organ ischemia [69–72].

In the emergency department, epinephrine is most useful as a primary agent for the treatment of anaphylaxis and as a secondary agent for the treatment of sepsis and severe bronchospasm. At doses of 2 to 10 μg/min, epinephrine's beta receptor stimulation predominates [67,73]. Epinephrine's $\beta_1$ stimulation causes an increase in heart rate (chronotropy) and an increase in stroke volume (inotrope) with a resultant increase in CO and cardiac oxygen consumption. At this dose, epinephrine also induces some $\beta_2$ stimulation that results in vasodilation in skeletal muscle arterioles offsetting some of its alpha-induced vasoconstriction. The end product of this predominant beta activity results in an increased CO, a decreased SVR, and variable effects on MAP [67,73]. At doses above 10 μg/min, alpha receptor stimulation results in generalized vasoconstriction and an increased MAP mediated through an increased SVR [67]. At variable doses, epinephrine also stimulates a number of important metabolic responses and directly stimulates the kidney, which produces renin. Through activation of the renin-angiotensin system, epinephrine indirectly causes additional vasoconstriction.

Ephedrine is a sympathomimetic agent with a structure similar to the other synthetic derivatives of epinephrine. Ephedrine acts on alpha and beta receptors with less potency than epinephrine and also stimulates the release of norepinephrine accounting for additional indirect alpha and beta effects [73]. Ephedrine's combined receptor activity causes an increase in systolic blood pressure and a modest inotropic effect. It has been shown to improve coronary and cerebral blood flow, but also has been linked to decreased renal and splanchnic blood flow [73]. Ephedrine is rarely used in a continuous infusion and its clinical use is mainly limited to treatment of hypotension associated with spinal anesthesia. Consequently, it is not likely to be useful in an emergency department setting.

Phenylephrine has pure alpha activity and results in veno and arteriolar vasoconstriction with minimal direct effects on inotrope or chronotropy [73,74]. It causes an increase in systolic, diastolic, and MAP and can lead to reflex bradycardia [73,75]. Phenylephrine has little effect on heart rate or contractility, so arrhythmia potentiation is minimal. CO may be decreased because of a marked increase in SVR (afterload), but most studies document normal CO maintenance [75,76]. The associated increased oxygen demand may induce coronary ischemia in vulnerable patients, although this is largely theoretic. Phenylephrine's vasoconstrictive effects have been associated with decreased renal and splanchnic perfusion [75,76].

The standard starting dose of phenylephrine is 10 to 20 μg/kg/min. In the emergency department, this agent may be clinically useful as a second-tier agent for the support of hyperdynamic vasodilatory shock (sepsis) [66]; in shock caused by central neurologic causes (neurogenic); and in other states where a low SVR is suspected and CO is not impaired [75]. It also may prove useful in hypotension caused by tachydysrhythmias because of its ability to stimulate reflex bradycardia.

Norepinephrine is the primary neurotransmitter of the postganglionic sympathetic nerves. It acts on both α- and β-adrenergic receptors producing potent vasoconstriction and a less pronounced increase in CO [66,73]. The potent vasoconstrictor effects act to increase venous return and improve cardiac preload. Norepinephrine's vasoconstriction is primarily seen as a disproportionate increase in systolic blood pressure over diastolic pressure that can lead to a reflex bradycardia. This bradycardic response is often countered by norepinephrine's mild chronotropic effects, leaving the heart rate unchanged [73,77]. In low doses (2 μg/min), norepinephrine stimulates β-adrenergic receptors. In usual clinical doses (> 3 μg/min), norepinephrine stimulates alpha receptors promoting vasoconstriction.

In early theoretic work, norepinephrine was thought to negatively impact the pulmonary vascular beds causing vasoconstriction and potentiation of pulmonary hypertension [73], although this has been largely dismissed by later studies in animal models [78–80]. Like other agents that increase inotrope and afterload, norepinephrine increases myocardial oxygen demand [81]. This is generally offset by a relative perfusion balance created by the mixed alpha and beta activity, but should be considered in patients with coronary compromise [73]. Norepinephrine, like other vasoconstrictors, can induce ischemia. This is of particular concern within the renal [82–84] and splanchnic vascular beds [12,13,85], where profound vasoconstriction may cause unintended organ injury. Norepinephrine's negative effects on hepatosplanchnic perfusion has drawn great controversy [13,77] and in recent studies these negative effects have been questioned [70,72,85].

It is important to consider the results of studies in context to the treatment population. In the case with norepinephrine, most of the data available have been studied in a septic model that because of humoral and microcirculation abnormalities is unlike other shock states [12,49]. Several trends have been uncovered in the use of norepinephrine in septic shock. Norepinephrine has been shown to be more effective at improving blood pressure [86], has demonstrated mortality benefits over other agents [87], and has largely been adopted as the first-line agent of choice for the hemodynamic support of septic shock [12,13,29,66,88–90]. In an emergency department setting, norepinephrine should be the agent of choice for treating hypotension associated with sepsis. It can also serve as an adjunct to other vasodilatory conditions, such as anaphylaxis and neurogenic shock, and might prove useful in states with ventricular dysfunction [4,59].

Dopamine is the immediate precursor of norepinephrine in the catecholamine cascade. When administered intravenously, dopamine has a variety of dose-dependent effects mediated by direct and indirect adrenergic activity. Directly, dopamine stimulates $\alpha$- and $\beta$-adrenergic receptors and may be converted to norepinephrine. Indirectly, dopamine stimulates the release of norepinephrine from sympathetic nerves [59,73,91]. These indirect mechanisms and dose-dependent variability make predicting the hemodynamic effects of dopamine difficult.

At low infusion rates (0.5–2 µg/kg/min), dopamine stimulates $D_1$ receptors resulting in selective vasodilatation of the renal, splanchnic, cerebral, and coronary vasculature [73,91]. Even at low doses, some beta stimulation occurs, which may increase MAP and CO. At rates from 2 to 5 µg/kg/min, dopamine stimulates norepinephrine release and has mixed receptor activity. Infusions of 5 to 10 µg/kg/min stimulate $\beta_1$ receptors increasing stroke volume, heart rate, and CO [73,91]. At doses greater than 10 µg/kg/min, dopamine activates both $\beta_1$ and $\alpha$-adrenergic receptors [12]. With escalating doses (> 10 µg/kg/min), alpha effects predominate causing vasoconstriction in most vascular beds [73]. There is extensive overlap, however, especially in critically ill patients. Dopamine has been shown to produce a median increase MAP of 24% in volume-optimized patients who remain hypotensive. Stroke volume was the major contributor to increased MAP, with heart rate contributing to a lesser extent and minimal contribution from SVR [66,85].

Dopamine's broad range of receptor activity offers primary benefits and clinical disadvantages. Like other adrenergic agents, concerns over dopamine's effect on hepatosplanchnic perfusion have been raised [69,85] and studies have shown that dopamine's effects may be more profound than those of other agents [92,93]. Additionally, the renal protective mechanisms of dopamine have been questioned [93] and "reno-protection" has largely been rejected [94]. Tachydysrhythmias often limit the clinical predictability of dopamine [95].

Dopamine is stable in premixed form and in emergency medical applications; it often is the most readily available vasoactive agent. Either norepinephrine or dopamine is recommended as a first-line agent for the treatment of septic shock by the Surviving Sepsis Campaign [90]. It also has clinical use in treating neurogenic and other states where the stimulation of heart rate, contractility, and the ability to modulate vascular resistance is of benefit.

Dobutamine is a synthetic catecholamine that is viewed primarily as an inotropic agent. It is predominantly a $\beta_1$ agonist with only weak alpha and $\beta_2$ effects. The selective $\beta_1$ activity of dobutamine primarily increases the inotropic effect because of increased stroke volume and heart rate with a variable effect on blood pressure [66]. The end effect of dobutamine's stimulus response is an increased CO and a decreased SVR that result in a global reduction in ventricular wall tension, sympathetic cardiac stress, and myocardial oxygen consumption [96]. Dobutamine's typical therapeutic doses range from 2.5 to 10 µg/kg/min.

Dobutamine might be used by the emergency practitioner to augment inotropic activity and improve perfusion in septic shock patients with global myocardial dysfunction [90]. It is also a commonly used agent to support contractility and cardiac decompensation, although its long-term effect on morbidity has been questioned in congestive heart failure [59].

Isoproterenol, a catecholamine structurally similar to epinephrine, is primarily an inotropic agent that produces $\beta_1$ and $\beta_2$ stimulation. Isoproterenol stimulates inotropic and prominent chronotropic activity that increases contractility, heart rate, and oxygen consumption [73]. Isoproterenol's prominent $\beta_2$ activity causes vasodilatation and creates the potential to produce arrhythmias. Both can be limiting factors of its use in shock. Isoproterenol is generally used for its chronotropic effects and may be useful in the treatment of hypotension associated with bradycardia or heart block.

Vasopressin is an endogenous hormone with vasoconstrictive effects whose relative deficiency has been tied to refractory hypotension in vasodilatory shock [97]. There is support for using a low-dose continuous infusion (0.01–0.03 U/min) in conjunction with other agents to treat refractory vasodilatory shock [12]. Vasopressin's use in other vasodilatory states like those seen with profound cardiogenic shock has not been solidified [98]. Its use has been linked to the reduction of mesenteric and renal blood flow, although results regarding the effects are conflicting [98]. Many questions remain unanswered regarding vasopressin's clinical effect and the Surviving Sepsis Campaign recommends it not be used as a first-line agent [90].

Amrinone and milrinone are phosphodiesterase-3 inhibitors that lead to the accumulation of intracellular cAMP, affecting a similar chain of events in vascular and cardiac tissues seen with $\beta$-adrenergic stimulation [99,100]. The end result of this activity produces vasodilation and a positive inotropic response. These drugs lead to a short-term improvement in hemodynamic performance and an improvement in hemodynamic variables. Like dobutamine, they are used to improve cardiac function and treat refractory heart failure. These agents are largely limited in shock states because of their vasodilatory properties [99]. Although these drugs have been shown to provide short-term clinical hemodynamic improvements, studies have largely failed to translate these into long-term mortality benefits [100–104].

## Alternative agents

Glucagon, a polypeptide hormone, in large dose infusion is beneficial in the treatment of $\beta$-blocker overdose, tricyclic overdose, and calcium channel blocker overdose [105–114]. Glucagon is thought to have its own receptor that is separate from adrenergic receptors. Stimulation of this receptor stimulates increased intracellular cAMP, which promotes inotrope and chronotropy [108,110]. It is generally given as a 5-mg bolus followed by a 1 to 5 mg/h infusion, which can be titrated up to 10 mg/h to achieve the desired patient response. High-dose insulin is the most recently proposed remedy for cardiovascular support in drug toxicity [115–121]. Insulin has an intrinsic positive inotropic effect and seems to promote calcium entry into the cells by means of an unknown mechanism. Although the therapeutic efficiency of high-dose insulin has been effective in animal models, no randomized human trials have been performed [106]. Anecdotally, insulin given as a 0.5 units/kg intravenous bolus, then as 0.5 to 1 U/kg/h intravenous infusion with dextrose 10% solution, has been shown to be effective in calcium channel and β-blocker toxicity [106]. Calcium salts have been shown to increase blood pressure and CO without effecting heart rate by increasing the intracellular pool of calcium available for release during depolarization [122–124]. One gram of a 10% solution (10 mL) of calcium chloride administered as a slow intravenous push has shown some efficacy in treating β-blocker [122–124] and calcium channel antagonist toxicity [125,126].

## Clinical applications

Authors have penned opinions on vasoactive therapy selection for years. Many of these opinions are based on pharmacology modeling, animal studies, or limited design studies. One Cochran review [127] and a recent series review [128] evaluated the data supporting the selection of one vasoactive drug over another and both produced limited answers. They were able to find only eight studies that provided randomized, controlled data and based on the limitations of these data were unable "to determine whether a particular vasopressor is superior to other agents in the treatment of shock states" [127,128]. It is important to note that most of the evidence available on vasoactive drugs has been gathered through clinical treatment of hypotension in very specific shock states. It is beneficial to consider and choose agents based on specific evidence available for the individual shock state being treated. Several specific shock states are reviewed (Table 5).

## Anaphylactic shock

Anaphylaxis, initiated by an unregulated IgE-mediated hypersensitivity response [129], is associated with bronchospasm, systemic vasodilation, increased vascular permeability, and a loss of venous tone [130]. Anaphylactoid reactions are clinically indistinguishable responses that are not IgE-mediated [131]. In this disease, mast cells release histamine, triggering bronchial smooth muscle contraction, vascular smooth muscle relaxation, and an increase in the vascular bed capacitance, which is not adequately filled by the normal circulating blood volume [132]. Platelets are activated

Table 5
Vasoactive drugs for shock states

| Shock state | First-tier agents | Second-tier agents |
|---|---|---|
| Anaphylactic shock | Epinephrine, 1 mL of 1:10,000 solution (100 μg), can be given as a slow IV push, then as a 0.02 μg/kg/min infusion (5–15 μg/min) | Norepinephrine infused at 0.1–1 μg/kg/min (0.5–30 μg/min) |
| Cardiogenic shock, left ventricular | SBP <70, norepinephrine infused at 0.1–1 μg/kg/min (0.5–30 μg/min); SBP 70–90, dopamine infused at 15 μg/kg/min; SBP >90, dobutamine infused at 2–20 μg/kg/min | Amrinone, 0.75 mg/kg loading dose, then 5–10 μg/kg/min (not recommended post-MI); Milrinone, 50 μg/kg loading dose, then 5–10 μg/kg/min (not recommended post-MI) |
| Cardiogenic shock, pulmonary embolism | Dobutamine infused at 5 μg/kg/min; Norepinephrine infused at 0.1–1 μg/kg/min | Phenylephrine infused at 10–20 μg/kg/min |
| Hemorrhagic shock | Volume resuscitation | Dopamine infused at 5–15 μg/kg/min as a temporizing adjunct |
| Neurogenic shock | Dopamine infused at 5–15 μg/kg/min | Norepinephrine infused at 0.1–1 μg/kg/min; Phenylephrine infused at 10–20 μg/kg/min |
| Septic shock | Norepinephrine infused at 0.1–1 μg/kg/min; Dobutamine infused at 5 μg/kg/min | Dopamine infused at 5–15 μg/kg/min; Epinephrine infused at 0.02 μg/kg/min |
| Toxic drug overdose with shock | Norepinephrine infused at 0.1–1 μg/kg/min | Phenylephrine infused at 10–20 μg/kg/min; Glucagon given as a 5-mg IV bolus, then as a 1–5 mg/h infusion; Calcium salts: calcium gluconate, 0.6 mL/kg bolus, then a 0.6–1.5 mL/kg/h infusion; Insulin started at 0.1 units/kg/h IV and titrated to a goal of 1 unit/kg/h |

*Abbreviations:* IV, intravenous; MI, myocardial infarction; SBP, systolic blood pressure.

in this cascade and release platelet-activating factor, which amplifies peripheral vasodilation and has a role in coronary and pulmonary artery vasoconstriction. The combined effects result in a reduction in volume and cardiac preload, a reduction in inotrope, and the consequent decrease in effective output. Consequently, hypotension and tissue hypoperfusion ensue.

Death from anaphylactic reactions is most commonly linked to unresolved bronchospasm, upper airway collapse from edema, or cardiovascular collapse [133]. Shock occurs in 30% to 50% percent of cases [132,133]. Shock in anaphylaxis shares variable components with hypovolemic shock caused by capillary fluid leak, distributive shock caused by the loss of vasomotor tone, and cardiogenic shock caused by inotropic reductions [131–134]. Knowledge of this physiologic distribution is important to the emergency management of anaphylaxis and specifically to the selection of therapies.

## Treatment

Rapid assessment of the patient's airway and cardiopulmonary condition should be performed. Pharmacologic therapy for anaphylactic shock is generally guided by data from observational or animal studies. The balance of evidence is aimed at reversing the effects of anaphylactic mediators. Dependent on the severity of presenting symptoms, this generally involves treatment with intravenous fluids, early antihistamines, bronchodilators, steroids, and epinephrine [135–137]. Early fluid resuscitation is required to correct relative volume deficits and restore cardiac preload.

Epinephrine is the vasoactive drug of choice in anaphylactic shock [136,138,139]. Epinephrine's catecholamine effects counteract the vasodepression, bronchoconstriction, fluid transudation, and cardiac depression seen in anaphylaxis [138]. It is generally given to patients with early signs of angioedema, bronchospasm, or hypotension. Early administration is typically given subcutaneously or intramuscularly. Clinical guidelines [136] recommend giving 0.3 to 0.5 mL of a 1:1000 (1 mg/mL) solution of epinephrine intramuscularly into the anterior or lateral thigh because of evidence of more rapid absorption by intramuscular routes [140]. Repeated doses may be administered in conjunction with aggressive fluid resuscitation every 3 to 5 minutes based on the clinical severity or symptom response.

For refractory or profound hypotension, epinephrine may be administered by continuous infusion at 5 to 15 μg/min and titrated to effect. In the case of difficult intravenous access, epinephrine (3–5 mL of 1:10:000 dilution) can be delivered by an endotracheal tube with desired effects [141]. Supplementary vasoactive agents (dopamine, norepinephrine, or phenylephrine) can be used to alter venous capacitance in persistent hypotension [138,139]. Additionally, an intravenous bolus of 1 mg of glucagon repeated at 5-minute intervals, particularly in patients on β-blockers, has been shown to provide inotropic and chronotropic support in patients with refractory hypotension and bradycardia [142,143]. Vasopressin has also gained attention as a secondary agent for the treatment of severe anaphylaxis that is unresponsive to epinephrine [144].

## Neurogenic shock

Neurogenic shock is caused by the sudden loss of the autonomic nervous system signal to the smooth muscle in vessel walls and to the nodal centers of the heart as a result of severe central nervous system (brain or spinal cord) damage. With the sudden loss of background sympathetic stimulation, the vessels vasodilate causing a sudden decrease in peripheral vascular resistance (decreased MAP) and the heart experiences a predominant parasympathetic stimulus promoting bradycardia (decreased CO) [145].

### Treatment

Treatment of neurogenic shock with aggressive volume resuscitation and prompt hemodynamic augmentation results in improved outcomes [146–150]. The weight of evidence defending medical support strategies is limited and is largely based on case series. The collective experience suggests that maintenance of MAP at 85 to 90 mm Hg improves spinal cord perfusion and impacts neurologic outcome [150]. Vasoactive agents are typically started after or concomitantly with volume resuscitation. Typically, agents with mixed receptor activity and stronger beta agonism (dopamine, norepinephrine) are initiated before the addition of a pure alpha agonist (phenylephrine) to elevate the MAP and stimulate chronotropy [149,150].

## Cardiogenic shock with acute left ventricular dysfunction

Cardiogenic shock is a state of inadequate tissue perfusion caused by cardiac dysfunction and is most commonly associated with acute myocardial infarction with left ventricular failure [34]. Cardiogenic shock, defined by sustained hypotension with tissue hypoperfusion (oliguria, cool extremities) despite adequate left ventricular filling pressure, complicates approximately 6% to 7% of acute myocardial infarctions and has an associated mortality of 60% to 90% [151,152]. Support for aggressive therapy has been championed by several large trials (GUSTO-1 and SHOCK) [6,153]. The largest mortality benefits in these trials were seen with early support, timely revascularization, and intra-aortic balloon pump augmentation [6,153,154].

### Treatment

Prompt treatment of hypotension and hypoperfusion is essential to the management of cardiogenic shock. American College of Cardiology–American Heart Association guidelines for the management of patients with ST-elevation myocardial infarction recommend an empiric intravenous volume challenge of 250 mL of isotonic saline be given in patients with suspected cardiogenic shock when there is no evidence of volume overload (pulmonary congestion, venous distention, respiratory distress) [155]. The guidelines for early emergency department management of complicated ST-elevation myocardial infarction caution against vigorous fluid challenges in patients with extensive left ventricular infarction, particularly the elderly [155]. Aggressive fluid therapy might be indicated in right ventricular (RV) dysfunction caused by a RV infarction and is commonly required to compensate for the venodilation and hypotension associated with inferior myocardial infarction [33,155].

Sympathomimetic drugs remain first-line agents in the treatment of cardiogenic shock associated with acute ischemic left ventricular dysfunction [33,34]. The guidelines generally use systolic blood pressure to guide vasoactive management. In patients with a systolic blood pressure ranging from 70 to 100 mm Hg who are less sick and show no signs of shock, the guidelines generally recommend an intravenous dobutamine infusion (2–20 µg/kg/min) be initiated to help support stroke volume and reduce afterload. In shock states with signs of hypoperfusion, initial therapy should begin with a dopamine infusion (5–15 µg/kg/min) to provide inotropic and vasoconstrictive support. In profoundly hypotensive patients (systolic blood pressure <70 mm Hg) norepinephrine is recommended as a 0.5 to 30 µg/min infusion [155].

## Cardiogenic shock with right ventricular dysfunction

RV dysfunction can be classified into impaired RV contractility, RV pressure overload, and RV volume overload. Patients with acutely decompensated RV function, however, often suffer from a combination of all three entities [156].

RV function is better suited to volume overload than pressure overload compared with the left ventricle (LV) [157]. The thin-walled RV is compliant, but does not have the myocardial bulk and contractility to overcome elevated afterload, unless it is conditioned over time to gradual increases in pulmonary vascular resistance [158]. Depressed RV contractility, secondary to RV infarction, cardiomyopathy, and sepsis, leads to dilation of the normal chamber, impaired relaxation, and subsequent increased end-diastolic pressures. This causes a shift in the normal contour of the interventricular septum toward the LV and an increase in intrapericardial pressures that limit both RV and LV filling [159].

RV pressure overload, secondary to pulmonary artery obstruction (pulmonary, fat, and amniotic fluid embolism), pulmonic stenosis, or pulmonary hypertension (associated with lung disease hypercarbia and hypoxemia, left heart disease, chronic thromboembolic disease and acute respiratory distress syndrome), leads to increased RV wall tension, RV chamber dilatation, and impaired diastolic and systolic function [160]. With overload, the interventricular septum shifts inward on the LV chamber. The increased wall tension of pressure overload results in increased myocardial oxygen consumption, which when coupled with decreased coronary perfusion and decreased oxygen supply can lead to myocardial ischemia or infarction [161]. Even in compensated states, failure can result from abrupt changes in pulmonary resistance or increased volumes. All of these pathways for impaired RV dysfunction result in a similar cascade of depressed RV CO. This depressed RV CO leads to decreased LV preload, then depressed LV CO, and subsequent systemic hypotension. This cascade is further exacerbated by the dyskinesis of the interventicular septum. Systemic hypotension in turn lowers coronary perfusion pressure and the vicious cycle termed "autoaggravation" continues to worsen RV dysfunction [162–164].

*Treatment*

The treatment of RV failure is aimed at disrupting the autoaggravation cycle. The specific clinical therapies, thrombolysis, percutaneous intervention, and possible surgical interventions are determined by the etiology of the acutely decompensated RV. Emergency management should primarily focus on supportive therapy as a bridge to final correction. Determining if volume is needed in the setting of RV failure can be difficult, because in all of the settings of RV failure, there is some degree of RV dilatation. Ultimately, fluid challenges and monitoring heart rate, blood pressure, cardiac performance, and urine outputs direct the further management of RV failure. As with LV failure secondary to myocardial infarction, an initial fluid challenge may be advocated if frank signs of volume overload are clinically absent [161,165].

There are no absolute guidelines to direct appropriate use of vasopressors or inotropes in the setting of acute RV failure. Hemodynamic support often requires the use of vasopressors and inotropes in addition to volume resuscitation, or if the RV is deemed volume overloaded vasodilators are indicated [43,161,166]. Norepinephrine, epinephrine, phenylephrine, dopamine, and vasopressin are vasoactive agents that could be used to offset systemic hypotension that often occurs with RV failure. Increasing MAP and afterload may seem counterintuitive; however, the RV is perfused by the coronary arteries in both diastole and systole [167]. Maintaining a pressure head that increases RV myocardial perfusion can be advantageous in the setting of increased RV myocardial oxygen demand. The ideal agent increases systemic vasoconstriction without increasing pulmonary vascular resistance; however, there are no human data to advocate for one agent over another. Norepinephrine has been supported in animal models of pulmonary embolism, which have shown improved survival, CO, and coronary blood flow with minimal changes in pulmonary vasculature with its use [80]. Epinephrine has been advocated in case-based literature for therapy in shock complicating pulmonary embolism [168]. Vasopressin has been used in low doses to treat milrinone-induced hypotension without detriment to CO or pulmonary artery pressures [169]. Theoretically, norepinephrine, epinephrine, and dopamine have $\beta_2$ activity that can lead to decreased pulmonary vascular resistance to differing degrees. This benefit is lost, however, when alpha and $\beta_1$ activity targeted to increase CO overpowers the early $\beta_2$ effects and increases pulmonary vascular resistance and myocardial oxygen demand [164]. There are no outcome data to support one agent over another for hypotension in the setting of RV failure.

There is no selective inotropic agent for the RV. Inotropic support can augment cardiac contractility by $\beta_1$ activity (dobutamine-isoproterenol); phosphodiesterase inhibition (milrinone-amrinone); or calcium sensitization (levosimendan). There have been recent studies comparing inotropes in LV failure; however, there are no trials specifically isolating RV failure. The Levosimendan Infusion versus Dobutamine trial and Calcium Sensitizer or Inotrope or None in Low-Output Heart Failure trial both demonstrated increased survival with levosimendan over dobutamine or placebo [147,170,171]. Levosimendan is a calcium sensitizer. It increases contraction by increasing sensitivity of troponin C to calcium. The Survival of Patients with Acute Heart Failure in Need of intravenous Inotropic Support trial, however, failed to demonstrate a difference in survival between dobutamine and levosimendan [172]. Additionally, levosimendan, although available in other countries, is only available as an investigational drug in the United States.

Although dopamine, dobutamine, and milrinone-amrinone have historically been used in cardiogenic shock patients (LV dysfunction), there have not been studies specifically evaluating their use in isolated RV failure. The use of these agents can neither be supported nor refuted with the current available evidence for RV dysfunction. Contrastingly, isoproterenol, amrinone, and milrinone have been investigated in animal models of acute pulmonary embolism and have not been shown to be favorable [173,174]. Many questions remain unanswered regarding RV support and there is no clear front-runner for "agent of choice" in this clinical scenario.

### Summary

There are few studies that provide evidence for a particular vasopressor or inotropic strategy in the early emergency department management of shock. Most recommendations for vasoactive strategies are largely based on pharmacodynamic modeling, animal research, empiric experience, and limited human trials performed in a critical care environment. Despite these limitations, a basic knowledge of available evidence can help guide a best practice approach until large, prospective, randomized, and well-conducted studies are completed. Understanding the background physiology of shock states and the actions and limitations of individual vasoactive agents can help the emergency medicine physician to tailor therapy to specific patient presentations.

## References

[1] Mitchell RN. Shock. In: Kumar V, editor. Robins and Cotran: pathologic basis of disease. 6th edition. Philadelphia: Saunders; 2005. p. 134–8.

[2] Lambe S, Washington DL, Fink A, et al. Trends in the use and capacity of California's emergency departments, 1990–1999. Ann Emerg Med 2002;39:389.

[3] McCaig LF, Burt CW. National hospital ambulatory medical care survey: 2002 emergency department summary. Adv Data 2004;1.

[4] Jones AE, Kline JA. Shock. In: Marx J, editor. Rosen's emergency medicine: concepts and clinical practice, vol. 1. 6th edition. Philadelphia: Mosby; 2006. p. 230–42.

[5] Shoemaker WC, Peitzman AB, Bellamy R, et al. Resuscitation from severe hemorrhage. Crit Care Med 1996;24:S12.

[6] Hochman JS, Boland J, Sleeper LA, et al. Current spectrum of cardiogenic shock and effect of early revascularization on mortality. Results of an International Registry. SHOCK Registry Investigators. Circulation 1995;91:873–81.

[7] Shoemaker WC. Temporal physiologic patterns of shock and circulatory dysfunction based on early descriptions by invasive and noninvasive monitoring. New Horiz 1996;4:300.

[8] Angus DC, Linde-Zwirble WT, Lidicker J, et al. Epidemiology of severe sepsis in the United States: analysis of incidence, outcome, and associated costs of care. Crit Care Med 2001;29: 1303.

[9] Dellinger RP. Cardiovascular management of septic shock. Crit Care Med 2003;31:946.

[10] Osborn TM, Tracy JK, Dunne JR, et al. Epidemiology of sepsis in patients with traumatic injury. Crit Care Med 2004;32:2234.

[11] Prasad A, Lennon RJ, Rihal CS, et al. Outcomes of elderly patients with cardiogenic shock treated with early percutaneous revascularization. Am Heart J 2004;147:1066.

[12] Holmes CL. Vasoactive drugs in the intensive care unit. Curr Opin Crit Care 2005;11:413–7.

[13] Kellum JA, Pinsky MR. Use of vasopressor agents in critically ill patients. Curr Opin Crit Care 2002;8:236–41.

[14] Otero RM, Nguyen HB, Huang DT, et al. Early goal-directed therapy in severe sepsis and septic shock revisited: concepts, controversies, and contemporary findings. Chest 2006;130: 1579.

[15] Parrilo JE. Approach to the patient with shock. In: Goldman L, Ausiello DA, editors. Cecil textbook of medicine. 22nd edition. Philadelphia: W.B. Saunders Company; 2004. p. 609.

[16] Rivers EP, Ander DS, Powell D. Central venous oxygen saturation monitoring in the critically ill patient. Curr Opin Crit Care 2001;7:204.

[17] Barber AE. Cell damage after shock. New Horiz 1996;4:161.

[18] Abou-Khalil B, Scalea TM, Trooskin SZ, et al. Hemodynamic responses to shock in young trauma patients: need for invasive monitoring. Crit Care Med 1994;22:633.

[19] Abramson D, Scalea TM, Hitchcock R, et al. Lactate clearance and survival following injury. J Trauma 1993;35:584.

[20] Blow O, Magliore L, Claridge JA, et al. The golden hour and the silver day: detection and correction of occult hypoperfusion within 24 hours improves outcome from major trauma. J Trauma 1999;47:964.

[21] Scalea TM, Maltz S, Yelon J, et al. Resuscitation of multiple trauma and head injury: role of crystalloid fluids and inotropes. Crit Care Med 1994;22:1610.

[22] Ander DS, Jaggi M, Rivers E, et al. Undetected cardiogenic shock in patients with congestive heart failure presenting to the emergency department [In Process Citation]. Am J Cardiol 1998;82:888.

[23] Jaggi M, McGeorge FT, Charash DS, et al. Occult cardiogenic shock in end-stage heart failure patients presenting to the emergency department. Clin Intensive Care 1995;6(2): 104.

[24] Rady M, Jafry S, Rivers E, et al. Characterization of systemic oxygen transport in end-stage chronic congestive heart failure. Am Heart J 1994;128:774.

[25] Rady MY, Edwards JD, Rivers EP, et al. Measurement of oxygen consumption after uncomplicated acute myocardial infarction. Chest 1993;104:930.

[26] Donnino M, Nguyen B, Rivers EP. Severe sepsis and septic shock: a hemodynamic comparison of early and late phase sepsis. Chest 2002;122:5S.

[27] Donnino MW, Nguyen HB, Jacobsen G, et al. Cryptic septic shock: a sub-analysis of early goal-directed therapy. Chest 2003;124:90S.

[28] Nguyen HB, Rivers EP, Knoblich BP, et al. Early lactate clearance is associated with improved outcome in severe sepsis and septic shock. Crit Care Med 2004;32:1637.

[29] Rivers E, Nguyen B, Havstad S, et al. Early goal-directed therapy in the treatment of severe sepsis and septic shock. N Engl J Med 2001;345:1368.

[30] Knoblich BRE, Nguyen B, Rittinger W, et al. Lactic acid clearance (Lactime) in the emergency department: implications for the development of multisystem organ failure and death. Acad Emerg Med 1999;6:479.

[31] Rady M, Rivers EP. The response of blood pressure, heart rate, shock index, central venous oxygen saturataion and lactate to resuscitation in the emergency department. Crit Care Med 1995;A138.

[32] Rady MY, Rivers EP, Nowak RM. Resuscitation of the critically ill in the ED: responses of blood pressure, heart rate, shock index, central venous oxygen saturation, and lactate. Am J Emerg Med 1996;14:218–25.

[33] Rodgers KG. Cardiovascular shock. Emerg Med Clin North Am 1995;13:793.

[34] Moscucci M, Bates ER. Cardiogenic shock. Cardiol Clin 1995;13:391.

[35] Landry DW, Oliver JA. The pathogenesis of vasodilatory shock. N Engl J Med 2001;345: 588–95.

[36] Riddez L, Hahn RG, Brismar B, et al. Central and regional hemodynamics during acute hypovolemia and volume substitution in volunteers. Crit Care Med 1997;25:635.

[37] Wo CC, Shoemaker WC, Appel PL, et al. Unreliability of blood pressure and heart rate to evaluate cardiac output in emergency resuscitation and critical illness. Crit Care Med 1993; 21:218–23.

[38] Rivers E. Mixed vs central venous oxygen saturation may be not numerically equal, but both are still clinically useful. Chest 2006;129:507.

[39] Trzeciak S, Rivers EP. Clinical manifestations of disordered microcirculatory perfusion in severe sepsis. Crit Care 2005;9(Suppl 4):S20.

[40] Shoemaker WC. Oxygen transport and oxygen metabolism in shock and critical illness: invasive and noninvasive monitoring of circulatory dysfunction and shock. Crit Care Clin 1996;12(4):939–69.

[41] Verdant C, De Backer D. How monitoring of the microcirculation may help us at the bedside. Curr Opin Crit Care 2005;11(3):240–4.

[42] Shoemaker WC, Kram HB, Appel PL. Therapy of shock based on pathophysiology, monitoring and outcome prediction. Crit Care Med 1990;18:S19.

[43] Michard F, Teboul JL. Predicting fluid responsiveness in ICU patients: a critical analysis of the evidence. Chest 2002;121:2000.

[44] Shoemaker WC, Wo CC, Yu S, et al. Invasive and noninvasive haemodynamic monitoring of acutely ill sepsis and septic shock patients in the emergency department. Eur J Emerg Med 2000;7:169–75.

[45] Pinsky MR. Assessment of indices of preload and volume responsiveness. Curr Opin Crit Care 2005;11:235.

[46] Gunn SR, Pinsky MR. Implications of arterial pressure variation in patients in the intensive care unit. Curr Opin Crit Care 2001;7:212.

[47] Magder S. Clinical usefulness of respiratory variations in arterial pressure. Am J Respir Crit Care Med 2004;169:151.

[48] Porter JM, Ivatury RR. In search of the optimal end points of resuscitation in trauma patients: a review. J Trauma 1998;44:908.

[49] Hinshaw LB. Sepsis/septic shock: participation of the microcirculation. An abbreviated review. Crit Care Med 1996;24(6):1072–8.

[50] Hayes MA, Timmins AC, Yau HS, et al. Elevation of systemic oxygen delivery in the treatment of critically ill patients. N Engl J Med 1994;330:1717.

[51] Ruffolo RR Jr, Nichols AJ, Stadel JM, et al. Pharmacological and therapeutic applications of alpha2-adrenoceptor subtypes. Annu Rev Pharmacol Toxicol 1993;32:243–79.

[52] Bourgoin A, Leone M, Delmas A, et al. Increasing mean arterial pressure in patients with septic shock: effects on oxygen variables and renal function. Crit Care Med 2005;33(4):780–6.

[53] LeDoux D, Astiz ME, Carpati CM, et al. Effects of perfusion pressure on tissue perfusion in septic shock. Crit Care Med 2000;28:2729–32.

[54] Nagashima M, Hattori Y, Akaishi Y, et al. Alpha 1-adrenoceptor subtypes mediating inotropic and electrophysiological effects in mammalian myocardium. Am J Phys 1996; 271:H1423–32.

[55] Fedida D, Bouchard RA. Mechanisms for the positive inotropic effect of alpha 1-adreno-ceptor stimulation in rat cardiac myocytes. Circ Res 1992;71:673–88.

[56] Grupp IL, Lorenz JN, Walsh RA, et al. Over expression of alpha 1B adrenergic receptor induces left ventricular dysfunction in the absence of hypertrophy. Am J Physiol 1998; 275:H1338–50.

[57] Ishibashi Y, Duncker DJ, Bache RJ. Endogenous nitric oxide masks alpha 2-adrenergic coronary vasoconstriction during exercise in the ischemic heart. Circ Res 1997;80: 196–207.

[58] Huang L, Tang W. Vasopressor agents: old and new components. Curr Opin Crit Care 2004;10:183–7.

[59] Steele A, Bihari D. Choice of catecholamine: does it matter? Curr Opin Crit Care 2000;6: 347–53.

[60] Girault J, Greengard P. The neurobiology of dopamine signaling. Arch Neurol 2004;61(5): 641–4.

[61] Jose P, Eisner G, Felder R. Regulation of blood pressure by dopamine receptors. Nephron Physiol 2003;95(2):19–27.

[62] Ricci A, Mignini F, Tomassoni D, et al. Dopamine receptor subtypes in the human pulmonary arterial tree. Auton Autacoid Pharmacol 2006;126(4):361–9.

[63] Holmes CL, Landry DW, Granton JT. Science review: vasopressin and the cardiovascular system. Part 1. Receptor physiology. Crit Care 2003;7(6):427–34.

[64] Vincent JL. Vasopressin in hypotensive and shock states. Crit Care Clin 2006;2:187–97.

[65] Holmes CL, Granton JT, Landry DW. Science review: vasopressin and the cardiovascular system. Part 2. Clinical physiology. Crit Care 2004;8:15–23.

[66] Hollenberg SM, Ahrens TS, Annane D, et al. Practice parameters for hemodynamic support of sepsis in adult patients: 2004 update. Crit Care Med 2004;32:1928–48.

[67] Di Giantomasso D, Bellomo R, May CN. The haemodynamic and metabolic effects of epinephrine in experimental hyperdynamic septic shock. Intensive Care Med 2005;31:454–62.

[68] Clutter WE, Bier D, Shah SD, et al. Epinephrine plasma metabolic clearance rates and physiologic thresholds for metabolic and hemodynamic actions in man. J Clin Invest 1980;66:94–101.

[69] De Backer D, Creteur J, Silva E, et al. Effects of dopamine, norepinephrine, and epinephrine on the splanchnic circulation in septic shock: which is best? Crit Care Med 2003;31: 1659.

[70] Levy B, Bollaert PE, Charpentier C, et al. Comparison of norepinephrine and dobutamine to epinephrine for hemodynamics, lactate metabolism, and gastric tonometric variables in septic shock: a prospective, randomized study. Intensive Care Med 1997;23:282–7.

[71] Meier-Hellmann A, Reinhart K, Bredle DL, et al. Epinephrine impairs splanchnic perfusion in septic shock. Crit Care Med 1997;25:399–404.

[72] Duranteau J, Sitbon P, Teboul JL, et al. Effects of epinephrine, norepinephrine, or the combination of norepinephrine and dobutamine on gastric mucosa in septic shock. Crit Care Med 1999;27:893–900.

[73] Zaritsky AL, Chernow B. Catecholamines, sympathomimetics. In: Chernow B, Lake CR, editors. The pharmacologic approach to the critically ill patient. Baltimore (MD): Williams & Wilkins; 1983. p. 481–549.

[74] Williamson KL, Broadley KJ. Characterization of the alpha-adrenoreceptors mediating positive inotropy of rat left atria by use of selective agonists and antagonists. Arch Int Pharmacodyn Ther 1987;285:181–98.

[75] Gregory JS, Bonfiglio MF, Dasta JF, et al. Experience with phenylephrine as a component of the pharmacologic support of septic shock. Crit Care Med 1991;19:1395–400.

[76] Yamazaki T, Shimada Y, Taenaka N, et al. Circulatory responses to afterloading with phenylephrine in hyperdynamic sepsis. Crit Care Med 1982;10:432.

[77] Nasraway SA. Norepinephrine: no more "leave 'em dead"? Crit Care Med 2000;28: 3096–8.

[78] Angle MR, Molloy DW, Penner B, et al. The cardiopulmonary and renal hemodynamic effects of norepinephrine in canine pulmonary embolism. Chest 1989;95:1333–7.

[79] Mathru M, Venus B, Smith RA, et al. Treatment of low cardiac output complicating acute pulmonary hypertension in normovolemic goats. Crit Care Med 1986;14:120–4.

[80] Hirsch LJ, Rooney MW, Wat SS, et al. Norepinephrine and phenylephrine effects on right ventricular function in experimental canine pulmonary embolism. Chest 1991;100: 796–801.

[81] Russell JA, Phang PT. The oxygen delivery/consumption controversy. Am J Respir Crit Care Med 1994;149:533.

[82] Schaer GL, Find MP, Parrillo JE. Norepinephrine alone versus norepinephrine plus low-dose dopamine: enhanced renal blood flow with combination pressor therapy. Crit Care Med 1985;13:492.

[83] Redl-Wenzl EM, Armbruster C, Edelmann G, et al. The effects of norepinephrine on hemodynamics and renal function in severe septic shock states. Intensive Care Med 1993;19:151.

[84] Desjars P, Pinaud M, Bugnon D, et al. Norepinephrine therapy has no deleterious renal effects in human septic shock. Crit Care Med 1989;17:426–9.

[85] Marik PE, Mohedin M. The contrasting effects of dopamine and norepinephrine on systemic and splanchnic oxygen utilization in hyperdynamic sepsis. JAMA 1994;272:1354.

[86] Martin C, Papazian L, Perrin G, et al. Norepinephrine or dopamine for the treatment of hyperdynamic septic shock? Chest 1993;103:1826–31.

[87] Martin C, Viviand X, Leone M, et al. Effect of nor-epinephrine on the outcome of septic shock. Crit Care Med 2000;28:2758–65.

[88] Morimatsu H, Singh K, Uchino S, et al. Early and exclusive use of norepinephrine in septic shock. Resuscitation 2004;62:249.

[89] Baele RJ, Hollenberg SM, Vincent JL, et al. Vasopressor and inotropic support in septic shock: an evidence based review. Crit Care Med 2004;32(Suppl):S455–65.

[90] Dellinger RP, Levy MM, Carlet JM, et al. Surviving Sepsis Campaign guidelines for management of severe sepsis and septic shock: 2008. Crit Care Med 2008;36(1):296–327.

[91] Goldberg LI. Dopamine: clinical uses of an endogenous catecholamine. N Engl J Med 1974; 291:707.

[92] Guerin JP, Levraut J, Samat-Long C, et al. Effects of dopamine and norepinephrine on systemic and hepatosplanchnic hemodynamics, oxygen exchange, and energy balance in vasoplegic septic patients. Shock 2005;23:18–24.

[93] Kellum JA, Decker JM. The use of dopamine in acute renal failure: a metaanalysis. Crit Care Med 2001;29:1526–31.

[94] Holmes CL, Walley KR. Bad medicine: low-dose dopamine in the ICU. Chest 2003;123: 1266–75.

[95] MacGregor DA, Smith TE, Prielipp RC, et al. Pharmacokinetics of dopamine in healthy male subjects. Anesthesiology 2000;92:338.

[96] Al-Hesayen A, Azevedo ER, Newton GE, et al. The effects of dobutamine on cardiac sympathetic activity in patients with congestive heart failure. J Am Coll Cardiol 2002;39:1269.

[97] Landry DW, Levin HR, Gallant EM, et al. Vasopressin deficiency contributes to the vasodilation of septic shock. Circulation 1997;95:1122–5.

[98] Dunser MW, Mayr A, Ulmer HR, et al. The effects of vasopressin on systemic hemodynamics in catecholamine-resistant septic and postcardiotomy shock: a retrospective analysis. Anesth Analg 2001;93:7–13.

[99] Lollgen H, Drexler H. Use of inotropes in the critical care setting. Crit Care Med 1990;18: S56.

[100] Honerjager P. Pharmacology of bipyridine phosphodiesterase III inhibitors. Am Heart J 1991;121:1939–44.

[101] Packer M, Carver JR, Rodeheffer RJ, et al. Effect of oral milrinone on mortality in severe chronic heart failure: The PROMISE Study Research Group. N Engl J Med 1991;325: 1468–75.

[102] Milfred-LaForest SK, Shubert J, Mendoza B, et al. Tolerability of extended duration intravenous milrinone in patients hospitalized for advanced heart failure and the usefulness of uptitration of oral angiotensin-converting enzyme inhibitors. Am J Cardiol 1999;84:894–9.

[103] Hatzizacharias A, Makris T, Krespi P, et al. Intermittent milrinone effect on long-term hemodynamic profile in patients with severe congestive heart failure. Am Heart J 1999; 138:241–6.

[104] Silver MA. Intermittent inotropes for advanced heart failure: inquiring minds want to know. Am Heart J 1999;138:191–2.

[105] Pollack CV. Utility of glucagon in the emergency department. J Emerg Med 1993;11: 195–205.

[106] Kerns W. Treatment of beta adrenergic blocker and calcium channel antagonist toxicity. Emerg Med Clin North Am 2007;25:309–31.

[107] Holger JS, Engebretsen KM, Obetz CL, et al. A comparison of vasopressin and glucagon in beta-blocker induced toxicity. Clin Toxicol 2006;44:45–51.

[108] Love JN, Sachdeva DK, Bessman ES, et al. A potential role for glucagon in the treatment of drug-induced symptomatic bradycardia. Chest 1998;114:323–6.

[109] Love JN, Howell JM, Litovitz TL, et al. Acute beta blocker overdose: factors associated with the development of cardiovascular morbidity. J Toxicol Clin Toxicol 2000;38:275–81.

[110] Chernow B, Zaloga GP, Malcolm D, et al. Glucagon's chronotropic action is calcium dependent. J Pharmacol Exp Ther 1987;241(3):833–7.

[111] Doyon S, Roberts JR. The use of glucagon in a case of calcium channel blocker overdose. Ann Emerg Med 1993;22(7):1229–33.

[112] Mahr NC, Valdes A, Lamas G. Use of glucagon for acute intravenous diltiazem toxicity. Am J Cardiol 1997;79(11):1570–1.

[113] Papadopoulos J, O'Neil MG. Utilization of a glucagon infusion in the management of a massive nifedipine overdose. J Emerg Med 2000;18:453–5.

[114] Sensky PR, Olczak SA. High dose intravenous glucagon in severe tricyclic poisoning. Postgrad Med J 1999;75:611–2.

[115] Kline JA, Tomaszewski CA, Schroeder JD, et al. Insulin is a superior antidote for cardiovascular toxicity induced by verapamil in the anesthetized canine. J Pharmacol Exp Ther 1993;267(2):744–50.

[116] Farah AE, Alousi AA. The actions of insulin on cardiac contractility. Life Sci 1981;29: 975–1000.

[117] Boyer EW, Duic PA, Evans A. Hyperinsulinemia/euglycemia therapy for calcium channel blocker poisoning. Pediatr Emerg Care 2002;18:36–7.

[118] Boyer EW, Shannon M. Treatment of calcium-channel-blocker intoxication with insulin infusion. N Engl J Med 2001;344:1721–2.

[119] Marques M, Gomes E, de Oliviera J. Treatment of calcium channel blocker intoxication with insulin infusion: case report and literature review. Resuscitation 2003;57:211–3.

[120] Reith DM, Dawson AH, Epid D, et al. Relative toxicity of beta blockers in overdose. J Toxicol Clin Toxicol 1996;34:273–8.

[121] Kerns W, Schroeder D, Williams C, et al. Insulin improves survival in a canine model of acute beta-blocker toxicity. Ann Emerg Med 1997;29:748–57.

[122] Haddad LM. Resuscitation after nifedipine overdose exclusively with intravenous calcium. Am J Emerg Med 1996;14:602–3.

[123] Pertoldi F, D'Orlando L, Mercante WP. Electromechanical dissociation 48 hours after atenolol overdose: usefulness of calcium chloride. Ann Emerg Med 1998;31:777.

[124] Love J, Hanfling D, Howell JM. Hemodynamic effects of calcium chloride in a canine model of acute propranolol intoxication. Ann Emerg Med 1996;28:1.

[125] Isbister GK. Delayed asystolic cardiac arrest after diltiazem overdose: resuscitation with high dose intravenous calcium. Emerg Med J 2002;19:355.

[126] Lam YM, Tse HF, Lau CP. Continuous calcium chloride infusion for massive nifedipine overdose. Chest 2001;119:1280.

[127] Mullner M, Urbanek B, Havel C, et al. Vasopressors for shock. Cochrane Database Syst Rev 2008;2:CD003709.

[128] Jones AE. What vasopressors should be used to treat shock? Ann Emerg Med 2007;49(3): 367–8.

[129] Sampson HA, Munoz-Furlong A, Bock SA, et al. Symposium on the definition and management of anaphylaxis: summary report. J Allergy Clin Immunol 2005;115:584.

[130] Silverman HJ, Van Hook C, Haponik EF. Hemodynamic changes in human anaphylaxis. Am J Med 1984;77(2):341–4.

[131] DeJarnatt AC, Grant JA. Basic mechanisms of anaphylaxis and anaphylactoid reactions. Immunol Allergy Clin North Am 1992;12:501.

[132] Brown GA. The pathophysiology of shock in anaphylaxis. Immunol Allergy Clin North Am 2007;27:165–75.

[133] Pumphrey RS. Lessons for management of anaphylaxis from a study of fatal reactions. Clin Exp Allergy 2000;30(8):1144–50.

[134] Wasserman SI. The heart in anaphylaxis. J Allergy Clin Immunol 1986;77:663.

[135] Chamberlain D. Emergency medical treatment of anaphylactic reactions. Project Team of the Resuscitation Council (UK). J Accid Emerg Med 1999;16:243.

[136] Lieberman P, Kemp S, Oppenheimer J, et al. The diagnosis and management of anaphylaxis: an updated practice parameter. J Allergy Clin Immunol 2005;115:S483.

[137] Sampson HA, Munoz-Furlong A, Campbell RL, et al. Second symposium on the definition and management of anaphylaxis: summary report–Second National Institute of Allergy and Infectious Disease/Food Allergy and Anaphylaxis Network Symposium. J Allergy Clin Immunol 2006;117:391.

[138] Fisher M. Treating anaphylaxis with sympathomimetic drugs. BMJ 1992;305:1107–8.

[139] Heytman M, Rainbird A. Use of alpha-agonists for management of anaphylaxis occurring under anaesthesia: case studies and review. Anaesthesia 2004;59(12):1210–5.

[140] Simons FE, Gu X, Simons KJ. Epinephrine absorption in adults: intramuscular versus subcutaneous injection. J Allergy Clin Immunol 2001;108:871.

[141] Raymondos K, Panning B, Leuwer M, et al. Absorption and hemodynamic effects of airway administration of adrenaline in patients with severe cardiac disease. Ann Intern Med 2000;132:800.

[142] Zaloga GP, Delacey W, Holmboe E, et al. Glucagon reversal of hypotension in a case of anaphylactoid shock. Ann Intern Med 1986;105:65.

[143] Thomas M, Crawford I. Best evidence topic report: glucagon infusion in refractory anaphylactic shock in patients on beta blockers. Emerg Med J 2005;22(4):272–3.

[144] Schummer W, Schummer C, Wippermann J, et al. Anaphylactic shock: is vasopressin the drug of choice? Anesthesiology 2004;101(4):1025–7.

[145] Tator CH. Experimental and clinical studies of the pathophysiology and management of acute spinal cord injury. J Spinal Cord Med 1996;19(4):206–14.

[146] Tator CH, Fehlings MG. Review of the secondary injury theory of acute spinal cord trauma with emphasis on vascular mechanisms. J Neurosurg 1991;75:15–26.

[147] Levi L, Wolf A, Belzberg H. Hemodynamic parameters in patients with acute cervical cord trauma: description, intervention, and prediction of outcome. Neurosurgery 1993;33(6): 1007–17.

[148] Isaac L, Pejic L. Secondary mechanisms of spinal cord injury. Surg Neurol 1995;43:484–5.

[149] Vale FL, Burns J, Jackson AB, et al. Combined medical and surgical treatment after acute spinal cord injury: results of a prospective pilot study to assess the merits of aggressive medical resuscitation and blood pressure management. J Neurosurg 1997;87:239–46.

[150] Amar AP, Levy ML. Pathogenesis and pharmacological strategies for mitigating secondary damage in acute spinal cord injury. Neurosurgery 1999;44(5):1027–40.

[151] Goldberg RJ, Gore JM, Alpert JS, et al. Cardiogenic shock after acute myocardial infarction. Incidence and mortality from a community wide perspective, 1975 to 1988. N Engl J Med 1991;325:1117.

[152] Goldberg RJ, Gore JM, Thompson CA, et al. Recent magnitude of and temporal trends (1994–1997) in the incidence and hospital death rates of cardiogenic shock complicating acute myocardial infarction: The second National Registry of Myocardial Infarction. Am Heart J 2001;141:65.

[153] Berger PB, Holmes DR, Stebbins AL, et al. Impact of an aggressive invasive catheterization and revascularization strategy on mortality in patients with cardiogenic shock in the Global Utilization of Streptokinase and Tissue Plasminogen Activator for Occluded Coronary Arteries (GUSTO-I) trial. Circulation 1997;96:122.

[154] Sanborn TA, Sleeper LA, Bates ER, et al. Impact of thrombolysis, intra-aortic balloon pump counterpulsation, and their combination in cardiogenic shock complicating acute myocardial infarction: a report from the SHOCK Trial Registry. Should we emergently revascularize occluded coronaries for cardiogenic shock? J Am Coll Cardiol 2000;36:1123.

[155] Anbe DT, Armstrong PW, Bates ER, et al. ACC/AHA guidelines for the management of patients with ST-elevation myocardial infarction. Available at: http://www.cardiosource.com/guidelines/guidelines/stemi/index.pdf. Accessed December 15, 2007.

[156] Piazza F, Goldhaber SZ. The acutely decompensated right ventricle: pathways for diagnosis and management. Chest 2005;128:1836–52.

[157] Brieke A, DeNofrio D. Right ventricular dysfunction in chronic dilated cardiomyopathy and heart failure. Coron Artery Dis 2005;16:5–11.

[158] Cecconi M, Johnston E, Rhodes A. What role does right side of the heart play in circulation? Crit Care 2006;10(Suppl 3):S5.

[159] Goldstien JA. Pathophysiology and management of the right heart ischemia. J Am Coll Cardiol 2002;40:841–53.

[160] Goldhaber SZ, Elliott CG. Acute pulmonary embolism. Part I. Epidemiology, pathophysiology and diagnosis. Circulation 2003;108:2726–9.

[161] Woods J, Monteiro P, Rhodes A. Right ventricular dysfunction. Curr Opin Crit Care 2007; 13:532–40.

[162] Louie EK, Lin SS, Rehnertson SI, et al. Pressure and volume loading of the right ventricle have opposite effects on left ventricular ejection fraction. Circulation 1995;92:819–24.

[163] Budev M, Arroliga A, Wiedemann H, et al. Cor pulmonale: an overview. Semin Respir Crit Care Med 2003;24:233–44.

[164] Mebazaa A, Karpati P, Renaud E, et al. Acute right ventricular failure: from pathophysiology to new treatments. Intensive Care Med 2004;30:185–96.

[165] Pfisterer M. Right ventricular involvement in myocardial infarction and cardiogenic shock. Lancet 2003;362:392–4.

[166] Mercat A, Diehl JL, Meyer G, et al. Hemodynamic effects of fluid loading in acute massive pulmonary embolism. Crit Care Med 1999;27:540–4.

[167] Lee FA. Hemodynamics of the right ventricle in normal and disease states. Cardiol Clin 1992;10:59.

[168] Boulain T, Lanotte R, Legras A, et al. Efficacy of epinephrine therapy in shock complicating pulmonary embolism. Chest 1993;104:300–2.

[169] Gold J, Cullinane S, Chen J, et al. Vasopressin in the treatment of milrinone-induced hypotension in sever heart failure. Am J Cardiol 2000;85:506–8, A511.

[170] Follath F, Cleland JG, Just H, et al. Efficacy and safety of intravenous levosimendan compared with dobutamine in sever low-output heart failure (the LIDO study). Lancet 2002;360:196–202.

[171] Zairis MN, Apostolatos C, Anastasiadis P, et al. The effect of calcium sensitizer or an inotrope or none in the chronic low output decompensated heart failure: results from the Calcium Sensitizer or Inotrope or None in Low Output Heart Failure Study (CASINO) [Abstract 835–836]. J Am Coll Cardiol 2004;43:206A.

[172] Mebazza A, Nieminen M, Packer M, et al. Levosimendan vs dobutamine for patients with acute decompensated heart failure: the SURVIVE Randomized Trial. JAMA 2007;297:1883–91.

[173] Smith HJ, Oriol A, Morch J, et al. Hemodynamic studies in cardiogenic shock: treatment with isoproterenol and metaraminol. Circulation 1967;35:1084.

[174] Tanak J, Tajimi K, Matsumoto A, et al. Vaso dilatory effects of milrinone on pulmonary vasculature in dogs with pulmonary hypertension due to pulmonary embolism: a comparison with those of dopamine and dobutamine. Clin Exp Pharmocol Physiol 1990;17:681.

ELSEVIER
SAUNDERS

Emerg Med Clin N Am
26 (2008) 787–812

EMERGENCY
MEDICINE
CLINICS OF
NORTH AMERICA

# Emergency and Critical Care Imaging

## J. Christian Fox, MD, RDMS*, Zareth Irwin, MD, MS

*Division of Emergency Ultrasound, Department of Emergency Medicine,
University of California Irvine Medical Center, 101 The City Drive,
Rt. 128-01, Orange, CA 92868, USA*

A complete discussion of the applications and techniques available for patient imaging in emergency and critical care settings is beyond the scope of this article. In this article the authors highlight traditional modalities and recent advances that allow rapid diagnosis of conditions requiring urgent intervention in critically ill patients. This overview emphasizes modalities that can be performed rapidly at the bedside (ultrasound andradiography) as well as CT and CT angiography (CTA), that provide a wealth of information in a relatively short time.

## Bedside ultrasound in the critically ill patient

Ultrasound allows instantaneous imaging of the organs and vessels and is being used increasingly in critical care settings to improve diagnostic capability and guide invasive procedures. A diagnostic approach to unexplained hypotension might include ultrasound of the heart for cardiac tamponade, left ventricular failure, and right ventricular outflow obstruction and examination of the abdomen for evidence of intraperitoneal hemorrhage, decreased preload in the inferior vena cava, and abdominal aortic aneurysm (AAA). Similarly, sonographic evaluation of unexplained dyspnea might include evaluation of the heart, both hemithoraces for pneumothorax, hemothorax, or effusion, and the lower extremities for proximal deep venous thrombosis.

Ultrasound is unique in its portability and its ability to provide real-time imaging with an absence of ionizing radiation. Commonly performed resuscitative procedures such as arterial and venous cannulation, paracentesis,

---

\* Corresponding author.

*E-mail address:* jchristianfox@gmail.com (J.C. Fox).

0733-8627/08/$ - see front matter © 2008 Elsevier Inc. All rights reserved.
doi:10.1016/j.emc.2008.05.003        *emed.theclinics.com*

thoracentesis, pericardiocentesis, and placing and confirming cardiac capture with transcutaneous or transvenous pacing may be facilitated with ultrasound guidance. This guidance allows nearly instantaneous treatment of many of the conditions diagnosed with sonographic evaluation.

### Cardiac ultrasound

Cardiac ultrasound (echocardiography or "echo") is a powerful diagnostic tool in the evaluation of critically ill patients and is an integral part of the focused assessment with sonography in trauma (FAST) examination [1–5]. Perhaps the most dramatic indications for echocardiography are evaluations of patients who have severe hypotension [6,7] or pulseless electrical activity. In these cases echocardiography may help distinguish between left ventricular dysfunction, volume depletion, cardiac tamponade, and right ventricular outflow obstruction. Ultrasound also may guide treatment decisions in the setting of pulseless electrical activity, because mortality rates approach 100% for patients who have visualized cardiac standstill even in the setting of an organized electrical rhythm [8,9].

Cardiac ultrasound should be considered in any patient who has chest pain, tachycardia, hypotension, or dyspnea to evaluate for pericardial effusion and impending tamponade [10,11]. In cases of pulmonary embolism, echocardiography helps stratify a patient's risk, provides prognostic information, and aids in deciding whether to administer thrombolytic therapy [12–16]. In the setting of acute coronary syndrome, information about left ventricular function also may provide overall prognostic information [17]. Recent research demonstrates the usefulness of echocardiography as an aid in the evaluation of sepsis, specifically in assessing preload and left ventricular function to help guide fluid resuscitation and the choice of vasopressors [18,19]. Although echocardiography has a high negative predictive value for pericardial effusion/tamponade and acute valvular emergencies, its low sensitivity for acute coronary syndrome, pulmonary embolism, and thoracic aortic aneurysm/dissection limits the usefulness of negative studies for these conditions [12,20,21].

### Diagnostic capabilities

Because comprehensive echocardiography requires significant expertise, the authors recommend that the novice sonographer focus primarily on identifying cardiac standstill, the presence and extent of pericardial effusions, global left ventricular function, and right ventricular strain. Cardiac standstill is seen simply as an absence of cardiac motion during visualization of the heart. Pericardial effusions are evidenced by an anechoic area between the epicardium and pericardium. Cardiac tamponade results from extrinsic compression of the right side of the heart, with sonographic signs including diastolic collapse of the right atrium and/or ventricle (Fig. 1) and increased respiratory variation in the Doppler signal of mitral inflow (the

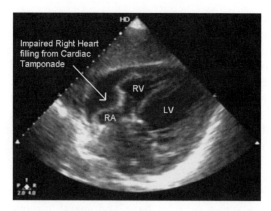

Fig. 1. Subxiphoid view demonstrating a moderate to large effusion with evidence of diastolic right atrial collapse.

echocardiographic equivalent of pulsus paradoxicus) in the setting of a pericardial effusion.

Global left ventricular function typically is measured with ejection fraction, with the reference standard for ejection fraction being nuclear studies or cardiac catheterization. Although formulas exist for calculating ejection fraction based on echo measurements, most cardiologists use a visual estimation. The authors recommend that the novice sonographer avoid attempting to quantify ejection fraction and instead describe the myocardial contractility qualitatively as hyperdynamic (high-outflow states), generally normal, or hypokinetic (low-outflow states).

Although many chronic conditions may result in right ventricular dilatation and/or hypertrophy, signs of right ventricular strain including right ventricular dilatation (Fig. 2) or hypokinesis, paradoxical septal motion,

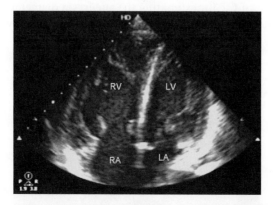

Fig. 2. Apical four-chamber view of a patient who has right ventricular dilatation secondary to right ventricular outflow obstruction in the setting of a large pulmonary embolus. Note that he right ventricle (RV) is larger than the left ventricle (LV). LA, left atrium; RA, right atrium.

and tricuspid regurgitation may suggest massive pulmonary embolism in critically ill patients [12,14,16]. In the presence of acute right ventricular outflow obstruction, right ventricular dilatation increases the right ventricular:left ventricular ratio beyond the normal 0.7:1. In the right clinical setting, when the right ventricular approaches or surpasses the size of the left ventricle, the clinician can infer the presence of right ventricular outflow obstruction, consistent with a large pulmonary embolism. Although the specificity of this finding is high, the low sensitivity prevents exclusion of this diagnosis when right ventricular dilatation is absent [12].

*Imaging limitations and pitfalls*

For mechanical reasons, subxiphoid views may be unobtainable in patients who are obese or who have abdominal trauma or distension. Hyperexpansion of the lungs (eg, in patients who have obstructive pulmonary disease or who are mechanically ventilated) may prevent the acquisition of parasternal images because of gas scatter artifact. Fortunately, in most patients at least one view allows adequate visualization of the heart. A common pitfall is misinterpretation of what may be physiologic pericardial fluid and/or epicardial fat as a significant pericardial effusion. Differentiating between these conditions may be difficult; signs that favor epicardial fat include the presence of gray-scale echoes that move with the heart and are less than 1 cm thick and the lack of effect on myocardial contractility.

*Abdominal aorta ultrasound*

An AAA is defined by a diameter greater than 3 cm or more than 1.5 times the diameter of the proximal uninvolved segment (Fig. 3). Ultrasound is the imaging test of choice for initial detection and measurement of AAA because it is sensitive and risk free, accurately estimates aneurismal diameter, and can be performed at the bedside. The accuracy of ultrasound is similar to that of CT for estimating the aneurysm diameter, and the ultrasound assessment can be performed rapidly and accurately with 95% to

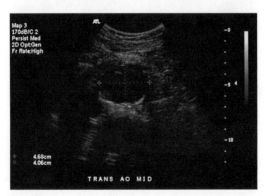

Fig. 3. Abdominal aortic aneurysm, transverse view.

98% sensitivity for AAA even when performed by sonographers who have minimal experience [22–24].

### Imaging limitations and pitfalls

Although sonography is sensitive for identification of AAA, signs of rupture, including extraluminal blood and retroperitoneal hematoma with or without displacement of the ipsilateral kidney, may be absent. For this reason, abnormal findings in stable patients warrant follow-up abdominal CT studies, and unstable patients require emergent surgical evaluation. Bedside ultrasound is useful for evaluation of AAA in most patients, but image acquisition is hindered by bowel gas and obesity, which prevent successful bedside evaluation in approximately 10% of emergency department patients [25]. As a result, clinicians may be forced to rely on the physical examination and abdominal radiographs (for signs of calcification) in unstable patients and on CT scanning in stable patients when AAA is among the differential diagnoses and sonographic visualization is obscured.

### Trauma ultrasound

The FAST examination traditionally focused on findings of hemoperitoneum (Fig. 4) and hemopericardium (see Fig. 1) in blunt thoracoabdominal trauma. Recently an extended FAST examination has been used as a more thorough assessment of the thorax in blunt and penetrating trauma and to evaluate also for pneumothorax (Fig. 5) and hemothorax (Fig. 6), allowing noninvasive diagnosis of most life-threatening thoracoabdominal injuries (hemoperitoneum, hemopericardium, cardiac tamponade, pneumothorax, and hemothorax) at the bedside.

### Diagnostic capabilities

Reported accuracies of the FAST examination for hemoperitoneum vary, with sensitivities ranging from 86% to 94% and specificities as high as 98%

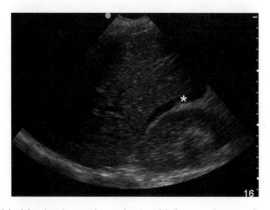

Fig. 4. Free fluid in Morrison's pouch consistent with hemoperitoneum in a trauma patient. The asterisk indicates free fluid.

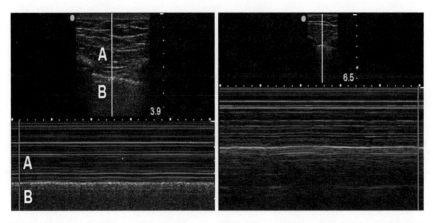

Fig. 5. (*Left panel*) Absence of pneumothorax on M-mode as evidenced by the normal "sand on the beach" sign, which is generated by the interface of the subcutaneous tissue (A) and lung parenchyma (B). (*Right panel*) Presence of pneumothorax on M-mode as evidenced by the stratosphere sign (lack of "sand on the beach" sign), resulting from loss of the normal interface between subcutaneous tissue and lung parenchyma.

for detection of intra-abdominal injury [26,27]. The use of intravenous (IV) contrast (stabilized microbubbles) may improve the detection of solid-organ injury in blunt abdominal trauma. A recent study demonstrated 91% sensitivity and 100% specificity in this setting [28]. The FAST examination is specific (94%) and has a reasonably high positive predictive value (90%) for free fluid in penetrating trauma, but its low sensitivity (46%) necessitates additional evaluation when the suspicion of injury remains [29].

Ultrasound is particularly useful for identification of life-threatening thoracic injuries. In the setting of penetrating trauma, cardiac ultrasound allows faster disposition to surgery [30] with sensitivities and specificities

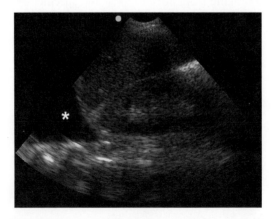

Fig. 6. Fluid above the diaphragm with loss of the normal mirror-image artifact in a patient who has a hemothorax (*asterisk*) secondary to trauma.

for hemopericardium approaching 100% [31]. The extended FAST is highly sensitive and specific for hemothorax (97.5% and 99.7%, respectively) [32] and pneumothorax (98% and 99%, respectively) [33]. Given the critical nature of these findings, it may be appropriate to evaluate the thorax before the abdomen during the initial assessment of airway, breathing, and circulation in unstable trauma patients.

Research suggests that sonographic measurement of optic nerve sheath diameter (ONSD) allows detection of papilledema (Fig. 7) in the setting increased intracranial pressure [34–41]. An ONSD greater than 5 mm is up to 100% sensitive and 95% specific for identifying increased intracranial pressure when compared with head CT [34]. Studies using intracranial pressure monitors to relate ONSD directly to intracranial pressure are ongoing. The usefulness of ocular ultrasound in trauma has yet to be determined, but the technique may prove useful in triaging patients awaiting CT scanning or in mass casualty settings when CT is unavailable.

*Imaging limitations and pitfalls*

Small amounts of intra-abdominal free fluid may be missed on ultrasound, especially when they do not form discrete collections. Placing patients in the Trendelenburg position improves the detection of hemoperitoneum by concentrating free fluid in dependent areas within the abdomen. A distended bladder also may improve detection of intra-abdominal free fluid by providing a sonographic window to improve imaging of the pelvis. For this reason the initial FAST examination should be completed before urethral catheterization, when possible.

Thoracoabdominal sonography may be hindered by adipose tissue, bowel gas, subcutaneous emphysema, pneumoperitoneum, and rib shadows. Parasternal cardiac imaging is affected adversely by rib shadows, emphysematous lungs, and subcutaneous emphysema, whereas subxiphoid cardiac

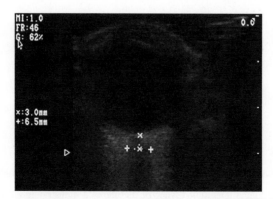

Fig. 7. Papilledema as evidenced by of an enlarged optic nerve sheath diameter (6.5 mm) in a patient who has an increased intracranial pressure. The arrowhead is the focal point of the sound beam. It is optimizing the image by narrowing the sound beam at that level.

imaging may be challenging in patients who have protuberant and/or painful abdomens. For this reason it is necessary to be familiar with the acquisition and interpretation of views from both approaches.

## Pelvic ultrasound

Pelvic ultrasound is invaluable in the diagnosis of gynecologic and obstetric emergencies. All unstable female patients of childbearing age should undergo bedside transabdominal and/or transvaginal pelvic ultrasound to look for the presence, location, (intrauterine versus ectopic), and viability of a pregnancy unless this possibility has been excluded [42]. In critically ill patients, early detection of an intrauterine or ectopic gestation helps guide resuscitative efforts and expedites involvement of an obstetrician. The presence of an intrauterine gestation (Fig. 8 A and B) may be an indication for specific laboratory tests (eg, disseminated intravascular coagulation screen, Kleihauer-Betke test) and play a role in diagnostic decision making such as need for fetal monitoring and judicious radiation exposure. A stable patient who has an ectopic pregnancy (Fig. 9) requires obstetric consultation, whereas an unstable patient mandates laparotomy.

## Diagnostic capabilities

In female trauma patients, ultrasound may demonstrate abruption, uterine rupture, and fetal distress or death. Pelvic ultrasound also is appropriate to evaluate for ovarian torsion and tubo-ovarian abscess in nonpregnant patients who have pelvic or lower abdominal pain. In the critical care setting the authors recommend that novice sonographers focus solely on making the diagnosis of live intrauterine pregnancy, abnormal intrauterine pregnancy, fetal demise, ectopic pregnancy, and/or free fluid on pelvic ultrasound.

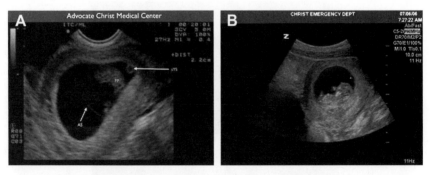

Fig. 8. (A) Transvaginal longitudinal view of the uterus demonstrating an intrauterine pregnancy. The amniotic sac (AS) (short arrow), which frequently is seen between the ninth and twelfth gestational week, is visualized also. (B) Transabdominal longitudinal view of the uterus showing an intrauterine pregnancy. FP, fetal pole.

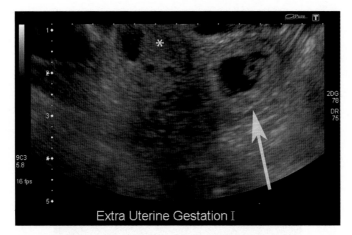

Fig. 9. Ectopic pregnancy: transvaginal view of the pelvis with evidence of an extrauterine gestation (*arrow*) adjacent to the ovary (*asterisk*).

## Imaging limitations and pitfalls

Obesity and the presence of bowel gas may inhibit image acquisition during transabdominal pelvic ultrasound. Although a distended bladder is helpful for transabdominal pelvic imaging, because it provides an acoustic window, a full bladder moves the uterus farther from the probe and results in artifact and image degradation during transvaginal scanning. Therefore, when both transvaginal and transabdominal scanning are performed on the same patient, it is preferable for the patient to have a full bladder for the abdominal approach and to void before the transvaginal approach.

## CT

### CT of the head

Head CT detects most pathology requiring emergent intervention in patients who have head trauma, altered mental status, and other acute neurologic abnormalities.

Unexplained neurologic abnormalities and altered mental status generally necessitate emergent head CT [43], but criteria regarding the indications for CT may be helpful in patients presenting with minor head trauma, headache, or suspected intracranial infection [43–47].

### Diagnostic capabilities

Third-generation CT scanners are fast and sensitive for the detection of bony injury (Fig. 10) and most acute hemorrhages (Fig. 11 A–C). Extracranial lesions, such as hematomas and soft tissue edema, also are distinguished easily. Although CT does not demonstrate all intracranial space-occupying

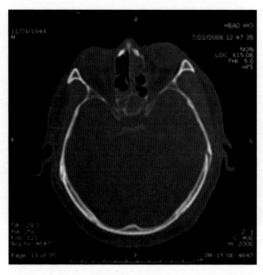

Fig. 10. Skull fracture. Fractures of the skull can be classified as linear, depressed, basal, or diastatic. In this image there is a fracture of the left temporal bone seen with the bone window.

lesions, it readily identifies those requiring urgent intervention because of size or mass effect.

*Imaging limitations and pitfalls*

In the setting of ischemic stroke, head CT lacks the sensitivity to detect abnormalities in most patients presenting early after the event. Nonetheless, an emergent initial CT is appropriate in this setting to rule out the presence

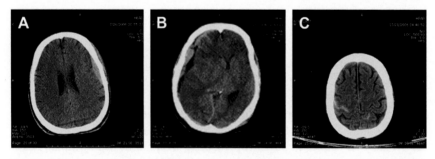

Fig. 11. (*A*) Left-sided epidural hematoma with the characteristic lenticular shaped collection of blood. This type of hematoma may occur with or without an associated skull fracture. (*B*) Right-sided subdural hematoma. Subdural fluid collections are crescent shaped and do not cross the midline but rather invaginate inward alongside the falx cerebri and the tentorium cerebelli. They also are associated with a greater degree of underlying brain edema. (*C*) Traumatic subarachnoid hemorrhage. Blood can be seen invaginating between the cerebral convolutions in both of these examples of traumatic subarachnoid hemorrhage. On the right, blood can be seen in the left Sylvian fissure.

of hemorrhage, masses, and other pathologies and may show evidence that a stroke is older than the clinical presentation suggests. Although CT is sensitive for most acute hemorrhages, minute amounts of blood may not be visualized. For this reason many practitioners advocate that a negative CT in the setting of suspected subarachnoid hemorrhage should be followed by a lumbar puncture to evaluate for blood and/or xanthochromia in the spinal fluid.

CT is insensitive for early signs of axonal and cellular injury. Small-mass lesions and intracranial abscess may not be visualized on CT, especially in the absence of IV contrast, but the mass effect and edema that result from sizable space-occupying lesions and abscesses generally are evident. Beam-hardening artifact from the adjacent skull base may obscure identification of basilar artery occlusion or aneurysm and may necessitate additional imaging when these pathologies are suspected.

*CT angiography of the head and neck*

Multimodal CT techniques that use noncontrast CT, CTA, and/or CT perfusion imaging (CTP) provide rapid imaging of vascular anatomy and tissues of the head and neck and allow physicians to streamline the care of the hyperacute patient. In addition to identifying the site and severity of stenosis, occlusion (Fig. 12 A–C), or trauma, CTA of the head and neck provides vital information regarding tissue injury and perfusion (location, size, and degree of reversibility or hypoperfusion). Although the choice of imaging modality is patient- and disease-specific, continuing improvements in CTA and magnetic resonance angiography (MRA) and the relative ease of acquisition of these studies has resulted in these studies largely replacing digital subtraction angiography (Fig. 13 A and B) in the evaluation of cervico-cranial vascular disorders.

CTA of the head and neck may be indicated in the management of patients who present with signs of acute stroke when the use of IV

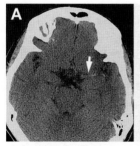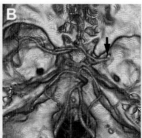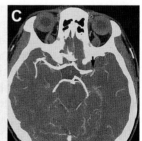

Fig. 12. (*A*) Nonconrast CT scan reveals a hyperdense left middle cerebral artery (*arrow*) suggesting the presence of a clot. (*B*) CT angiography reveals complete occlusion of the distal left middle cerebral artery (*arrow*). (*C*) Axial multiplanar reconstruction of CT angiography again showing occlusion of the middle cerebral artery (*arrow*).

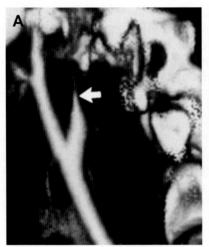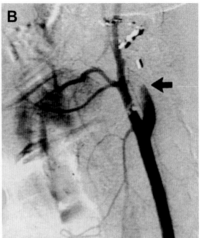

Fig. 13. (*A*) Parasagittal CT angiography image reconstruction demonstrating left internal carotid arterial occlusion (*arrow*). (*B*) Lateral digital subtraction angiogram again showing left internal carotid arterial occlusion (*arrow*).

recombinant tissue plasminogen activator is being considered, and in the management of patients suspected of having intracranial aneurysm rupture or subarachnoid hemorrhage, penetrating neck injuries for which surgical management is being debated, suspected vertebrobasilar disease, and in the management of patients who have unexplained neck pain with or without neurologic symptoms. In these settings CTA provides rapid information regarding early ischemic changes, hypoperfusion/ischemic penumbra, and location of vascular lesions, allowing triage of patients to appropriate therapies quickly, when the benefit from acute therapies is greatest.

*Diagnostic capabilities*

CTA is accurate for carotid artery and circle of Willis stenosis [48–50]. The rapid acquisition of three-dimensional data (Fig. 14) and the potential for assessment of whole-brain perfusion are clear advantages over catheter angiography. CTA also provides visualization of the vessel wall, improving detection of intramural dissection and thrombosed aneurysms. CTA relies on venous rather than arterial access, reducing the risk of complication compared with conventional angiography.

The three-dimensional reconstructions produced by CTA are similar to those obtained with MRA. Although MRI/MRA may be more sensitive for detection of ischemia and provide improved soft tissue contrast, CTA better demonstrates calcifications within atherosclerotic plaques and is superior for delineating the relationship of intracranial aneurysms to adjacent bony structures. CTA may be more readily obtainable and is indispensable when a rapid work-up is needed or there is a contraindication to MRI such as implanted ferromagnetic material or patient intolerance.

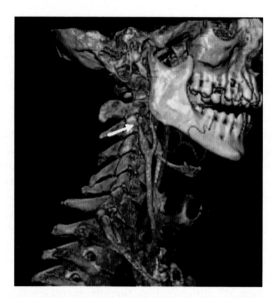

Fig. 14. Contrast-enhanced three-dimensional reconstruction of a CT image of a patient who has a right internal carotid artery occlusion (*arrow*).

CTA and CTP can be performed immediately after conventional CT scanning while the patient is still in the scanner. Although the techniques still are evolving, CTP offers the advantages of assessing both reversible and irreversible ischemia through map generation of cerebral blood volume, cerebral blood flow, and mean contrast transit time. CTP can be used to differentiate the core infarcted area from ischemic penumbra and to predict tissue outcome [51]. CTA and CTP may aid the physician in identifying the regions of salvageable brain tissue that may be amenable to reperfusion therapy.

*Imaging limitations and pitfalls*

The accuracy and speed of CTA is influenced by technical factors such as slice thickness, length of coverage, kilovolt and milliampere settings, and contrast bolus delay time. Although the radiation dose administered during CTA generally is considered safe for adults, the iodinated contrast may be dangerous in patients who have contrast allergy or renal failure. Care also should be exercised in children and pregnant women, for whom the long-term effects of radiation exposure are largely unknown.

*CT of the chest*

CT scanning of the chest with and without IV contrast provides a wealth of information for the evaluation of many life-threatening conditions. CTA provides a detailed evaluation of the coronary and pulmonary arteries, as well as the thoracic aorta, allowing rapid evaluation of coronary artery disease, pulmonary embolism, and aortic dissection. It is postulated that in the future patients presenting with chest pain may undergo a "triple rule-out" in which all three of these conditions are addressed with a single, high-resolution CTA of the chest.

### Diagnostic capabilities

Coronary heart disease is the leading cause of death in the United States, responsible for about 817,000 deaths each year [52]. CTA of the coronary arteries is highly sensitive for both obstructive and nonobstructive coronary artery disease (Fig. 15) [53,54]. Scanners using multidetector technology with 16 or more slices and cardiac gating enable visualization of the lumen and vessel wall of the coronary arteries in a matter of seconds. Studies using 64-slice CT scanners demonstrate sensitivities and specificities exceeding 95% for the diagnosis of significant coronary artery disease [55].

Pulmonary embolism (Fig. 16 A and B) is relatively common, with an annual incidence of 25 to 70 cases per 100,000 patients. Prompt diagnosis and administration of anticoagulant therapy increases favorable clinical outcomes. CTA of the pulmonary arteries is the diagnostic test of choice for the evaluation of acute pulmonary embolism [56,57], and the improved spatial and temporal resolution of multidetector CT (MDCT) enables visualization of the pulmonary arteries in less than 10 seconds. The sensitivity and specificity of CTA for the detection of pulmonary embolism exceeds 90%, and a negative CT is associated with a good prognosis when anticoagulation is withheld [58].

Aortic dissection (Fig. 17) is uncommon, with a peak incidence of 3 to 5 cases per 1 million people per year. The mortality of untreated aortic dissection involving the ascending aorta (Stanford Type A) approaches 1% to

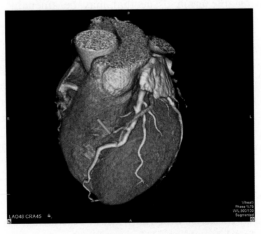

Fig. 15. Contrast-enhanced three-dimensional reconstruction of a CT image demonstrating a nonobstructing stenosis of the left anterior descending artery (*arrow*).

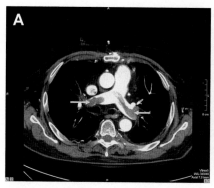
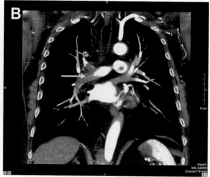

Fig. 16. (*A*) Axial maximum intensity projection of thoracic multidetector CT imaging with contrast performed in a 60-year-old man who had known coronary artery disease (status post coronary artery bypass graft) and who presented with severe central chest discomfort. The images show two large filling defects in the left and right main pulmonary arteries (*arrows*), consistent with acute massive pulmonary embolism. (*B*) Coronal maximum intensity projection of the thoracic multidetector CT performed in the same patient who had severe central chest discomfort. The images again show a large filling defect in the right main and segmental pulmonary arteries (*arrow*), consistent with acute pulmonary embolism.

2% per hour after symptom onset [59,60], emphasizing the need for prompt diagnosis and treatment. MDCT enables rapid visualization of the entire aorta, localizing the site of intimal tear and the extent of anatomic involvement. The sensitivity and specificity of MDCT approach 100% for the diagnosis of aortic dissection [61].

*Imaging limitations and pitfalls*

CT coronary angiography relies on technical expertise and specific patient characteristics. Patients should be capable of an 8- to 9-second

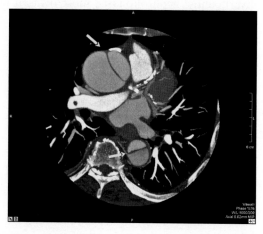

Fig. 17. Contrast-enhanced axial CT scan of the chest demonstrating a Stanford type A aortic dissection affecting both the ascending and descending portions of the thoracic aorta (*arrows*).

respiratory pause, and a relatively slow heart rate is required to avoid motion artifact during image acquisition. Beta-blockers or other rate-controlling agents may be required to control heart rate. CT pulmonary angiography is affected strongly by the timing of the administration of the intravenous contrast relative to image acquisition, and subsegmental pulmonary emboli may be missed in lower resolution scanners. CT studies for aortic dissection may yield false-positive results when motion artifact from the aorta mimics an intimal flap.

## CT of the abdomen

CT scanning has emerged as the primary diagnostic imaging modality for patients presenting with abdominal or pelvic pain and to evaluate for intra-abdominal injury in the stable trauma patient. Studies show CT sensitivities of 69% to 95% and specificities of 95% to 100% for the diagnosis of bowel and mesenteric injuries [62], with higher sensitivities for diagnosis of solid-organ injuries. CT scanning for bowel obstruction (Fig. 18) is highly sensitive and helps delineate the location, severity, and underlying cause. The administration of oral water-soluble contrast may be therapeutic and diagnostic because of increased intraluminal absorption of water and diminution of bowel wall edema. The ability to generate reconstructions in different planes with MDCT assists the clinician in identifying closed-loop obstructions.

### Diagnostic capabilities

Right upper quadrant pathology that may be diagnosed by CT includes pancreatitis, cholecystitis, ascending cholangitis, perforated hollow viscous injury, and hepatic tumor or abscess. Right lower quadrant pathology readily imaged by CT includes appendicitis, mesenteric adenitis, ectopic pregnancy, hernia, diverticulitis, nephrolithiasis, most ovarian pathology, and

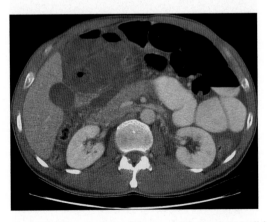

Fig. 18. Contrast-enhanced CT scan of the abdomen demonstrating small bowel obstruction with failure of the oral contrast to pass into the distal small bowel.

psoas abscess. Left upper quadrant pathologies seen on CT include pancreatitis, splenic infarct or abscess, peptic ulcer disease, hiatal hernias, and gastric malignancy. Most disorders of the left lower quadrant also are visualized on CT and include diverticulitis, ectopic pregnancy, ovarian pathology, hernia, psoas abscess, and nephrolithiasis. Causes of diffuse abdominal pain also often found on CT include small bowel obstruction, abdominal aortic aneurysm, pancreatitis, mesenteric ischemia, aortic dissection, and urosepsis.

The use of MDCT scanners allows rapid image acquisition, reduced motion artifact, and decreased distance between CT slices. These factors result in improved visualization of intra-abdominal organs and are particularly important in diagnosing appendiceal and pancreatic pathology, because these are small organs that can cause significant illness.

CT scanning without contrast allows rapid image acquisition but provides limited data. Thus, the use of oral and IV contrast may improve diagnostic accuracy for some conditions. Oral contrast helps elucidate the degree and location of bowel obstruction and may aid in the diagnosis of intra-abdominal abscesses. IV contrast is avoided in the setting of renal insufficiency or suspected nephrolithiasis but is indicated in most other settings. Rectal contrast is warranted for evaluation of suspected colonic perforation from penetrating abdominal, flank, or back trauma and may aid the diagnosis in common diseases such as appendicitis or diverticulitis. It often is not necessary in nontrauma settings, however, and may cause patient discomfort. Overall, the decision to administer oral and/or rectal contrast is dictated largely by physician preference and departmental policy.

*Imaging limitations and pitfalls*

Because fat planes are less developed in children, CT scanning is less effective in this population. The added concern about radiation exposure in pediatric patients has led many practitioners to try to avoid CT scanning in this population. The relative diagnostic yield of abdominal CT in obese patients is debated because increased adipose tissue results in scatter of the beams and poorer resolution, but increased fat stranding may assist in recognition of pathology. In general, CT scanning is severely hindered by obesity only when the patient exceeds the weight limit of the scanner.

*CT angiography of the abdomen*

Transitioning from axial abdominal imaging with single-detector CT scanners to volumetric imaging with MDCT scanners has revolutionized vascular studies. Arterial and venous structures now can be visualized in three-dimensional reconstructions and rotated to see an aneurysm's full contour. The emergent use of MDCT angiography of the abdomen in the ICU is in the early stages, but MDCT promises to be a powerful tool for evaluation of a patient in whom a vascular catastrophe is suspected.

*Diagnostic capabilities*

Embolic disease, thrombosis (Fig. 19), hemorrhage, aortoduodenal fistulas, arteriovenous malformations, aortic aneurysms (Fig. 20), and dissections are potentially life-threatening intra-abdominal processes that can be evaluated with CTA. Computer-generated reconstructions enable visualization of the size and location of such lesions and of the site of the leakage in aortic rupture. In the setting of trauma, vascular data are supplemented quickly and accurately with information on solid organs and skeletal injuries. Thrombi in the inferior vena cava or its tributaries from the pelvis and proximal lower extremities are visualized easily, and this information can be useful in guiding therapy involving thrombolysis and stent placement.

*Imaging limitations and pitfalls*

CTA requires the administration of iodinated IV contrast and is relatively contraindicated in patients who have renal failure. The large radiation exposure also necessitates that this technology be used judiciously. Patients must be stable enough to leave the critical care environment and be able to lie supine and motionless during the examination.

## Radiography

*Radiography of the chest*

Although radiography lacks the resolution and sensitivity of CT scans in evaluating thoracic pathology, it does provide a wealth of information and

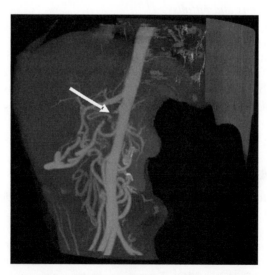

Fig. 19. Superior mesenteric artery thrombus resulting in partial occlusion (*arrow*) seen in this sagittal view.

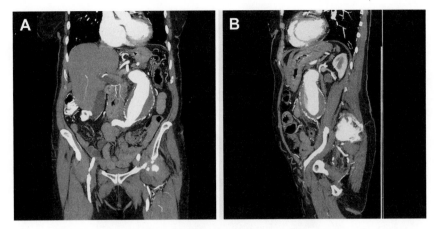

Fig. 20. (*A*) A coronal image demonstrating a large aneurysm of the distal abdominal aorta, 6.1 × 5.7 cm in diameter and 10.1 cm in length, with extensive thrombus formation and wall calcifications. The true lumen measures 3 cm. Note the tortuous nature of the aorta. (*B*) Sagittal image demonstrating the abdominal aortic aneurysm seen in Fig. 20 A. Note the significant amount of calcification surrounding the false lumen in both images.

allows the diagnosis of many life-threatening conditions. The portability and rapidity with which radiographic studies can be obtained make it invaluable in patients who have chest pain, dyspnea, hypotension, thoracic trauma, or known pulmonary pathology, in patients requiring serial evaluations, and in those too unstable to undergo CT scanning. It also is commonly indicated in fever of unclear source and altered mental status.

*Diagnostic capabilities*

Life-threatening conditions that may be diagnosed with chest radiography include tension pneumothorax (Fig. 21), hemothorax, pneumonia, congestive heart failure, pulmonary edema, moderate to large pericardial effusions, pulmonary contusions, and thoracic aortic dissection.

*Imaging limitations and pitfalls*

Chest radiography lacks the sensitivity to find mild or early cases of many of the conditions listed in the previous section and lacks the specificity to determine the causes of many abnormal findings. It has low sensitivity for pulmonary embolism and is affected significantly by patient positioning. For these reasons, it should be considered an initial screening examination but should not be used to exclude dangerous diseases definitively when a high clinical suspicion exists.

*Radiography of the abdomen*

Abdominal radiography lacks the sensitivity of CT scans but allows rapid imaging of many acute conditions and does not require the administration

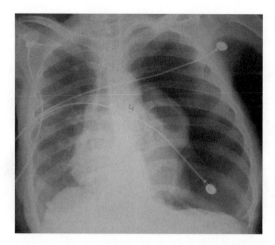

Fig. 21. Tension pneumothorax. The absence of lung markings extending out from the hilum on the patient's left side is consistent with pneumothorax. The hyperinflation of the left hemithorax and rightward shift of the trachea and mediastinum are demonstrative of tension pneumothorax.

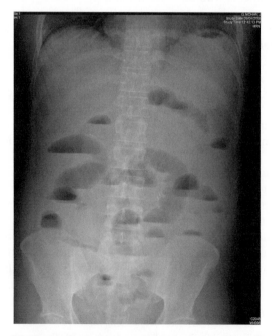

Fig. 22. Upright abdominal radiograph of a patient who has small bowel obstruction as evidenced by multiple air/fluid levels and an absence of air in the rectum.

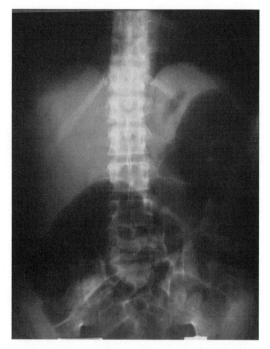

Fig. 23. Large bowel obstruction. This patient has a dilated air-containing large bowel. Note the prominent haustra.

of oral or IV contrast. Unlike CT scanning, the portability of radiography allows patients to remain in the critical care setting, and patients do not have to tolerate lying motionless in a supine position. A single view of the kidneys, ureters, and bladder or an acute abdominal series may be an appropriate initial imaging study in select patients presenting with abdominal pain, vomiting, or constipation.

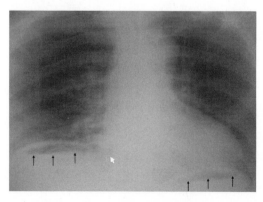

Fig. 24. Upright chest radiograph of a patient who has a perforated hollow viscous injury resulting in free air under both hemidiaphragms (*arrows*).

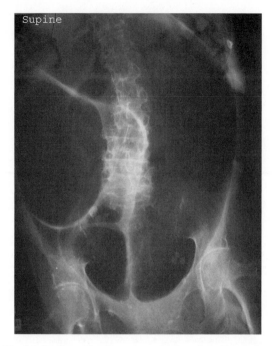

Fig. 25. Radiograph of a patient who has sigmoid volvulus.

*Diagnostic capabilities*

Abdominal radiography readily demonstrates high-grade bowel obstruction (Fig. 22 A and B), perforated hollow viscous injury (Fig. 23), volvulus (Fig. 24), and pneumatosis intestinalis (Figs. 25 and 26). Additional findings include but are not limited to renal, biliary, and appendiceal lithiasis, vascular disease/calcification, ileus, intussusception, soft tissue masses, and metastatic disease.

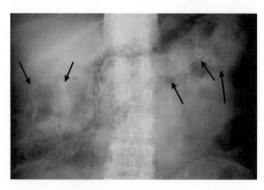

Fig. 26. Pneumatosis intestinalis. Note the free air within the bowel wall of the small bowel (*arrows*).

*Imaging limitations and pitfalls*

Abdominal radiography has poor sensitivity for many of the disease processes for which it is used. It should not be used as a definitive study for the exclusion of high-risk diagnoses when clinical suspicion remains. Plain films are used most appropriately as an initial imaging study for specific intra-abdominal pathologies. When nondiagnostic, they should be followed with abdominal CT in critically patients when abdominal pathology is suspected.

## Summary

Recent advances in medical imaging have increased portability, decreased image acquisition time, improved data resolution, and increased the use of noninvasive studies. As imaging technologies develop, appropriate studies for the evaluation of specific pathologies in emergency and critical care settings change. Although the choice of imaging is influenced by patient and practice environment factors, it is imperative to have a general knowledge of the strengths and limitations of particular imaging tests to maximize diagnostic efficiency and improve patient care.

This article is not intended to be an exhaustive discussion of all imaging modalities available to critical care practitioners or of all applications of the modalities covered. The authors have attempted to highlight the use of portable, noninvasive imaging (bedside ultrasound and radiography) and studies available for rapid acquisition of high-quality data (CT and CTA) that are appropriate in the evaluation of time-sensitive diagnoses in critically ill patients. As current technologies improve and new technologies are discovered, it is likely that novel applications and techniques will be discovered and used in the care of critically ill patients.

## References

[1] Cardenas E. Limited bedside ultrasound imaging by emergency medicine physicians. West J Med. 1998;168(3):188–9.
[2] Chizner MA. The diagnosis of heart disease by clinical assessment alone. Curr Probl Cardiol 2001;26(5):285–379.
[3] Hauser AM. The emerging role of echocardiography in the emergency department. Ann Emerg Med. 1989;18(12):1298–303.
[4] Kimura BJ, Bocchicchio M, Willis CL, et al. Screening cardiac ultrasonographic examination in patients with suspected cardiac disease in the emergency department. Am Heart J 2001;142(2):324–30.
[5] Plummer D, Brunette D, Asinger R, et al. Emergency department echocardiography improves outcome in penetrating cardiac injury. Ann Emerg Med 1992;21(6):709–12.
[6] Bocka JJ, Overton DT, Hauser A. Electromechanical dissociation in human beings: an echocardiographic evaluation. Ann Emerg Med 1988;17(5):450–2.
[7] Tayal VS, Kline JA. Emergency echocardiography to detect pericardial effusion in patients in PEA and near-PEA states. Resuscitation 2003;59(3):315–8.

[8] Amaya SC, Langsam A. Ultrasound detection of ventricular fibrillation disguised as asystole. Ann Emerg Med 1999;33(3):344–6.

[9] Blaivas M, Fox JC. Outcome in cardiac arrest patients found to have cardiac standstill on the bedside emergency department echocardiogram [comment]. Acad Emerg Med 2001; 8(6):616–21.

[10] Blaivas M. Incidence of pericardial effusion in patients presenting to the emergency department with unexplained dyspnea. Acad Emerg Med 2001;8(12):1143–6.

[11] Shabetai R. Pericardial effusion: hemodynamic spectrum. Heart 2004;90(3):255–6.

[12] Nazeyrollas P, Metz D, jolly D, et al. Use of transthoracic Doppler echocardiography combined with clinical and electrocardiographic data to predict acute pulmonary embolism. Eur Heart J 1996;17:779–86.

[13] Grifoni S, Olivotto I, Cecchini P, et al. Utility of an integrated clinical, echocardiographic, and venous ultrasonographic approach for triage of patients with suspected pulmonary embolism. Am J Cardiol 1998;82:1230–5.

[14] Johnson ME, Furlong R, Schrank K. Diagnostic use of emergency department echocardiogram in massive pulmonary emboli. Ann Emerg Med 1992;21(6):760–3.

[15] Kasper W, Konstantinides S, Geibel A, et al. Prognostic significance of right ventricular afterload stress detected VY echocardiography in patients with clinically suspected pulmonary embolism. Heart 1997;77:346–9.

[16] Ribiero A, Lindmarker P, Juhlin-Dannfelt A, et al. Echocardiography Doppler in pulmonary embolism: right ventricular dysfunction as a predictor of mortality rate. Am Heart J 1997;134(3):479–87.

[17] Sabia P, Abbott RD, Afrookteh A, et al. Importance of two-dimensional echocardiographic assessment of left ventricular systolic function in patients presenting to the emergency room with cardiac-related symptoms. Circulation 1991;84(4):1615–24.

[18] Jones AET, Tayal VS, Sullivan, et al. Randomized controlled trial of immediate vs. delayed goal-directed ultrasound to identify the etiology of nontraumatic hypotension in emergency department patients. Acad Emerg Med 2004;11(5):445–6.

[19] Moore CL, Rose GA, Tayal VS, et al. Determination of left ventricular function by emergency physician echocardiography of hypotensive patients. Acad Emerg Med 2002;9(3):186–93.

[20] Peels CH, Visser CA, Kupper AJ, et al. Usefulness of two-dimensional echocardiography for immediate detection of myocardial ischemia in the emergency room. Am J Cardiol 1990; 65(11):687–91.

[21] Roudaut RP, Billes MA, Gosse P, et al. Accuracy of M-mode and two-dimensional echocardiography in the diagnosis of aortic dissection: an experience with 128 cases. Clin Cardiol 1988;11:553–62.

[22] Miller J, Grimes P. Case report of an intraperitoneal ruptured abdominal aortic aneurysms diagnosed with bedside ultrasonography. Acad Emerg Med 1999;6:662–3.

[23] Johansen K, Kohler RT, Nicholls SC, et al. Ruptured abdominal aortic aneurysms: the Harborview experience. J Vasc Surg 1991;13:240–7.

[24] Shuman WP, Hastrup W Jr, Kohler TR, et al. Suspected leaking abdominal aortic aneurysm: use of sonography in the emergency room. Radiology 1988;168:117–9.

[25] Blaivas M, Theodoro D. Frequency of incomplete abdominal aorta visualization by emergency department bedside ultrasound. Acad Emerg Med 2004;11:103–5.

[26] Dolich MO, McKenney MG, Varela JE, et al. 2,576 ultrasounds for blunt abdominal trauma. J Trauma 2001;50(1):108–12.

[27] Lingawi SS, Buckley AR. Focused abdominal US in patients with trauma. Radiology 2000; 217(2):426–9.

[28] Valentino M, Serra C, Zironi G, et al. Blunt abdominal trauma: emergency contrast-enhanced sonography for detection of solid organ injuries. AJR Am J Roentgenol 2006; 186(5):1361–7.

[29] Udobi KF, Rodriguez A, Chiu WC, et al. Role of ultrasonography in penetrating abdominal trauma: a prospective clinical study. J Trauma 2001;50(3):475–9.

[30] Rozycki GS, Feliciano DV, Ochsner MG, et al. The role of ultrasound in patients with possible penetrating cardiac wounds: a prospective multicenter study. J Trauma 1999; 46(4):543–51.

[31] Meyer DM, Jessen ME, Grayburn PA. Use of echocardiography to detect occult cardiac injury after penetrating thoracic trauma: a prospective study. J Trauma 1995;39(5):902–7.

[32] Sisley AC, Rozycki GS, Ballard RB, et al. Rapid detection of traumatic effusion using surgeon-performed ultrasonography. J Trauma 1998;44(2):291–6.

[33] Blaivas M, Lyon M, Duggal S. A prospective comparison of supine chest radiography and bedside ultrasound for the diagnosis of traumatic pneumothorax. Acad Emerg Med 2005; 12(9):844–9.

[34] Blaivas M, Theodoro D, Sierzenski P. Elevated intracranial pressure detected by bedside emergency ultrasonography of the optic nerve sheath. Acad Emerg Med 2003;10(4): 376–81.

[35] Girisgin AS, Kalkan E, Kocak S, et al. The role of optic nerve ultrasonography in the diagnosis of elevated intracranial pressure. Emerg Med J 2007;24:251–4.

[36] Ahmad S, Kampondeni S, Molyneux E. An experience of emergency ultrasonography in children in a sub-Saharan setting. Emerg Med J 2006;23:335–40.

[37] Ashkan AM, Bavarian S, Mehdizadeh M. Sonographic evaluation of optic nerve diameter in children with raised intracranial pressure. J Ultrasound Med 2005;24:143–7.

[38] Newman WD, Hollman AS, Dutton GN, et al. Measurement of optic nerve sheath diameter by ultrasound: a means of detecting acute raised intracranial pressure in hydrocephalus. Br J Ophthalmol 2002;86:1109–13.

[39] Geeraerts T, Launey Y, Martin L, et al. Ultrasonography of the optic nerve sheath may be useful for detecting raised intracranial pressure after severe brain injury. Intensive Care Med [serial online]. 2007;33(10). Available at: http://www.springerlink.com/content/p0488540814208n4/fulltext.html. Accessed October 4, 2003.

[40] Tayal VS, Neulander M, Norton HJ, et al. Emergency department sonographic measurement of optic nerve sheath diameter to detect findings of increased intracranial pressure in adult head injury patients. Ann Emerg Med 2007;49:508–14.

[41] Kimberly H, Shah S, Marill K, et al. Correlation of optic nerve sheath diameter with direct measurement of intracranial pressure. Acad Emerg Med 2008;15(2):201–4.

[42] Thorsen MK, Lawson TL, Aiman EJ, et al. Diagnosis of ectopic pregnancy: endovaginal vs transabdominal sonography. AJR Am J Roentgenol 1990;(155):307–10.

[43] American College of Emergency Physicians. Clinical policy: critical issues in the evaluation and management of patients presenting to the emergency department with acute headache. Ann Emerg Med 2002;39:108–22.

[44] Haydel MJ, Preston GA, Mills TJ, et al. Indications for computed tomography in patients with minor head injury. N Engl J Med 2000;343:100–5.

[45] Mower WR, Hoffman JR, Herbert M, et al. Developing a decision instrument to guide computed tomographic imaging of blunt head injury patients. J Trauma 2005;59:954–9.

[46] Stiell IG, Wells GA, Vandemheen K, et al. The Canadian CT head rule for patients with minor head injury. Lancet 2001;357:1391–6.

[47] Hasbun R, Abrahams J, Jekel J, et al. Computed tomography of the head before lumbar puncture in adults with suspected meningitis. N Engl J Med 2001;345:1727–33.

[48] Wardlaw JM, Chappell FM, Best JJ, et al. Non-invasive imaging compared with intra-arterial angiography in the diagnosis of symptomatic carotid stenosis: a meta-analysis. Lancet 2006;367(9521):1503–12.

[49] Koelemay MJ, Nederkoorn PJ, Reitsma JB, et al. Systematic review of computed tomographic angiography for assessment of carotid artery disease. Stroke 2004;35(10):2306–12.

[50] Katz DA, Marks MP, Napel SA, et al. Circle of Willis–evaluation with spiral CT angiography, MR-angiography, and conventional angiography. Radiology 1995;195(2):445–9.

[51] Parsons MW, Pepper EM, Chan V, et al. Perfusion computed tomography: prediction of final infarct extent and stroke outcome. Ann Neurol 2005;58(5):672–9.

[52] Rosamond W, Flegal K, Friday G, et al. Heart disease and stroke statistics—2007 update: a report from the American Heart Association Statistics Committee and Stroke Statistics Subcommittee. Circulation 2007;115:e69–171.

[53] Achenbach S. Computed tomography coronary angiography. J Am Coll Cardiol 2006;48: 1919–28.

[54] Johnson TR, Nikolaou K, Wintersperger BJ, et al. ECG-gated 64-MDCT angiography in the differential diagnosis of acute chest pain. AJR Am J Roentgenol 2007;188:76–82.

[55] Raff GL, Gallagher MJ, O'Neill WW, et al. Diagnostic accuracy of noninvasive coronary angiography using 64-slice spiral computed tomography. J Am Coll Cardiol 2005;46:552–7.

[56] Schoepf UJ. Diagnosing pulmonary embolism: time to rewrite the textbooks. Int J Cardiovasc Imaging 2005;21:155–63.

[57] Schoepf UJ, Goldhaber SZ, Costello P. Spiral computed tomography for acute pulmonary embolism. Circulation 2004;109:2160–7.

[58] Quiroz R, Kucher N, Zou KH, et al. Clinical validity of a negative computed tomography scan in patients with suspected pulmonary embolism: a systematic review. JAMA 2005; 293:2012–7.

[59] Hagan PG, Nienaber CA, Isselbacher EM, et al. The International Registry of Acute Aortic Dissection (IRAD): new insights into an old disease. JAMA 2000;283:897–903.

[60] Hirst AE Jr, Johns VJ Jr, Kime SW Jr. Dissecting aneurysm of the aorta: a review of 505 cases. Medicine (Baltimore) 1958;37:217–79.

[61] Hayter RG, Rhea JT, Small A, et al. Suspected aortic dissection and other aortic disorders: multi-detector row CT in 373 cases in the emergency setting. Radiology 2006;238:841–52.

[62] Brofman N, Atri M, Hanson JM, et al. Evaluation of mesenteric and bowel blunt trauma with multi-detector CT. Radiographics 2006;26:1119–31.

ELSEVIER
SAUNDERS

Emerg Med Clin N Am
26 (2008) 813–834

EMERGENCY
MEDICINE
CLINICS OF
NORTH AMERICA

# Antibiotics in the Intensive Care Unit: Focus on Agents for Resistant Pathogens

David F. Volles, PharmD*,
Trisha N. Branan, PharmD

*Department of Pharmacy Services, University of Virginia Health System,
P.O. Box 800674, Charlottesville, VA 22908-0674, USA*

Antimicrobial therapy for the critically ill has increasingly become more complicated and challenging because of escalation in the rates of antimicrobial resistance and increases in patients' severity of illness and overall complexity. Rates of nosocomial infection and antibiotic resistance are much higher in the intensive care unit (ICU) compared with other units in the hospital. Nosocomial infections affect up to 30% of patients in the ICU, and they are 5–10 times greater than non-ICU patients [1,2]. Numerous surveillance studies have documented both the increase in the incidence of infections in the ICU and the increase in antimicrobial resistance rates. Up to 70% of nosocomial infections are now caused by organisms resistant to one or more drugs [1,3–5]. Several factors may account for this increase including: use of more invasive procedures and techniques such as endotracheal tubes and intravenous catheters; poor hand hygiene; lapses in aseptic technique; antibiotic selective pressure due to inappropriate use; patient transfers within the hospital; and patient specific factors including severe underlying disease, extremes of age, malnutrition, and immunosuppression [2].

Microbial resistance in the acutely ill is increasing for both gram-positive organisms, including methicillin-resistant *Staphylococcus aureus* (MRSA), vancomycin-resistant *Enterococcus* species (VRE), and gram-negative organisms such as multidrug resistant *Pseudomonas aeruginosa*, *Acinetobacter* species, and extended-spectrum beta-lactamase (ESBL) producing strains of *Escherichia coli* and *Klebsiella* [2,6,7]. Medical personnel are more commonly facing organisms that are resistant to most broad spectrum agents. Inadequate initial empiric treatment of these resistant pathogens has been documented in several studies to result in worse patient outcomes including

---

* Corresponding author.
*E-mail address:* dfv3q@virginia.edu (D.F. Volles).

0733-8627/08/$ - see front matter © 2008 Elsevier Inc. All rights reserved.
doi:10.1016/j.emc.2008.04.006

increased mortality [8–11]. In one study, the most common reasons for what was deemed "inadequate coverage" included a failure to include antibiotics with activity against MRSA and agents active against gram-negative pathogens resistant to third generation cephalosporins [9] Unfortunately, the rapid rise in resistant organisms has outpaced the development of novel, effective, well-tolerated antimicrobial agents by the major pharmaceutical companies. This has forced medical providers to reconsider older, potentially more toxic therapies for these organisms such as the polymyxins [12]. It is therefore crucial that physicians attempt to use currently available antibiotics in a rational, judicious way to preserve their utility for future, critical infections. Because of the known risks of worse outcomes associated with inadequate empiric treatment and the potential for development of bacterial resistance with inappropriate overuse of antibiotics, clinicians have the difficult task of carefully balancing between providing adequate initial coverage for resistant pathogens while at the same time avoiding excessive, unnecessary antibiotic use that will lead to resistance [11]. This article discusses some of the general principles of rational antibiotic use in the acute setting; it also reviews the pharmacology and clinical utility of select antibiotics that may be used for common resistant bacterial pathogens including: vancomycin, linezolid (Zyvox), daptomycin (Cubicin), quinupristin/dalfopristin (Synercid), colistin, tigecycline (Tygacil), carbapenems, extended spectrum antipseudomonal penicillins, and fourth generation cephalosporins.

## General principles of antibiotic use in the ICU

For most serious infections in the ICU, it is appropriate to start with very broad spectrum, aggressive therapy to ensure coverage for possible resistant pathogens, with a narrowing of antibiotic coverage when culture and susceptibility data are known. An accurate diagnosis is important when deciding on appropriate antimicrobial therapy, and the noninfectious possibilities (eg, noninfectious pancreatitis, colonization, contamination) should be eliminated to avoid unnecessary treatment with antibiotics. Knowledge of the site of infection helps predict the most likely pathogens that would need to be targeted with empiric treatment. See Table 1 for antibiotic options for common infections encountered in the emergency department. Source control (ie, draining of abscess or fluid collection and surgical debridement) may be the primary treatment for certain infections with antibiotics providing supportive treatment. An understanding of antibiotic penetration into various sites of infection is also crucial when considering difficult to treat infections such as meningitis, osteomyelitis, and endocarditis.

On a national level, bacterial antimicrobial resistance continues to increase as MRSA rates are approximately 60% and *Pseudomonas aeruginosa* resistant to imipenem, third generation cephalosporins, and fluoroquinolones are 21%, 32%, and 30% respectively [4,13]. There are wide regional variations in the incidence of each resistant pathogen and these epidemiologic factors must be considered when making decisions about empiric antibiotics. Clinicians should rely on updated institution specific information highlighting local antibiotic susceptibility and resistance patterns. Local outbreaks of resistant organisms alter the specific pathogens that may require coverage with empiric therapy. Specifically, ESBL producing strains of *Escherichia coli* and *Klebsiella* species, multidrug-resistant *Pseudomonas aeruginosa* and *Acinetobacter baumannii*, and the resistant gram positive organisms, MRSA and VRE, are the organisms causing great concern and may require empiric coverage depending on hospital specific or ICU specific antibiograms. Despite the need for broad spectrum coverage initially for empiric coverage, it is appropriate to de-escalate the antibiotic regimen based on culture and susceptibility reports, or even reasonable to discontinue antibiotics if an infectious process is no longer suspected [14]. Timing issues are also important when treating infections in the critically ill. Decreasing the time it takes for patients to receive appropriate antibiotic therapy is important; consensus guidelines for the treatment of septic shock and pneumonia highlight this parameter [15–17]. Timely and appropriate antibiotic administration, within the first hour of hypotension, in septic shock patients improved survival by an estimated 79.9%. Every hour delay of antibiotic delivery after hypotension recognition during the first 6 hours resulted in a 7.9% increased mortality [17]. Durations of antibiotic therapy should also be defined in an effort to limit antibiotic regimens to the shortest possible course to avoid unnecessary use (ie, 8 days for hospital acquired pneumonia), but for many infections, unfortunately, this is not adequately defined [18].

Use of combination therapy, involving two agents from different classes (ie, usually a beta lactam agent plus an aminoglycoside or fluoroquinolone) to provide synergy or additive effects is often done for empiric treatment for serious infections and for select pathogens such as *Pseudomonas aeruginosa*, but combination therapy is a controversial topic. Most studies evaluating the benefit of combination therapy have not found any mortality or other benefits over monotherapy for gram-negative infections [19]. One meta-analysis did identify a mortality benefit in a subgroup of patients with *Pseudomonas*, but not in patients with other gram-negative organisms [20]. Combination therapy may be appropriate for empiric treatment of severe infections such as sepsis and ventilator-associated pneumonia if drug resistant strains are suspected [15,16,20]. Despite not being associated with a mortality benefit, double coverage may be employed initially to increase the chance of at least having one drug on board with activity against the offending pathogen [16]. In many circumstances, it may be appropriate to initiate combination therapy, but to discontinue one of the agents after a 5–7 day course or even less time if drug-resistant pathogens are not identified.

Pharmacokinetic and pharmacodynamic principles must be taken into account when designing antimicrobial regimens as it has become increasingly clear that suboptimal antibiotic concentrations at the site of infection

Table 1
Antibiotic option for common infection encountered in the emergency department

| Site | Common organisms | Antibiotic options |
|---|---|---|
| **Head** | | |
| Bacterial meningitis | S. pneumoniae<br>N. meningitides<br>H. influenza | Ceftraxone 2g q12h **or** Cefotaxime 2g q4h **or** Meropenem 2g q8h<br>Any of the above **plus** Vancomycin 1g q12hr (15mg/kg q 12hr)<br>If Listeria monocytogenes is suspected, add Ampicillin 2g q4h<br>If viral encephalities is suspected, add Acyclovir 10–15mg/kg q8h |
| After neurosurgery<br>or after head trauma<br>meningitis | S. aureus<br>P. aeruginosa<br>Enterobacteraceae<br>S. pneumoniae | Cefepime 2g q8h **or** Ceftazidime 2g q8h **or** Meropenem 2g q8h<br>Any of the above **plus** Vancomycin 1g q12h (15mg/kg q12h) |
| **Lung** | | |
| CAP without HCAP<br>risk factors | S. pneumoniae<br>H. influenzae<br>Atypical pathogens (Mycoplasma<br>pneumoniae or Chlamydia) | Ceftriaxone 1g q24h **or** Cefotaxime 2g q8h **or** Ampicillin/<br>Sulbactam 3g q6h<br>Any of the above **plus** Azithromycin 500mg q24h **or** Levofloxacin<br>750mg q24h **or** Moxifloxacin 400mg q24h pneumoniae<br>(Quinolone monotheraphy) |
| Pneumonia with HCAP<br>risk factors | Usual CAP pathogens<br>plus MRSA, drug-resistant<br>gram-negative organisms<br>including P. aeruginosa | Cefepime 2g q12h **or** Piperacillin/Tazobactam 4.5g q6h **or** Ceftazidime<br>2g q8h **or** Meropenem 1g q8h **or** Imipenem 500mg q6h<br>Any of the above **Plus** Vancomycin 1g q12h (15mg/kg q12h)<br>**or** Linezolid 600mg q12h |
| **Abdomen** | | |
| Primary peritonitis | Enterobacteriaceae gram negatives<br>(ie, E. coli, Klebsiella species)<br>S. pneumoniae, Enterococcus<br>faecalis | Ceftriaxone 1g q24h **or** Cefotaxime 2g q8h **or** Ampicillin/<br>Sulbactam 3g q6h **or** Ertapenem 1g q24h<br>If resistant gram negatives suspected, consider Meropenem 1g q8h<br>**or** Imipenem 500mg q6h **or** Ciprofloxacin 400mg q12h<br>**or** Moxifloxacin 400mg q24h **or** Levofloxacin 750mg q24h |

| | |
|---|---|
| Secondary peritonitis (ie, bowl perforation) Complicated intra-abdominal infection | Enterobacteriaceae gram negatives, anaerobic bacteria including *Bacteroides fragilis, Enterococcus* species | Piperacillin/Tazobactam 3.375g q6h **or** Ticarcillin/clavulanic acid 3.1g q6h **or** Ertapenem 1g q24h **or** Tigecycline 50mg q12h (after a 100mg loading dose) **or** Meropenem 1g q8h **or** Imipenem 500mg q6h **or** Moxifloxacin 400mg q24h **or** Cefepime 2g q12h **plus** Metronidazole 500mg q8h **or** Ciprofloxacin 400mg q12hr **plus** Metronidazole 500mg q8h **or** Levofloxacin 750mg **plus** Metronidazole 500mg q8h |

**Genital tract**

| Urinary tract | *E. coli* and other gram negatives *Staphylococcus saprophyticus Enterococcus* species | Trimethoprim/Sulfamethoxazole DS q12h **or** Ciprofloxacin 250mg PO q12h **or** Levofloxacin 250mg PO q24h **or** Cephalexin 500mg q6hr If C. trachomatic is suspected, add Doxycycline 100mg PO q12h **or** Azithromycin 1g PO single dose |

| Severely ill urosepsis | Enterobacteriaceae *P. aeruginosa Enterococcus* species *Staphylococcus* species | Piperacillin/Tazobactam 3.375g q6h **or** Meropenem 1g q8h **or** Imipenem 500mg q6h **or** Ciprofloxacin 400mg q12h **or** Levofloxacin 500mg q24h **or** Ertapenem 1g q24h **or** Ampicillin/ Sulbactam 3g q6h **or** Ceftriaxone 1g q24h **or** Ampicillin 2g q4h **plus** Gentamicin 2mg/kg q12h |

**Blood**

| Severe sepsis Septic shock | *E. coli S. aureus P. aeruginosa S. pneumoniae* Other resistant gram negatives | In general, treatment based on presumed source (lung, abdomen, genital tract, etc.) For unknown source, consider broad spectrum initially: Piperacillin/ Tazobactam 4.5g q6h **or** Meropenem 1g q8h **or** Cefepime 2g q12h **or** Imipenem 500mg q6h **or** Ceftriaxone 2g q24h **or** Ciprofloxacin 400mg q12h **or** Levofloxacin 750mg q24h Any of the above **plus** Vancomycin 1g q12h (15mg/kg q12h) **or** Linezolid 600mg q12h If suspect Bacteremia with **or** without Endocarditis from a resistant gram-positive, add Daptomycin 6mg/kg q24h in place of vancomycin **or** linezolid |

(continued on next page)

Table 1
(continued)

| Site | Common organisms | Antibiotic options |
|---|---|---|
| **Skin and extremities**<br>Skin and soft tissue | S. aureus<br>Stretococcus species<br>Gram-negatives<br>Anaerobic species | Clindamycin 600mg q6h **or** Ceftriaxone 1g q24h **plus** Metronidazole 500mg q8h **or** Ertapenem 1g q24h **or** Ampicillin/Sulbactam 3g q6h **or** Moxifloxacin 400mg q24h **or** Ciprofloxacin 400mg q12h **plus** Metronidazole 500mg q8h **or** Tigecycline monotherapy 50mg q12h (after 100mg loading dose)<br>Any of the above (except Tigecycline) **plus** Vancomycin 1g q12h (15mg/kg q12h) **or** Linezolid 600mg q12h |
| Necrotizing fasciitis | Group A Streptococcus<br>Clostridium perfringens<br>S. aureus | Piperacillin/Tazobactam 4.5g q6h **plus** Clindamycin 900mg q8h **or** Imipenem 500mg q6h **plus** Clindamycin 900mg q8h **or** Meropenem 1g q8h **plus** Clindamycin 900mg q8h<br>Any of the above **plus** Vancomycin 1g q12h (15mg/kg q12h) **or** Linezolid 600mg q12h **or** Daptomycin 4–6mg/kg q24h |

*Abbreviations:* CAP, community acquired pneumonia; HCAP, health care associated pneumonia.
*Data from Refs.* [11,16,62–65].

may contribute to increased microbial resistance and treatment failures [21–23]. In general, antibiotics can be divided into drugs that possess concentration-dependent killing of pathogens, which refers to faster eradication of bacteria pathogens with higher concentrations (ie, high peak), and concentration-independent killing, referring to maximal efficacy associated with maintaining concentrations above the pathogens minimum inhibitory concentration (MIC). For drugs with concentration-dependent killing, such as aminoglycosides, colistin, and fluoroquinolones, maximal efficacy is associated with giving larger doses less frequently, but for many drugs the dose given is limited by toxicity and clinical experience. The efficacy for drugs that possess concentration-independent killing, such as penicillins, carbapenems, and cephalosporins, can be maximized by more frequent administration in an effort to keep the concentration above the MIC for at least 40%–70% of the dosing interval [21–23]. Due to rising MICs for common pathogens, many standard doses used for nonacute patients may be inadequate for these more resistant bacterial species encountered in the critically ill [24]. It is often prudent to use the most aggressive tolerated dose until cultures and susceptibilities are known. Even in patients with renal insufficiency or failure, aggressive initial doses can be used for the first 24 hours and then adjusted accordingly based on organ function and patient's clinical response.

## Agents for gram-positive pathogens

### Vancomycin

Vancomycin is a bactericidal glycopeptide drug that inhibits bacterial wall synthesis by blocking glycopeptide polymerization through binding tightly to the D-alanyl-D-alanine portion of the cell wall precursor. Its spectrum of activity includes most aerobic and anaerobic gram-positive infections, including more resistant strains such as MRSA, resistant *Streptococcus* pneumoniae, the *Enterococcus* species, and *Clostridium difficile* [25].

With the increased use of vancomycin in recent years, several resistance mechanisms have emerged. Some bacterial strains have inducible resistance to high levels of vancomycin, while other strains have an acquired resistance. These resistant strains are the result of multiple gene transformations. In vancomycin-susceptible strains, vancomycin is able to bind to D-alanyl-D-alanine and inhibit bacterial synthesis. In vancomycin-resistant strains, the peptidoglycan intermediates are altered to D-alanyl-D-lactate or D-alanyl-D-serine; both have decreased affinity for vancomycin, resulting in higher MICs for these organisms. More recently, "vancomycin-intermediate *S. aureus*" (VISA) strains have been isolated with MICs ranging from 4–8 µg/mL. Excessive amounts of noncross-linked D-alanyl-D-alanine are produced that trap vancomycin molecules and prevent them from reaching their intended site of action. Although rarely isolated, infections due to

VISA are associated with treatment failure. Perhaps more important than VISA, there has been a recent increase in the number of heteroresistant strains of MRSA. These organisms have an MIC within an acceptable range, usually ≤ 4 µg/mL, but these patients exhibit a reduced susceptibility to vancomycin. These strains may potentially be precursors to VISA. There is also concern for the potential of resistance transmission across bacterial strains, for example from a resistant *Enterococcus* strain passed to a *Staphylococcus* organism. Enterococci contain plasmids and transposons that allow the transfer of genetic material from one bacterial strain to another. This has been observed in several case reports of patients with vancomycin-resistant *Staphylococcus aureus* who were colonized with VRE [25,26].

The recommended dose from the package insert for vancomycin is 2 g per day. The IDSA/ATS guidelines recommend 30 mg/kg/day in two divided doses for patients with normal renal function based on pharmacokinetic and pharmacodynamic properties of the drug [27]. Vancomycin undergoes a complex 2- or 3-compartment pharmacokinetic profile and is eliminated primarily through the kidneys. Vancomycin penetrates most body tissue, including CSF and lung tissue, although the penetration into these tissues is variable and may be dependent on the degree of inflammation present. It exhibits moderate protein binding, approximately 10–50%. Because elimination of vancomycin occurs primarily through the kidneys, in the presence of renal dysfunction the dose should be adjusted and trough levels of drug obtained. Standardized trough levels have not been established, but the general consensus recommends trough levels of 10–15 g/mL for most infections and higher goal trough levels of 15–20 g/mL for other infections, such as pneumonia, endocarditis, osteomyelitis, and CNS infections [25–28].

Acutely ill patients often exhibit different pharmacokinetic and pharmacodynamic properties than infected, stable patients. These factors should be considered carefully when dosing and monitoring vancomycin. Critically ill patients may have an altered volume of distribution, for example edematous patients will have an increased volume of distribution, and therefore may require an increased amount of drug. Although vancomycin is moderately protein-bound, protein levels will be decreased in critical illness that may increase the amount of free drug. Renal function is also typically altered in acutely ill patients who may require intermittent dialysis or continuous renal replacement therapy, both of which require dose modifications of vancomycin [25–28].

Although early toxicity of vancomycin could be attributed to impurities from the manufacturing process, several serious toxicities associated with therapy still exist. There is little evidence linking specific serum concentrations of vancomycin with efficacy or toxicity. There have been rare associations with vancomycin treatment linked to ototoxicity and nephrotoxicity. Reported incidences of vancomycin-associated nephrotoxicity range 1%–5%. The overall incidence of nephrotoxicity appears to be low and most clinicians do not believe this drug to be nephrotoxic. One reaction unique to vancomycin has been associated with rapid infusion rates. The "red man" or "red neck" syndrome is characterized by erythema, pruritis, hypotension, and angioedema and occurs as part of a histamine-like response to rapid infusion. This syndrome can be alleviated by slowing the infusion rate of the drug and also by the administration of antihistamines, such as diphenhydramine or hydroxyzine [25,26,28].

Vancomycin continues to be the drug of choice for the treatment of serious infections due to resistant gram-positive infections, such as MRSA and coagulase-negative staphylococci. It may also be used in patients with serious infections that are susceptible to penicillin in patients who are intolerant of penicillins or cephalosporins. Vancomycin is also used to treat infections due to some strains of *Enterococcus*, resistant *Streptococcus*, and orally for the treatment of *Clostridium difficile*. In the critically ill patient who has unspeciated gram positive cocci from a gram stain or is suspected of having a drug resistant gram-positive organism, vancomycin is typically used in combination with an anti–gram-negative drug as empiric treatment and may be continued until drug resistant species have been ruled out.

### Linezolid

Linezolid is a bacteriostatic, synthetic oxazolidinone that inhibits the initiation of protein synthesis at the 50S ribosome [27,29,30]. Its spectrum of activity includes aerobic gram-positive organisms, including MRSA, *S. epidermidis*, *Enterococcus* species, and streptococci. It also shows activity against aerobic and anaerobic gram-positive cocci, some gram-negative aerobes, *Nocardia* species, and *Mycobacteria* species [30]. Currently, linezolid is FDA-approved for the treatment of complicated skin and skin-structure infections, nosocomial pneumonia, and infections due to vancomycin-resistant *Enterococcus faecium* [29,30].

It was originally thought that linezolid would not experience the development of drug resistance mechanisms for several reasons. Linezolid is completely synthetic and there should be a low probability of pre-existing or naturally occurring resistance mechanisms. Also, previous studies have demonstrated that oxazolindinones inhibit bacterial ribosomal synthesis and are not susceptible to cross-resistance from existing resistance mechanisms to other ribosomal agents. Lastly, in vitro studies have shown that selection for linezolid-resistant mutants of various species is difficult. Despite this reasoning, there have been case reports of linezolid resistance, most commonly with the *Enteroccocus* species, but a few reports involving *Staphylococcus* species. The mechanism for resistance from these case reports all describe mutations in the 23S rRNA genes, which theoretically decrease the likelihood of transferable resistance. The increased use of this agent to treat a growing number of multiresistant gram-positive infections allows transfer of linezolid-resistant infections to occur. Linezolid resistance is likely to continue to increase in the future even without the presence of selective pressure [30].

The recommended dose for adults is 600 mg given twice daily and can be given intravenously or orally [31,32]. Oral administration results in rapid and complete bioavailability of the drug. Linezolid penetrates well into most body tissues and is useful in bacteremia, pneumonia, and skin and soft tissue infections. Animal models have shown good penetration into the meninges. Metabolism primarily occurs through oxidation of the morpholine ring to form two inactive carboxylic metabolites. Current data do not demonstrate involvement of the CYP450 enzyme system in metabolism. Because metabolism does not occur via the renal or hepatic system, dose adjustments in patients with renal or hepatic impairment are not necessary. One exception to this is in patients undergoing intermittent hemodialysis, resulting in an increased clearance of linezolid. In these patients, the dose should be given post-dialysis or a supplemental dose of 200 mg should be given at the end of dialysis [31].

Linezolid is generally well tolerated with mild adverse events, including nausea, headache, diarrhea, rash, and altered taste. Nervous system effects, such as peripheral neuropathy, have also been noted. Linezolid is a weak, reversible, nonselective inhibitor of monoamine oxidase and may interact with other serotenergic agents, such as selective serotonin reuptake inhibitors, to precipitate serotonin syndrome. Myelosuppression, particularly thrombocytopenia, has been associated with linezolid treatment. Platelet counts should be monitored in patients who are at increased risk for a bleeding event, or who have thrombocytopenia before initiation of linezolid. Several case studies have suggested that the incidence of thrombocytopenia may occur earlier in therapy, or in a larger proportion of patients than was originally reported [31,32].

Linezolid is an alternative agent to standard therapy with vancomycin for multidrug-resistant gram-positive infections. In contrast to vancomycin, linezolid offers an oral option for the treatment of these infections. In the ICU setting, linezolid may be used as an alternative agent to vancomycin as empiric therapy to cover multidrug-resistant gram-positive infections and may be continued based upon susceptibility results detailing resistance to vancomycin [31,32].

## Daptomycin

Daptomycin is a bactericidal cyclic lipopeptide that has a unique mechanism of action. It is hypothesized that the drug undergoes calcium-dependent oligomerisation and binding to the bacterial cell membrane, without penetration into the cytoplasm. This action results in an alteration of the bacterial cell membrane impairing potassium-dependent macromolecular synthesis, which leads to cell death. Its spectrum of activity includes most aerobic gram-positive infections, including MRSA and VRE. Currently, daptomycin is approved for use in complicated skin and skin-structure infections and *S. aureus* bacteremia with or without right-sided infective endocarditis [33–35].

Daptomycin resistance, although rare, has been reported in the literature. The resistance mechanism is not fully understood, but there are several theories. One theory suggests that the absence of specific cytoplasmic membrane proteins may contribute resistance to daptomycin. The mutant selection window is another theory that may explain daptomycin resistance; the theory suggests suboptimal antibacterial dosing is associated with the emergence of bacterial resistance. It is hypothesized that continued exposure of daptomycin at a low area under the curve (AUC) to MIC ratio allows for the emergence of resistant mutant organisms [35].

The recommended dose of daptomycin in skin or skin-structure infections is 4 mg/kg every 24 hours for patients with normal renal function. For *S. aureus* bacteremia with or without infective endocarditis, the recommended dose is 6 mg/kg every 24 hours in patients with normal renal function. Daptomycin disperses mainly into plasma and interstitial fluid and is preferentially distributed into highly vascularized organs. The drug does not appear to cross cell membranes, for example, daptomycin does not readily cross the blood-brain barrier in healthy individuals. In an animal model, daptomycin was able to cross inflamed meninges at a concentration that was sufficient to clear the infection [33]. In contrast to the other antibiotics discussed, daptomycin should not be used to treat pneumonia as the drug may be inactivated by pulmonary surfactants. Like vancomycin, daptomycin exhibits moderate protein binding, approximately 80% [34]. Daptomycin is not metabolized by the CYP450 enzyme system and does not inhibit or induce any of the isoenzymes. For this reason, there are no clinically significant drug interactions with daptomycin. It is eliminated primarily via the renal system. Dose reductions are recommended in patients with creatinine clearance < 30 mL/min, including patients receiving hemodialysis or continuous renal replacement therapy [33]. In these patients, the recommended dose should be administered every 48 hours rather than every 24 hours [33–35].

Comparable to linezolid, daptomycin is also generally well tolerated. The most common reported adverse events were gastrointestinal upset, such as constipation, diarrhea, nausea, and vomiting, and CNS symptoms, such as headache and insomnia. Other important adverse events reported were peripheral neuropathy and muscle myalgia. Muscle weakness was observed more frequently in studies using higher doses of daptomycin given twice daily. Newer dosing strategies using once daily dosing appear to have decreased the incidence of myopathy. It is recommended to check a baseline creatinine phosphokinase (CPK) level and then at least once weekly thereafter during therapy with daptomycin. More frequent monitoring of CPK levels may be necessary in patients with baseline renal insufficiency or when drugs also known to elevate CPK levels, such as statins, are being administered. Patients on daptomycin should be monitored for signs of muscle weakness or peripheral neuropathy especially in the distal extremities [33,34].

Typically, daptomycin is used as directed therapy after cultures and susceptibilities have been obtained. Because of its limited indications and its inability to treat infections in the lungs, daptomycin should not be used as empiric therapy. Daptomycin should be reserved for: gram-positive skin and skin-structure infections; bloodstream infections with or without infective endocarditis that are resistant to vancomycin; or for patients who are intolerant of vancomycin and linezolid [33–35]. There are also case reports of successful treatment of osteomyelitis with daptomycin [36].

## Quinupristin/dalfopristin

Quinupristin/dalfopristin is a streptogrammin antibacterial agent composed of a 30: 70 (w/w) ratio of two semisynthetic pristinamycin derivatives. Although each component exhibits bacteriostatic activity, the synergistic combination often is bactericidal [32,37]. Its spectrum of activity covers most aerobic gram-positive organisms, including *S.aureus*, MRSA, *E. faecium*, vancomycin-resistant *E. faecium*, *S. pneumoniae*, and other streptococci. However, quinupristin/dalfopristin does not cover infections due to *E. faecalis*, and it will be discussed in more detail later. Quinupristin/dalfopristin is FDA-approved for treatment of adult patients with serious infections due to vancomycin-resistant *Enterococcus faecium* associated with bacteremia and for complicated skin and skin-structure infections due to group A streptococci or methicillin-susceptible *S. aureus* [32,37,38].

There are several mechanisms by which resistance to quinupristin/dalfopristin occurs. The most commonly recognized resistance mechanism is $MLS_B$ resistance conferred through *erm* genes, which encode an enzyme that dimethylates an adenine residue in the 23S rRNA. This action results in decreased binding of macrolides, lincosamides, and streptogrammins B. Because quinupristin/dalfopristin is a combination of a streptogrammin A (dalfopristin) and streptogrammin B (quinupristin), it would be expected that quinupristin/dalfopristin would retain activity against $MLS_B$ positive organisms. Enterococcus faecalis is resistant to quinupristin/dalfopristin through a mechanism that has not been completely identified, but which is thought to occur due to active efflux of antibiotic. Other mechanisms of resistance include enzymatic modification of the antibiotic and alteration of the target site [32,37,38].

The recommended dose of quinupristin/dalfopristin is 7.5 mg/kg administered every 8 or 12 hours. In animal models, the drug has been shown to distribute into tissues and fluids associated with metabolism and elimination, including liver, kidneys, and gastrointestinal tract. Other animal models have shown good drug penetration into cardiac vegetations present in endocarditis. Dalfopristin has one active metabolite while quinupristin has two active metabolites, although in vivo activity of these metabolites has not been determined. Protein binding ranges from moderate for quinupristin (55%–78%) and mild for dalfopristin (11%–26%). Pharmacokinetic properties do not appear to be altered by age, gender, obesity, renal insufficiency (including dialysis), and severe hepatic dysfunction. Dose adjustments in these patient populations are not necessary. Of note, studies have shown that quinupristin/dalfopristin inhibits biotransformation of CYP450 isoenzyme 3A4 substrates, including nifedipine, midazolam, terfenadine, and cyclosporine. Quinupristin/dalfopristin increased the AUC of these drugs when coadministered [37,38].

The most common adverse events associated with quinupristin/dalfopristin are related to IV administration of the drug. Venous-related events are common especially if the drug is administered via a peripheral line. Reported events include pain and/or inflammation, atrophy, edema, burning, and thrombophlebitis. Adverse events can be limited through drug administration in a larger volume of fluid or administration through a central line. Hydrocortisone or diphenhydramine does not improve venous tolerability. Other adverse events include myalgias and arthralgias, gastrointestinal upset, and rash. Laboratory abnormalities have also been associated with quinupristin/dalfopristin, including increases in hepatic transaminases, hyperbilirubinemia, decreases in platelets, hemoglobin, hematocrit, and red blood cell count [37,38].

Typically, quinupristin/dalfopristin is used as a last-line therapy for serious gram-positive infections in which other treatment options have failed. The use of this drug should be weighed against its tolerability and drug interaction profile. In patients who have failed or are unresponsive to other therapies, quinupristin/dalfopristin may be considered an alternate treatment [37].

## Agents for gram-negative pathogens

### Colistin

Colistin is an old drug which was first introduced in 1952 and was used routinely until the 1970s when its use was replaced by less toxic cephalosporins and extended spectrum penicillins [39]. The emergence of multiresistant strains of *Pseudomonas* and *Acinetobacter* has generated a renewed interest in this compound as colistin has retained very good activity against these pathogens [40,41]. Colistin (polymyxin E) is administered systemically as the colistimethate sodium salt. Colistin is a polycationic peptide compound that acts as a detergent by disrupting the lipopolysaccharide membrane, resulting in bacterial cell leakage through the damaged bacterial cell membrane [42]. Colistin possesses concentration-dependent, bactericidal activity against a broad variety of gram-negative organisms, including multidrug resistant strains, however it appears to be less active against *Serratia* species, *Providencia* species, and *Proteus mirabilis* [43]. Resistance to colistin has been described in case reports and resistance is thought to be related to changes in the bacterial outer cell membrane or other adaptive changes. Colistin dosing is confusing because of recommendations being made in both international units (IU) and in milligrams (mg) as well as because of differences in dosing regimens between the United States and Europe. However, for the colistimethate salt, 2.5–5 mg/kg/day (divided in 2 to 4 doses) is recommended by the manufacturer. A dosing regimen of 2.5 mg/kg every twelve hours is the most commonly used dose for treatment of gram-negative pathogens. To take advantage of the concentration-dependent killing properties of the drug, larger doses given less frequently appear optimal. Following IV administration, colistin distributes well to most tissues in the body, except the blood–brain barrier where there is little penetration. Elimination of the drug occurs through the renal route and doses must be adjusted for kidney dysfunction. The primary toxicities associated with colistin are nephrotoxicity and neurotoxicity; both are thought to be dose related and reversible upon discontinuation. Despite early reports describing very high rates of toxicity, more recent data has suggested the rate of nephrotoxicity is not as high as initially thought. Many studies examining toxicity involved higher doses than are currently used and other causes for renal failure were not controlled for. The exact incidence for toxicity is difficult to assess, but appears to be 10%–25%. Toxicity is affected by the presence of pre-existing renal dysfunction and correlates well with total colistin dose. In earlier clinical trials the incidence of neurotoxicity was approximately 10%, but more recent studies have found the incidence to be lower than this [7]. The neurotoxicity usually occurs in patients with decreased renal function and may include a broad variety of symptoms such as dizziness, weakness, facial and distal paresthesia, confusion, visual disturbances, and, very rarely, a severe neuromuscular blockade that may lead to respiratory depression [44]. Due to the potential toxicity of this agent, the drug is generally reserved for multidrug-resistant strains of *Pseudomonas*, *Klebsiella*, and *Acinetobacter* when few other options are available. The drug has been given in combination with other gram-negative agents and also as monotherapy. The drug has not been studied in a randomized, controlled, clinical trial for these drug resistant pathogens, but observational studies demonstrate clinical utility and good clinical outcomes for these difficult to treat bacteria [42,44].

*Tigecycline*

Tigecycline is a glycylcycline compound that is a derivative of minocycline (a tetracycline antibiotic) and is unique in its broad coverage of both resistant gram-negative and gram-positive organisms. It has activity against gram-positive organisms such as MRSA and VRE as well as gram-negative bacteria, such as ESBL-producing *Klebsiella* species, and *Acinetobacter* species [45]. Additionally, it has good activity against anaerobic species including *Bacteriodes fragilis*. Despite its broad spectrum gram-negative activity, it is generally not active against *Pseudomonas*, *Morganella*, and *Providencia* species; that limits its usefulness as an empiric agent in the critically ill due to concerns with *Pseudomonas*. Tigecycline is bacteriostatic and inhibits bacterial protein synthesis by binding to the 30s ribosomal subunit [46,47]. It avoids the usual mechanisms of tetracycline resistance that generally include tetracycline efflux pumps and ribosomal protection by the bacteria. The mechanism of resistance to tigecycline is not completely understood, but is thought to be related to broad spectrum efflux pumps. It is approved as monotherapy for treatment of skin and skin structure infections and complicated intra-abdominal infections due to its broad coverage of gram-negative, gram-positive, and anaerobic pathogens. Dosing for tigecycline is 50 mg every 12 hours after a 100 mg initial loading dose. The drug distributes extensively to most tissues after administration and, as a result, it has a low peak plasma concentration. The low maximum plasma concentration following an IV dose is lower than the MICs for certain bacterial pathogens, which is concerning when treating patients who have bacteremia and sepsis [34]. Tigecycline is eliminated as both unchanged drug and inactive metabolites mainly in the bile and feces, and approximately 32% of the drug is excreted unchanged in the urine [34]. The pharmacokinetics of the drug is not significantly altered for patients with renal dysfunction and no dosing changes are required in this population. The dose should be reduced in patients with severe hepatic impairment (ie, Child Pugh C) to 25 mg every 12 hours following a 100 mg loading dose. The drug is generally well tolerated with nausea and vomiting the most common side effects reported in the pivotal clinical trials. Due to the similarities with the tetracycline class of antibiotics, precautions and warnings related to tetracycline use should be considered: photosensitivity, dental staining in children, pseudotumour cerebri, azotemia, and acute pancreatitis. The drug has clinical utility for patients with penicillin allergies or renal dysfunction for the treatment of the approved infections (ie, intra-abdominal infections and skin and skin structure infections) where other drugs may be problematic. In addition, due to its activity against multiple resistant pathogens including MRSA, VRE, *Acinetobacter* species, and ESBL producing strains of *Klebsiella*, tigecycline is a useful agent for infections caused by these pathogens. Case reports however, have described mixed results when treating drug resistant *Acinetobacter* species as treatment failures have been reported [7]. This may be due to the low plasma levels of the drug when treating blood stream infections. It is important to be aware of the low plasma concentrations and consider alternative agents or combination therapy when using tigecycline for bacteremia or septic shock [7,34].

## Carbapenems: meropenem, imipenem, ertapenem, doripenem

The carbapenem drugs are beta lactam agents that have the broadest spectrum antimicrobial activity of all the drug classes. Carbapenems, in general, have bactericidal activity against a broad range of gram-negative organisms, gram-positive organisms, and anaerobes including some of the more resistant pathogens such as *Pseudomonas*, *Acinetobacter* and ESBL producing strains of *Klebsiella* [48–51]. *Stenotrophomonas maltophilia*,

MRSA, and *Enterococcus faecium* are species that demonstrate general resistance to the carbapenems. There are differences also between individual agents as meropenem has slightly better activity against gram-negative organisms while imipenem has better activity for gram-positive pathogens. Additionally, ertapenem lacks coverage for *Pseudomonas* and *Enterococcus* species and therefore is not useful for empiric ICU nosocomial infections when multidrug-resistant pathogens are suspected. Doripenem is the newest agent and is more active against *Pseudomonas* species compared with the other drugs, but the clinical utility of doripenem for *Pseudomonas* resistant to other carbapenems remains to be determined [7]. The mechanism of action for carbapenems is similar to other beta lactam agents: it binds to penicillin binding proteins and prevents cell wall cross link, destabilizing the cell wall. Imipenem must be administered with cilastatin, which inhibits the rapid breakdown of the drug by dehydropeptidase, an enzyme in the proximal renal tubule cells. The other agents, meropenem, ertapenem, and doripenem are not affected by this enzyme and can be administered alone, without cilastatin. In general, these drugs are very resistant to the effects of most beta lactamases (ie, AmpC beta-lactamases, ESBLs), but when antimicrobial resistance occurs, it is due to very broad spectrum carbapenemases and also due to changes in porin channels in the bacterial cell wall [49]. Outbreaks of *Klebsiella* species resistant to carbapenems (KPC) have been reported and these are due to very broad spectrum carbapenemases making these bacteria resistant to most drugs [52]. The carbapenems have very good penetration into most body sites and meropenem specifically has adequate penetration into cerebrospinal fluid and is useful for patients with meningitis. The carbapenems are primarily eliminated renally and doses must be adjusted for renal impairment. Doses for imipenem are generally 500 mg every 6 hours or 1 g every 8hr, for meropenem 1 g every 8 hours is used (2 g every 8 hours for meningitis), for ertapenem 1 g every 24 hours is approved and for doripenem 500 mg every 8 hours is indicated. The most common adverse effects with theses drugs includes irritation at the injection site, diarrhea, rash, nausea, vomiting, and pruitis that are all usually mild and self-limiting [49]. Of note, these agents also have the potential to lower the seizure threshold and cause seizures that appears more commonly with imipenem than with other agents [49]. These agents are useful for a variety of polymicrobial infections where resistant pathogens are expected including sepsis, nosocomial pneumonia, intra-abdominal infections, febrile neutropenia, and skin and soft tissue infections. Unfortunately, because of their broad spectrum and overall good safety profile, these agents have been overused resulting in higher rates of resistance to common gram-negative bacteria such as *Pseudomonas*. These agents should be reserved for infections with known or suspected multiresistant organisms such as ESBL producing gram-negative pathogens (ie, *Klebsiella species* or *E. coli*) or AmpC producing beta-lactamase organisms resistant to other agents (ie, *Pseudomonas* and *Enterobacter* species) De-escalation to a less broad spectrum agent should occur whenever possible if carbapenems are empirically used in an effort to prevent bacterial resistance.

## Extended spectrum anti-pseudomonal penicillins (piperacillin-tazobactam)

Manipulations of the basic side chain of penicillin (6-aminopenicillanic acid) have lead to the creation of broader spectrum antibacterial agents. Piperacillin is a ureido, semisynthetic penicillin derivative with broad spectrum bactericidal activity against many common gram-negative and gram-positive organisms including penicillin susceptible *Streptococcal* species, penicillin susceptible *Enterococcus*, methicillin-susceptible *Staphylococcus*, *Pseudomonas*, *Enterobacter*, and *Serratia* species [53,54] The drug does not have activity against MRSA or penicillin-resistant strains of *Enterococcus,* and it tends to be resistant to *Acinetobacter* (ie, only about 59% of strains are susceptible) and ESBL strains of *Klebsiella* species [7]. The mechanism of action is similar to other beta lactam antibiotics. The drug binds to penicillin binding proteins and then inhibits the synthesis of the bacterial cell wall by preventing peptidoglycan cross linking. Resistance mechanisms are similar to other beta lactams antibiotics and may primarily include alterations in penicillin binding proteins and inactivation by certain beta lactamases. The drug has a short half-life (1 hour) and must be given frequently to maintain adequate concentrations above the MIC [54]. It is primarily eliminated unchanged in the urine and undergoes minimal liver metabolism. Piperacillin does have substantial penetration into the billiary system and additionally, it achieves therapeutic levels in the cerebral spinal fluid and bone tissue [54]. Addition of the beta lactamase inhibitor, tazobactam, to piperacillin (piperacillin and tazobactam, Zosyn) expands the spectrum of the base compound to include anaerobes such as *Bacteroides fragilis* and provides better activity against methicillin-susceptible *Staphylococcus aureus*. Due to its broad spectrum against common gram-negative, gram-positive, and anaerobe pathogens, piperacillin is commonly employed as empiric broad spectrum therapy for mixed infections including pneumonia, sepsis, bacteremia, skin and soft tissue infections, and intra-abdominal infections. Usual doses are 3.375 g to 4.5 g every 6 hours with the higher dose used for more serious infections and for *Pseudomonas*, but some clinicians are using longer infusions to achieve higher continuous concentrations (ie, 3.375–4.5 g administered over 4 hours every 8 hours) [55]. Pipeacillin-tazobactam is well tolerated with adverse effects similar to other penicillin antibiotics including gastrointestinal complaints, allergic reactions such as rashes and pruitis, and more rarely thrombocytopenia, increased liver function tests, and azotemia [53,54].

## Fluoroquinolones (ciprofloxacin, levofloxacin, moxifloxacin)

Fluoroquinolones are synthetic compounds with activity against a broad spectrum of pathogens and each agent has a unique profile [56]. Ciprofloxacin is the most active against gram-negative organisms including *Pseudomonas*, but it is not active against *Streptococcus* species and therefore not useful for community acquired respiratory tract infections. Fluoroquinolones have marginal activity against *Staphylococcus* species and should not be relied upon for serious *Staphylococcal* infections. Additionally, there is a clear upward trend in ciprofloxacin resistance to *Pseudomonas* limiting its utility for this pathogen. In addition to increased fluoroquinolone resistance, overuse of these agents may also contribute to the incidence of MRSA and *Clostridium difficile* associated disease [6]. Ciprofloxacin targets mainly DNA gyrase, which accounts for its broad spectrum gram negative activity. The newer agents, such as levofloxacin and moxifloxacin, target both DNA gyrase and topoisomease IV, which accounts for their broader spectrum to include more gram-positive coverage including *Streptococcus pneumoniae* [57]. Ciprofloxacin and the other fluoroquinolones have excellent tissue penetration that allows for treatment of deep-seated infections such as intra-abdominal infections, osteomyelitis, and respiratory tract infections [56–58]. Due to coverage for *S. pneumoniae* (including penicillin resistant strains), in addition to atypical pathogens, moxifloxacin and levofloxacin are useful for treatment of community respiratory tract infections. Moxifloxacin also has activity against some anaerobe species such as *Bacteroides fragilis* making it an alternative monotherapy agent for intra-abdominal infections. Ciprofloxacin and levofloxacin require dosing adjustments in renal failure, although moxifloxacin does not. The most common side effects with fluoroquinolones include gastrointenstinal effects such as diarrhea, nausea, and vomiting. Nervous system adverse effects are also possible and may include dizziness, headache, insomnia, and very rarely more serious adverse events including delirium, hallucinations, or seizure. Certain fluoroquinolones may prolong the QT interval (the time between the start of the "Q" wave and the end of the "T" wave on the electrocardiogram) predisposing patients to arrhythmias such as torsades de pointes and these drugs should not be used in combination with agents that may prolong the QT interval (ie, amiodarone, procainamide, quinidine). For most indications, fluoroquinolones are useful as second line agents for patients with allergies or intolerance to first line drugs. In the acute setting, ciprofloxacin and levofloxacin may be considered for combination therapy for gram-negative pathogens in place of an aminoglycoside, but generally not for monotherapy unless the pathogen is known and highly susceptible. Due to the concentration dependent killing associated with the fluoroquinolones, dosages should be maximized when used for serious infections in the ICU (ie, ciprofloxacin 400 mg every 8 hour, levofloxacin 750 mg once daily).

## Fourth generation cephalosporins (cefepime)

Cephalosporins include a family of broad spectrum beta lactam drugs that have a favorable pharmacokinetic and safety profile. The drugs are classified into "generations" based on their spectrum of activity and generally, the drugs have improved gram negative coverage proceeding from first to fourth generation [59,60]. Cefepime is classified as a fourth generation cephalosporin due to its broad spectrum of action and enhanced gram-positive coverage compared with third generation cephalosporins. Cefepime has broad gram-negative coverage including *Pseudomonas* and *Enterobacter* in addition to activity against gram-positive bacteria such as methicillin susceptible strains of *Staphylococcus aureus* [60]. It is not active against MRSA; none of the current cephalosporins have activity against *Enterococcus* species. When cefepime is used for mixed infections where anaerobe species may be present, an anti-anaerobic drug such as metronidazole or clindamycin should be added. Like other beta lactams it acts by binding to penicillin binding proteins and interfering with bacterial cell wall cross linking. Resistance occurs through inactivation by bacterial beta lactamases, or by changes in penicillin-binding proteins. Cefepime penetrates well into most body tissue including the cerebrospinal fluid and is useful for a variety of serious infections including sepsis, pneumonia, soft tissue infections, meningitis, intra-abdominal infections, and febrile neutropenia. Cefepime is eliminated renally and does require dosage adjustment in patients with renal impairment. Cefepime is generally well tolerated and the most common side effects include headache, nausea, rash, and diarrhea. Cefepime doses range from 1–2 g every 8–12 hours. When treating serious infections in the critically ill patient, such as pneumonia, sepsis, or meningitis, the maximum dose of 2 g every 8 hours should be considered. Despite its clinical utility for a variety of infections, a meta-analysis review of the results from all the controlled clinical trials involving cefepime demonstrated a higher mortality in the patients who received cefepime compared with the comparator. The clinical significance of this review is not yet known, but it is concerning [61].

## Summary

Antibiotic resistance is increasing faster than the drug industry can develop and market new antibiotics. Specifically, medical personnel commonly must deal with the resistant gram-positive pathogens including MRSA and VRE, in addition to the problem gram-negative bacteria, *Pseudomonas*, *Acinetobacter*, and ESBL producing strains of *Klebsiella* and *E. coli*. These pathogens are not just encountered in the ICU, but are spilling out into the rest of the hospital and even the community (ie, community acquired MRSA). Clinicians should be familiar with treatment strategies for these resistant pathogens. Due to the lack of novel agents to treat resistant infections, clinicians must use antibiotics judiciously and appropriately to limit further development of resistance. When treating serious life-threatening infections, it is appropriate to cover very broadly (ie, gram-positive, gram-negative, anaerobes), initially using aggressive doses taking advantage of pharmacodynamic principles. Early, appropriate cultures of the blood, urine, sputum and suspected source, ideally obtained before antibiotic initiation, allow for future de-escalation of antibiotics, or the decision to discontinue antibiotics.

## Acknowledgment

David F. Volles: On the speaker's bureau for Wyeth and Cubist pharmaceutical companies. Trisha N. Branan: No conflict of interest to declare.

## References

[1] Eggimann P, Pittet D. Infection control in the ICU. Chest 2001;120(6):2059–93.
[2] Weber DJ, Raasch R, Rutala WA. Nosocomial infections in the ICU. Chest 1999;15(3): 35s–41s.
[3] Jones ME, Draghi DC, Thornsberry C, et al. Emerging resistance among bacterial pathogens in the intensive care unit: a European and North American surveillance study (2000–2002). Ann Clin Microbiol Antimicrob 2004;3(14):1–11.
[4] CDC NNIS System. National nosocomial infections surveillance (NNIS) system report, data summary from January 1992 through June 2004, issued October 2004. Am J Infect Control 2004;32:470–85.
[5] Karam GH, Heffner JE. Emerging issues in antibiotic resistance in blood-borne infections. Am J Respir Crit Care Med 2000;162:1610–6.
[6] Esposito S, Leone S. Antimicrobial treatment for intensive care unit (ICU) infections including the role of the infectious disease specialist. Int J Antimicrob Agents 2007;29:494–500.
[7] Nicasio AM, Kuti JL, Nicolau DP. The current state of multidrug-resistant gram-negative bacilli in North America. Pharmacotherapy 2008;28(2):235–49.
[8] Alvarez-Lerma F. Modification of empiric antibiotic treatment in patients with pneumonia acquired in the intensive care unit. Intensive Care Med 1996;22:387–94.
[9] Kollef MH, Sherman G, Ward S, et al. Inadequate antimicrobial treatment of infections: a risk factor for hospital mortality among critically ill patients. Chest 1999;115:462–74.
[10] Ibrahim EH, Sherman G, Ward S, et al. The influence of inadequate antimicrobial treatment of bloodstream infections on patient outcomes in the ICU setting. Chest 2000;118:146–55.
[11] Paterson DL, Rice LB. Empirical antibiotic choice for the seriously ill patient: are minimization of selection of resistant organisms and maximization of individual outcome mutually exclusive? Clin Infect Dis 2003;36:1006–12.
[12] Talbot GH, Bradley J, Edwards JE, et al. Bad bugs need drugs: an update on the development pipeline from the antimicrobial availability task force of the Infectious Diseases Society of America. Clin Infect Dis 2006;42:657–68.
[13] Fridkin SK, Gaynes RP. Antimicrobial resistance in intensive care units. Clin Chest Med 1999;20(2):303–16.
[14] Singh N, Rogers P, Atwood CW, et al. Short-course empiric antibiotic therapy for patients with pulmonary infiltrates in the intensive care unit: a proposed solution to indiscriminate antibiotic prescription. Am J Respir Crit Care Med 2000;162:505–11.
[15] Dellinger RP, Levy MM, Carlet JM, et al. Surviving sepsis campaign: international guidelines for management of severe sepsis and septic shock: 2008. Crit Care Med 2008; 36:296–327.
[16] Niederman MS, Craven DE. ATS/IDSA Guidelines for the management of adults with hospital-acquired, ventilator-associated, and healthcare associated pneumonia. Am J Respir Crit Care Med 2005;171:388–416.

[17] Kumar A, Roberts D, Wood KE, et al. Duration of hypotension before initiation of effective antimicrobial therapy is the critical determinant of survival in human septic shock. Crit Care Med 2006;34:1589–96.

[18] Chastre J, Wolff M, Fagon JY, et al. Comparison of 8 vs 15 days of antibiotic therapy for ventilator-associated pneumonia in adults: a randomized trial. JAMA 2003;290: 2588–98.

[19] Paul M, Silbiger I, Grozinsky S, et al. Beta lactam antibiotic monotherapy versus beta lactam-aminoglycoside antibiotic combination therapy for sepsis Cochrane Database Syst Rev 2006;25(1):CD003344.

[20] Safdar N, Handelsman J, Maki DG. Does combination antimicrobial therapy reduce mortality in gram-negative bacteraemia? A meta-analysis. Lancet Infect Dis 2004;4(8): 519–27.

[21] Burgess DS. Pharmacodynamic principles of antimicrobial therapy in the prevention of resistance. Chest 1999;115:19s–23s.

[22] Levison ME. Pharmacodynamics of antimicrobial drugs. Infect Dis Clin North Am 2004;18: 451–65.

[23] Scheetz MH, Hurt KM, Noskin GA, et al. Applying antimicrobial pharmacodynamics to resistant gram-negative pathogens. Am J Health Syst Pharm 2006;63:1346–60.

[24] Eagye KJ, Nicolau DP, Lockhart SR, et al. A pharmacodynamic analysis of resistance trends in pathogens from patients with infection in intensive care units in the United States between 1993 and 2004. Ann Clin Microbiol Antimicrob 2007;6:11. Available at: http:// www.ann-clinmicrob.com/content/6/1/11. Accessed January 15, 2008.

[25] Wilhelm M, Estes L. Vancomycin. Mayo Clin Proc 1999;74:928–35.

[26] Levine D. Vancomycin: a History. Clin Infect Dis 2006;42:S5–12.

[27] Maclayton D, Hall R. Pharmacologic treatment options for nosocomial pneumonia involving methicillin-resistant Staphylococcus aureus. Ann Pharmacother 2007;41:235–44.

[28] Rybak M. The pharmacokinetic and pharmacodynamic properties of vancomycin. Clin Infect Dis 2006;42:S35–9.

[29] Micek S. Alternatives to Vancomycin for the treatment of methicillin-resistant staphylococcus aureus infections. Clin Infect Dis 2007;45:S184–90.

[30] Meka V, Gold H . Antimicrobial resistance to linezolid. Clin Infect Dis 2004;39:1010–5.

[31] Perry C, Jarvis B. Linezolid: a review of its use in the management of serious gram-positive infections. Drugs 2001;61:525–51.

[32] Eliopoulos G. Quinupristin-dalfopristin and linezolid: evidence and opinion. Clin Infect Dis 2003;36:473–81.

[33] Hair P, Keam S. Daptomycin: a review of its use in the management of complicated skin and soft-tissue infections and *staphylococcus aureus* bacteraemia. Drugs 2007;67:1483–512.

[34] Ziglam H. Daptomycin and tigecycline: a review of clinical efficacy in the antimicrobial era. Expert Opin Pharmacother 2007;8(14):2279–92.

[35] Fenton C, Keating G, Curran M. Daptomycin. Drugs 2004;64:445–55.

[36] Lamp K, Friedrich L, Mendez-Vigo L, et al. Clinical experience with daptomycin for the treatment of patients with osteomyelitis. Am J Med 2007;120:S13–20.

[37] Lamb H, Figgitt D, Faulds D. Quinupristin/dalfopristin: a review of its use in the management of serious gram-positive infections. Drugs 1999;58:1061–97.

[38] Hershberger E, Donabedian S, Konstantinou K, et al. Quinupristin-dalfopristin resistance in gram-positive bacteria: mechanism of resistance and epidemiology. Clin Infect Dis 2004; 38:92–8.

[39] Kallel H, Bahloul M, Hergafi L, et al. Colistin as a salvage therapy for nosocomial infections caused by multidrug-resistant bacteria in the ICU. Int J Antimicrob Agents 2006; 28:366–9.

[40] Michalopoulos AS, Tsiodras S, Rellos K, et al. Colistin treatment in patients with ICU-acquired infections caused by multiresistant gram-negative bacteria: the renaissance of an old antibiotic. Clin Microbiol Infect 2005;11:115–21.

[41] Berlana D, Llop JM, Fort E, et al. Use of colistin in the treatment of multiple-drug-resistant gram-negative infections. Am J Health Syst Pharm 2005;62:39–47.

[42] Gilad J, Carmeli Y. Treatment options for multidrug-resistant Acinetobacter species. Drugs 2008;68(2):165–89.

[43] Li J, Nation RL, Turnidge JD, et al. Colistin: The re-emerging antibiotic for multidrug-resistant gram-negative bacterial infections. Lancet Infect Dis 2006;6(9):589–601.

[44] Zapantis A, Lopez M, Hoffman E, et al. The use of colistin in multidrug-resistant infections. Hosp Pharm 2007;42:1127–38.

[45] Fraise AP. Tigecycline: The answer to the beta-lactam and fluoroquinolone resistance? J Infect 2006;53(5):293–300.

[46] Nathwani D. Tigecycline: clinical evidence and formulary positioning. Int J Antimicrob Agents 2005;25(3):185–92.

[47] Livermore DM. Tigecycline: what is it, and where should it be used? J Antimicrob Chemother 2005;56(4):611–4.

[48] Hurst M, Lamb HM. Meropenem: a review of its use in patients in intensive care. Drugs 2000;59(3):653–80.

[49] Zhanel GG, Wiebe R, Dilay L, et al. Comparitive review of the carbapenems. Drugs 2007; 67(7):1027–52.

[50] Hellinger WC, Brewer NS. Symposium on antimicrobial agents part VII. Carbapenems and monobactams: imipenem, meropenem, and aztreonam. Mayo Clin Proc 1999;74:420–34.

[51] Jones RN, Huynh HK, Biedenbach DJ, et al. Doripenem (S-4661), a novel carbapenem: comparative activity against contemporary pathogens including bactericidal action and preliminary in vitro methods evaluations. J Antimicrob Chemother 2004;54:144–54.

[52] Lomaestro BM, Tobin EH, Shang W, et al. The spread of Klebsiella pneumoniae carbapenemase-producing K. pneumoniae to upstate New York. Clin Infect Dis 2006;43:26–8.

[53] Wright AJ. Symposium on antimicrobial agents-Part VI. The penicillins. Mayo Clin Proc 1999;74:290–307.

[54] Chambers HF. Penicillins. In: Mandell GL, Bennett JE, Dolin R, editors. Principles and practice of infectious diseases. 6th edition. Philadelphia: Elsevier; 2005. p. 281–93.

[55] Lodise TP Jr, Lomaestro B, Drusano GL. Piperacillin-tazobactam for pseudomonas aeruginosa infection: clinical implications of an extended-infusion dosing strategy. Clin Infect Dis 2007;44:357–63.

[56] Hooper DC. Quinolones. In: Mandell GL, Bennett JE, Dolin R, editors. Principles and practice of infectious diseases. 6th edition. Philadelphia: Elsevier; 2005. p. 451–73.

[57] Walker RC. Symposium on antimicrobial agents part XIII. The fluoroquinolones. Mayo Clin Proc 1999;74:1030–7.

[58] Khardori N. Antibiotics-past, present, and future. Med Clin North Am 2006;90:1049–76.

[59] Marshall WF, Blair JE. Symposium on antimicrobial agents. Part V. The cephalosporins. Mayo Clin Proc 1999;74:187–95.

[60] Hardin TC, Jennings TS. Cefepime. Pharmacotherapy 1994;14(6):657–68.

[61] Yahav D, Paul M, Fraser A, et al. Efficacy and safety of cefepime: s systemic review and meta-analysis. Lancet Infect Dis 2007;7:338–48.

[62] Talan DA, Moran GJ, Abrahamian FM. Severe sepsis and septic shock in the emergency department. Infect Dis Clin N Am 2008;22:1–31.

[63] Abrahamian FM, Talan DA, Moran GJ. Management of skin and soft-tissue infections in the emergency department. Infect Dis Clin N Am 2008;22:89–116.

[64] Abrahamian FM, Moran GJ, Talan DA. Urinary tract infections in the emergency department. Infect Dis Clin N Am 2008;22:73–87.

[65] Fitch MT, Abrahamian FM, Moran GJ, et al. Emergency department management of meningitis and encephalitis. Infect Dis Clin N Am 2008;22:33–52.

ELSEVIER
SAUNDERS

Emerg Med Clin N Am
26 (2008) 835–847

EMERGENCY
MEDICINE
CLINICS OF
NORTH AMERICA

# Noninvasive Positive Pressure Ventilation in the Emergency Department

Mei-Ean Yeow, MD[a], Jairo I. Santanilla, MD[a,b,*]

[a]Division of Critical Care Medicine, University of California San Francisco,
505 Parnassus Avenue, M-917 San Francisco, CA 94143-0624, USA
[b]Alameda County Medical Center, Highland Hospital, 1411 East 31st Street,
Oakland, CA 94602-1018, USA

Noninvasive ventilation is defined as the provision of ventilatory assistance to the respiratory system without an invasive artificial airway. Noninvasive ventilators consist of both negative and positive pressure ventilators. Because negative pressure ventilation is so rarely used today, discussion is limited here to positive pressure ventilation.

One of the earliest descriptions of a "pulmonary plus pressure machine" was in 1936 when Poulton described using an Electrolux or Hoover vacuum cleaner to supply air at positive pressure to treat patients with "cardiac and bronchial asthma". He also wisely cautioned that: "the machine should be run for some minutes first of all to get rid of the dust" [1].

Before the 1960s, the use of negative pressure ventilation in the form of the tank ventilator or the "iron lung" was the most common form of mechanical ventilation outside of the anesthesia suite. It was not until the 1952 polio epidemic in Copenhagen that anesthesiologist Bjorn Ibsen showed that he could improve the survival of patients who had respiratory paralysis by using invasive positive pressure ventilation.

Despite this, negative pressure or iron lungs were the mainstay of ventilatory support for patients who had chronic respiratory failure until as late as the mid-1980s. In the early 1980s, nasal continuous positive airway pressure (CPAP) was introduced to treat obstructive sleep apnea. These tight-fitting masks proved to be an effective means of assisting ventilation and noninvasive positive pressure ventilation (NPPV) quickly displaced

* Corresponding author.
*E-mail address:* mei_ean@hotmail.com (J.I. Santanilla).

0733-8627/08/$ - see front matter © 2008 Elsevier Inc. All rights reserved.
doi:10.1016/j.emc.2008.04.005                                *emed.theclinics.com*

traditional negative pressure ventilation as the treatment of choice for chronic respiratory failure in patients with neuromuscular and chest wall deformities. Current NPPV devices are able to provide a set respiratory rate, set tidal volume, and set amount of inspiratory oxygen. The use of NPPV has also been integrated into the acute inpatient setting where it is now used to treat acute respiratory failure [2].

This article reviews the indications for NPPV in the treatment of acute respiratory failure, the evidence for its application in the emergency department (ED), and some relative and absolute contraindications for NPPV. The use of high flow nasal cannulae and their potential treatment benefit in patients with respiratory distress is also discussed.

## Definitions

The current literature uses different definitions for NPPV. Although some authors use NPPV as umbrella terms that include CPAP and bilevel positive airway pressure, more recently other authors have used the term NPPV as synonymous with bilevel and consider CPAP a separate entity. The terms NPPV and noninvasive intermittent positive pressure ventilation (NIPPV) are often used interchangeably with bilevel.

As its name suggests, CPAP supplies continuous positive pressure via a tight-fitting facemask. NPPV or bilevel provides an inspiratory pressure (set as IPAP or inspiratory positive airway pressure) in addition to end-expiratory positive pressure (set as EPAP or expiratory positive airway pressure) and breaths are usually triggered by the patient. On many such devices, backup rates may be set, that deliver bilevel pressures even if patients fail to initiate a breath.

## Rationale for using noninvasive positive pressure ventilation

The most important advantage of NPPV is avoiding the complications associated with invasive mechanical ventilation. It has been well documented that invasive mechanical ventilation increases the incidence of airway and lung injury, and it augments the risk of nosocomial pneumonia. NPPV avoids these complications by keeping the upper airway defense mechanisms intact and allows the patient to retain the ability to eat, clear secretions, and communicate normally when NPPV is used intermittently [2]. NPPV has the potential to reduce the mortality of a selected group of patients with acute respiratory failure and may shorten hospital stay, thereby reducing costs. Specific to the ED, appropriate initiation of NPPV may avoid unnecessary intubation of selected patients, hence avoiding ICU admissions, reducing costs, decreasing complications, and improving mortality.

## Pathophysiological effects of noninvasive positive pressure ventilation

CPAP increases alveolar recruitment and size, enhancing the area available for gas exchange, and improves ventilation-perfusion relationship, thus improving hypoxemia. The term CPAP is synonymous with extrinsic PEEP (PEEPe) and the bilevel expiratory positive airway pressure (EPAP). It can also negate the effects of intrinsic positive end expiratory pressure (PEEPi) also referred to as auto-PEEP or dynamic hyperinflation. In patients with dynamic hyperinflation (asthma or chronic obstructive pulmonary disease [COPD]), an increased PEEPi increases the magnitude of the drop in airway pressure that the patient must generate to trigger a breath. This causes an increase in the work of breathing for the patient. Careful application PEEPe can reduce this gradient and decrease the patient's work of breathing. Positive pressure ventilation creates an increase in intrathoracic pressure. This causes preload to decrease due to diminished venous return and also decreases transmural pressures and afterload [1].

In NPPV or bilevel, the inspiratory positive airway pressure (IPAP) is similar to pressure support and, when combined with expiratory positive airway pressure (EPAP), further augments alveolar ventilation and allows some respiratory muscle rest during the inspiratory phase.

## Indications for initiating noninvasive position ventilation

*Acute exacerbation of chronic obstructive pulmonary disease*

Numerous studies have shown that NPPV can reduce the need for intubation, length of the hospital stay, and also in-hospital mortality rate in patients presenting with acute exacerbations of COPD. One of the earliest, prospective, randomized studies was done by Bott and colleagues [3] in 1993 where they reported a reduction in mortality with the use of nasal NPPV in patients who had COPD. This study was followed by a large multi-center, prospective, randomized trial by Brochard and colleagues [4], which confirmed selected patients who had acute COPD exacerbations did benefit from NPPV, compared with standard medical care alone. In this study, NPPV decreased intubation rates compared with standard medical treatment (11/43 [26%] versus 31/42 [74%]); hospital mortality was 9% in the NPPV group compared with 29% in the standard medical therapy group. Since then, several systematic reviews have confirmed that NPPV reduces in-hospital mortality and decreases the need for endotracheal intubation in patients who have acute, severe COPD exacerbations. A systematic review by Keenan suggested that the patients who benefited most from NPPV treatment were those with severe exacerbations as manifested by a pH of < 7.3 [5]. This finding, however, has not been borne out in other reviews [6].

Interestingly, Conti and colleagues [7] showed that if NPPV is started later, after the failure of medical treatment, the benefits conferred by

NPPV (hospital mortality, length of ICU stay, number of days on the ventilator, overall complications) are eliminated. This emphasizes the importance of initiating NPPV early, alongside standard medical therapy.

It is reasonable to consider early implementation NPPV in patients who present to the ED with an acute exacerbation of COPD.

### Asthma

In many ways, an acute asthmatic attack is similar to a COPD exacerbation. There is pronounced airway obstruction, significant dynamic hyperinflation and, increases in PEEPi. CPAP has been reported to have a bronchodilatory effect in asthma, unloading fatigued muscles, and improving gas exchange. The PEEPe from NPPV can also offset the PEEPi that occurs during an asthmatic attack as mentioned earlier [8].

Soroksky conducted a prospective, randomized, placebo-controlled study in 30 patients who presented to the ED with a severe asthma attack (excluding patients with signs of concurrent pneumonia). Half the patients were assigned to NPPV (for 3 hours) and conventional therapy, while the other half received conventional therapy and subtherapeutic pressures via a sham device.

He found that patients who received NPPV had significantly improved lung function test results. There was also a significant reduction in the need for hospitalization in the treatment group (17.6% versus 62.5%, $P = .0134$). Therefore in selected patients who have severe asthmatic attacks, the use of NPPV may be a useful adjuvant, which potentially alleviates the attacks faster and decreases the need for hospitalization [8].

### Acute cardiogenic pulmonary edema

The great majority of patients who have acute cardiogenic pulmonary edema (ACPE) present to the ED. When these patients do not respond to conventional medical treatment, ventilator assistance becomes necessary. CPAP ventilation has been shown to be efficacious in ACPE. An early systematic review by Pang and colleagues [9] revealed that CPAP could reduce the rate of intubation and led to a trend toward decreasing mortality. A later, pooled analysis by Collins and colleagues [10] suggested that CPAP and NPPV both reduced the risk of subsequent intubation in the ED, although the mortality benefits were less convincing.

The data for NPPV or bilevel has been mixed, with an early article by Mehta and colleagues [11] describing an increase rate of acute myocardial infarction in patients who have ACPE treated with NPPV. Since this study, there have been several trials that have refuted this increased risk of myocardial infarction. Most of these have been small studies, the largest being a multicenter trial randomizing 130 patients who have ACPE to either NPPV or conventional therapy. This study found that the patients treated with NPPV had faster improvements in oxygenation, respiratory rates, and sensation of dyspnea. No difference was noted between the two groups with regard to rates of intubation, hospital mortality, length of stay, or myocardial infarction [12]. More recently, Ferrari and colleagues [13] compared CPAP and NPPV head-to-head in 52 patients with ACPE. They found no significant difference in the rates of intubation and hospital stay. Both techniques were found to be effective in improving gas exchange and vital signs in patients who have ACPE. More importantly, no significant difference was observed in the rate of acute myocardial infarction in the two groups.

In the largest study of patients presenting with ACPE in the ED, author Newby has reported in *Chest Physician* (October 2007) that in his study of 1,069 UK patients, both CPAP and NPPV were effective in resolving patient's symptoms (eg, dyspnea), but the mortality rate at 7 and 30 days after treatment was similar in the three groups (CPAP, NPPV and passive oxygen therapy).

It seems that it is safe to use either CPAP or NPPV for patients who present with ACPE. Although it seems that neither therapy improves mortality, it does seem to improve symptoms and may decrease intubation rates in the ED, thus avoiding the associated complications of intubation and potentially avoiding an ICU admission.

## Hypoxemic respiratory failure

The data for NPPV in patients with acute hypoxemic respiratory failure is mixed. The largest study examined 105 patients who had acute hypoxemic respiratory failure ($PaO_2 < 60$ mmHg, $SpO_2 < 90\%$ on oxygen by facemask). Patients who had hypercapnia were excluded. These 105 patients were assigned randomly to NPPV or oxygen therapy. The authors reported marked reductions in rates of endotracheal intubation, septic shock, ICU and cumulative 90-day mortality in the patients who were treated with NPPV [14]. This group also included patients who had cardiogenic pulmonary edema.

Antonelli and colleagues [15] looked at whether NPPV could be beneficial in patients who had acute hypoxemic respiratory failure and who would otherwise need intubation. They studied 64 patients who presented with acute hypoxemic respiratory failure and excluded patients who had COPD. The authors found that NPPV was as effective as conventional ventilation in improving gas exchange, and NPPV was associated with fewer serious complications (particularly pneumonia and sinusitis) and resulted in shorter stays in the ICU. The etiology for the respiratory failure in this cohort of patients was variable, and included patients who had cardiogenic pulmonary edema.

For patients who have pneumonia causing acute respiratory failure, the evidence is even more controversial, with some papers suggesting a decrease in intubation rates, while others have found no difference in intubation rates or in-hospital mortality [16,17].

In summary, although some of the literature suggests that NPPV may be beneficial in the setting of acute hypoxemic respiratory failure, doubts still exist, in part due to the heterogeneity of patients included in previous studies. A large multicenter trial of NPPV in patients who have acute hypoxemic respiratory failure that excludes patients who have cardiogenic pulmonary edema and COPD may help to clarify the use of NPPV in this setting.

### Immunosuppressed patients

NPPV can also be useful in patients who are profoundly immunosuppressed, either due to solid organ transplantation or from hematological conditions. In these patients, mortality after endotracheal intubation is particularly high, therefore any attempts to avoid this procedure may result in improved survival.

One study randomized 40 patients with acute hypoxemic respiratory failure after solid organ transplant to conventional treatment, including oxygen via facemask or NPPV. The patients assigned to NPPV had a lower rate of endotracheal intubation, shorter ICU stays, and lower ICU mortality. In-house mortality did not differ significantly between the two groups [18].

Another study included immunosuppressed patients who had pulmonary infiltrates, fever, and acute respiratory failure. This study also included patients who were immunosuppressed from: chemotherapy; bone marrow transplantation for hematologic cancers; corticosteroid or cytotoxic therapy for a nonmalignant disease; or, AIDS. They found that in these patients, early initiation of NPPV was associated with significant reductions in the rates of endotracheal intubation and serious complications, with lower rates of death in the ICU and in the hospital [19]. Of note, all of the patients who developed ventilator-associated pneumonia died in the ICU, in both aforementioned studies (2/26 in the NPPV group; 6/26 in the standard treatment group in Hilbert's study). This emphasizes the potential dangers of intubation in this group of patients.

When faced with a severely immunosuppressed patient with acute hypoxemic respiratory failure in the ED, early initiation of NPPV may be beneficial in avoiding the serious complications of endotracheal intubation.

### Do not intubate patients

Although most studies of NPPV have focused on patients with acute respiratory failure who desire maximum life-prolonging treatment, there is an emerging interest in using NPPV for patients who have made the decision to forego endotracheal intubation (DNI). A recent review article on this topic suggests that with good patient–family–physician communication, NPPV can successfully be used in these patients on a trial basis [20].

In DNI patients willing to undergo NPPV, success would be measured by improved ventilation or oxygenation. NPPV can provide support for the patient while the underlying cause of the respiratory failure is treated. NPPV should be discontinued if it is not producing the desired response or if the patient is unable to tolerate it. In these circumstances, a decision should be made by the health care team, the patient, and their family to discontinue NPPV and make the transition toward comfort measures.

The authors suggest that in patients who have chosen to forego any life-prolonging therapy and are receiving comfort care measures only, NPPV might be used as a form of palliative care, in an attempt to reduce associated dyspnea. In this circumstance, the use of NPPV is considered successful if it alleviates the patient's symptoms. If it causes any discomfort to the patient, it should be discontinued because the primary goal is patient comfort. This use of NPPV is controversial and there are no studies that have assessed the benefits of NPPV in this group of patients [20]. Another use of NPPV in patients who have chosen comfort care measures is a time-limited trial of NPPV to achieve the goal of survival until the arrival of family and friends. In this situation, NPPV would be used to provide life support until friends and family can achieve closure.

Even if a patient with a known DNI advanced directive presents to the ED with acute respiratory failure of reversible etiology, it still can be beneficial discussing the use of NPPV with the patient and their family. In this situation, communication about expectations and goals of care is of utmost importance.

*Facilitation of weaning and extubation*

Recent studies have shown that NPPV can potentially be useful in the discontinuation of mechanical ventilation in patients when respiratory failure is due to COPD. A recent meta-analysis found that in those patients who have COPD who failed a spontaneous breathing trial, extubating to NPPV decreased mortality, hospital length of stay, incidence of ventilator-associated pneumonia, and total duration of mechanical ventilation [21]. Although it is rare to extubate a patient in the ED, one does sometimes encounter patients with exacerbations of their COPD who were prematurely intubated in the field, or who have improved remarkably since arrival to the ED. These patients can be considered for extubation to NPPV on a case-by-case basis if there are no contraindications to extubation, and only if the clinician is confident that the patient can be re-intubated if necessary.

**Feasibility of using noninvasive positive pressure ventilation in the emergency department**

Most of the earlier NPPV studies were performed in the ICU. With the growing clinical and fiscal pressures to avoid endotracheal intubation whenever feasible, there has been an increasing interest in using this technology in the ED. Pollock showed in his study that the use of NPPV was feasible and had the potential utility in the management of patients with respiratory distress [22]. This early intervention had the potential to avoid the risks and complications of endotracheal intubation and shorten or possibly eliminate intensive care admissions. There is very little literature on the safety of using NPPV in the ED, how to identify patients who would benefit from this treatment or how long these patients should be treated with NPPV in the ED. There is also controversy over which type of mask should be used.

Nasal masks had been traditionally used in the setting of chronic home therapy and they were initially the masks of choice in the acute setting. Because dyspneic patients tend to be mouth breathers, it is thought that face-masks are preferable for the treatment of acute respiratory failure in the ED [1]. Poponick and colleagues, as well as Merlani and colleagues, have sought to define and identify those patients who might benefit from NPPV and conversely, identify what factors would predict failure of NPPV in the ED. Poponick and colleagues [23] investigated factors associated with NPPV failure in the emergency setting in 58 patients receiving a 30 minute trial of bilevel. Lack of improvement of pH and $PaCO_2$ level were identified as indicators for endotracheal intubation. Merlani and colleagues [24] retrospectively analyzed a total of 104 patients admitted to the ED and found that factors associated with failure of NPPV in the univariate analysis included Glasgow Coma Scale $< 13$ at ED admission, or a RR $> 20$/min, or a pH $< 7.35$ after one hour of NPPV. In the multivariate analysis, pH $< 7.35$ and RR $> 20$/min after one hour of NPPV were independently associated with NPPV failure and subsequent intubation of these patients. Both these studies looked at patients who had acute respiratory failure and the studies included predominantly patients who had COPD and congestive heart failure.

These two studies emphasize the importance of close follow-up of patients who are started on NPPV in the ED. It is important to serially assess patient response as soon as 30 minutes after the initiation of NPPV. Those who are persistently tachypneic and acidemic should be considered for intubation sooner rather than later.

## Initiation of noninvasive positive pressure ventilation

There is no standard approach to the initiation of NPPV. Different methods have been used in clinical trials, yet these methods have never been compared. There are two main strategies: a high-low approach and a low-high approach.

In the high-low approach, one initially starts with a high IPAP (20–25 $cmH_2O$) and then lowers this if the patient is unable to tolerate such high pressures. In the low-high approach, one starts with a lower IPAP (8–10 $cmH_2O$). This is gradually increased as tolerated to achieve alleviation of dyspnea, decreased respiratory rate, increased tidal volume, and patient–ventilator synchrony. The EPAP is usually set at 3–4 $cmH_2O$, unless the patient has a significant amount of autopeep or PEEPi. In these patients, one would start with an EPAP between 4–8 $cmH_2O$. The $FiO_2$ is titrated to keep the pulse oximetry $\geq$ 90%. Much like conventional ventilation, the EPAP can be adjusted to improve oxygenation and the $\Delta$ IPAP-EPAP can be adjusted to create a higher minute ventilation and thus mitigate hypercapnia.

As mentioned in the previous section, it is imperative to closely observe the patient for deterioration. Blood gases should be checked within 1 to 2 hours after initiation of NPPV to assess treatment success or failure. Patients who do not improve clinically should be considered for intubation.

### Cautions for use of noninvasive positive pressure ventilation

Most studies involving NPPV have excluded patients who were hemodynamically unstable, had an altered level of consciousness, or were unable to protect their airway. This was based on the concern that a depressed sensorium would predispose the patient to aspiration. The International Consensus Conference in Intensive Care Medicine on Noninvasive Positive Pressure Ventilation in Acute Respiratory Failure held in April 2000 considered the presence of severe encephalopathy, as manifested by a GCS < 10 to be a contraindication for NPPV [25].

Other accepted contraindications to NPPV are listed below: (Box 1).

Recently there have been studies looking specifically at the use of NPPV in patients presenting with hypercapnic coma secondary to acute respiratory failure. This was based on the observation that some DNI patients who declined intubation had successful outcomes using NPPV therapy despite their initial comatose presentation. Diaz and colleagues [26] conducted an observational study and found that success rates were comparable between the comatose and noncomatose group. Scala and colleagues [27,28] performed two studies, both showing that NPPV could be used successfully in treating patients with COPD exacerbations with hypercapnic encephalopathy. Their 2007 study showed that the use of NPPV performed by an experienced team led to similar short-term and long-term survivals, fewer nosocomial infections, and shorter durations of hospitalization compared with patients who were placed on mechanical ventilation. Of note, the above

---

**Box 1. Contraindications to the use of noninvasive ventilation**

Impending cardiovascular collapse or respiratory arrest
Severe upper gastrointestinal bleeding
Facial surgery, trauma or deformity, limiting placement of the
  NPPV mask
Upper airway obstruction
Inability to cooperate/protect the airway, altered mental status
Inability to clear respiratory secretions
High risk for aspiration

studies were conducted in the ICU [26] or specialized respiratory care units [28], with a nursing ratio of at least 1:3. The patients were also very closely monitored by staff while they received NPPV. This high level of nursing to patient ratio may not be feasible in a busy ED.

The other key point in these studies was the rapid improvement in neurologic status that occurred 1–2 hrs after the initiation of NPPV. The importance of close monitoring of patients started on NPPV is crucial in identifying those who will fail this therapy.

### High flow nasal cannula

The high flow nasal cannula (HFNC) is a relatively new oxygen delivery system. Conventional nasal cannula uses a low flow system; at higher flows (>6 L/min), it can cause nasal dryness, epistaxis and patient discomfort. The HFNC system (Fig. 1) is a novel device, combining oxygen, pressurized air, and warm humidification to deliver tolerable flows of up to 40 L/min through a nasal cannula. The $FiO_2$ and flow rates can be adjusted. With higher flows, less air entrapment occurs and the higher flow rates match the dyspneic patient's increased minute ventilation.

Use of the HFNC has been more extensively studied in neonatal respiratory care where ongoing studies suggest that HFNC may be as effective as nasal CPAP in the preterm neonate [29]. One study looked at the effect

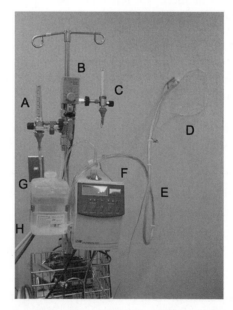

Fig. 1. High flow nasal cannula system. A) High flow flowmeter, B) oxygen blender, C) low flow flowmeter, D) nasal cannula, E) low compliance, heated-wire circuit, F) high flow humidifier, G) water reservoir, H) air/$O_2$ supply.

of HFNC on exercise performance in adults with COPD [30]. Currently, there are no published studies investigating the use of HFNC in patients who have acute respiratory failure. Anecdotally, this system has been used with some success in adults in the ICU, targeting immunosuppressed patients in hopes of avoiding intubation. It seems to be better tolerated than NPPV and, at higher flows, it is believed to provide a certain amount of continuous positive pressure. More studies will have to be performed before this technology becomes a mainstay treatment of patients with acute respiratory failure.

## Summary

NPPV has been shown to work well in patients with reversible conditions and acts as a bridge while allowing medical therapy (eg, bronchodilators, steroids, diuretics) to take effect, thus potentially avoiding the need for endotracheal intubation. Those with less reversible causes of their acute respiratory failure (ARDS, pneumonia) may be less likely to respond. With careful patient selection, NPPV can be safely initiated in the ED, giving time for the medical treatment to work, and potentially avoiding an ICU admission. Patients who are being considered for intubation should be evaluated for the potential use of NPPV.

Close monitoring and follow-up of patients placed on NPPV is crucial in determining whether the therapy has been successful or if further intervention is needed. Therefore, in EDs where the staff have been adequately trained, selected patients, even those who present in a hypercapnic coma can be considered for a short trial of NPPV, with the caveat that extreme diligence in monitoring these patients must be employed and if improvement is not seen in 1–2 hours, intubation should not be delayed.

## References

[1] Cross AM. Review of the role of non-invasive ventilation in the emergency department. J Accid Emerg Med 2000;17(2):79–85.
[2] Rajan T, Hill N. Noninvasive positive pressure ventilation. In: Fink M, Abraham E, Vincent JL, et al, editors. Textbook of critical care. 5th edition. Philadelphia: Elseiver Saunders; 2005. p. 519–26.
[3] Bott J, Carroll MP, Conway JH, et al. Randomised controlled trial of nasal ventilation in acute ventilatory failure due to chronic obstructive airways disease. Lancet 1993; 341(8860):1555–7.
[4] Brochard L, Mancebo J, Wysocki M, et al. Noninvasive ventilation for acute exacerbations of chronic obstructive pulmonary disease. N Engl J Med 1995;333(13):817–22.
[5] Keenan SP, Sinuff T, Cook DJ, et al. Which patients with acute exacerbation of chronic obstructive pulmonary disease benefit from noninvasive positive-pressure ventilation? A systematic review of the literature. Ann Intern Med 2003;138(11):861–70.
[6] Ram FS, Picot J, Lightowler J, et al. Non-invasive positive pressure ventilation for treatment of respiratory failure due to exacerbations of chronic obstructive pulmonary disease-Cochrane Database Syst Rev 2004;(3):CD004104.

[7] Conti G, Antonelli M, Navalesi P, et al. Noninvasive vs. conventional mechanical ventilation in patients with chronic obstructive pulmonary disease after failure of medical treatment in the ward: a randomized trial. Intensive Care Med 2002;28(12):1701–7.

[8] Soroksky A, Stav D, Shpirer I. A pilot prospective, randomized, placebo-controlled trial of bilevel positive airway pressure in acute asthmatic attack. Chest 2003;123(4):1018–25.

[9] Pang D, Keenan SP, Cook DJ, et al. The effect of positive pressure airway support on mortality and the need for intubation in cardiogenic pulmonary edema: a systematic review. Chest 1998;114(4):1185–92.

[10] Collins SP, Mielniczuk LM, Whittingham HA, et al. The use of noninvasive ventilation in emergency department patients with acute cardiogenic pulmonary edema: a systematic review. Ann Emerg Med 2006;48(3):260–9, 269. e261–4.

[11] Mehta S, Jay GD, Woolard RH, et al. Randomized, prospective trial of bilevel versus continuous positive airway pressure in acute pulmonary edema. Crit Care Med 1997;25(4):620–8.

[12] Nava S, Carbone G, DiBattista N, et al. Noninvasive ventilation in cardiogenic pulmonary edema: a multicenter randomized trial. Am J Respir Crit Care Med 2003;168(12):1432–7.

[13] Ferrari G, Olliveri F, De Filippi G, et al. Noninvasive positive airway pressure and risk of myocardial infarction in acute cardiogenic pulmonary edema: continuous positive airway pressure vs noninvasive positive pressure ventilation. Chest 2007;132(6):1804–9.

[14] Ferrer M, Esquinas A, Leon M, et al. Noninvasive ventilation in severe hypoxemic respiratory failure: a randomized clinical trial. Am J Respir Crit Care Med 2003;168(12):1438–44.

[15] Antonelli M, Conti G, Rocco M, et al. A comparison of noninvasive positive-pressure ventilation and conventional mechanical ventilation in patients with acute respiratory failure. N Engl J Med 1998;339(7):429–35.

[16] Confalonieri M, Potena A, Carbone G, et al. Acute respiratory failure in patients with severe community-acquired pneumonia. A prospective randomized evaluation of noninvasive ventilation. Am J Respir Crit Care Med 1999;160(5 Pt 1):1585–91.

[17] Wysocki M, Tric L, Wolff MA, et al. Noninvasive pressure support ventilation in patients with acute respiratory failure. A randomized comparison with conventional therapy. Chest 1995;107(3):761–8.

[18] Antonelli M, Conti G, Bufi M, et al. Noninvasive ventilation for treatment of acute respiratory failure in patients undergoing solid organ transplantation: a randomized trial. JAMA 2000;283(2):235–41.

[19] Hilbert G, Gruson D, Vargas F, et al. Noninvasive ventilation in immunosuppressed patients with pulmonary infiltrates, fever, and acute respiratory failure. N Engl J Med 2001;344(7):481–7.

[20] Curtis JR, Cook DJ, Sinuff T, et al. Noninvasive positive pressure ventilation in critical and palliative care settings: understanding the goals of therapy. Crit Care Med 2007;35(3):932–9.

[21] Burns KE, Adhikari NK, Meade MO. Noninvasive positive pressure ventilation as a weaning strategy for intubated adults with respiratory failure. Cochrane Database Syst Rev 2003;(4):CD004127.

[22] Pollack C Jr, Torres MT, Alexander L. Feasibility study of the use of bilevel positive airway pressure for respiratory support in the emergency department. Ann Emerg Med 1996;27(2):189–92.

[23] Poponick JM, Renston JP, Bennett RP, et al. Use of a ventilatory support system (BiPAP) for acute respiratory failure in the emergency department. Chest 1999;116(1):166–71.

[24] Merlani PG, Pasquina P, Granier JM, et al. Factors associated with failure of noninvasive positive pressure ventilation in the emergency department. Acad Emerg Med 2005;12(12):1206–15.

[25] International Consensus Conferences in Intensive Care Medicine: noninvasive positive pressure ventilation in acute respiratory failure. Am J Respir Crit Care Med 2001;163(1):283–91.

[26] Diaz GG, Alcaraz AC, Talavera JC, et al. Noninvasive positive-pressure ventilation to treat hypercapnic coma secondary to respiratory failure. Chest 2005;127(3):952–60.

[27] Scala R, Naldi M, Archinucci I, et al. Noninvasive positive pressure ventilation in patients with acute exacerbations of COPD and varying levels of consciousness. Chest 2005;128(3): 1657–66.

[28] Scala R, Nava S, Conti G, et al. Noninvasive versus conventional ventilation to treat hypercapnic encephalopathy in chronic obstructive pulmonary disease. Intensive Care Med 2007; 33(12):2101–8.

[29] Sreenan C, Lemke RP, Hudson-Mason A, et al. High-flow nasal cannulae in the management of apnea of prematurity: a comparison with conventional nasal continuous positive airway pressure. Pediatrics 2001;107(5):1081–3.

[30] Chatila W, Nugent T, Vance G, et al. The effects of high-flow vs low-flow oxygen on exercise in advanced obstructive airways disease. Chest 2004;126(4):1108–15.

ELSEVIER
SAUNDERS

Emerg Med Clin N Am
26 (2008) 849–862

EMERGENCY
MEDICINE
CLINICS OF
NORTH AMERICA

# Mechanical Ventilation

## Jairo I. Santanilla, MD[a,b,*], Brian Daniel, RRT[c], Mei-Ean Yeow, MD[a]

[a]Division of Critical Care Medicine, University of California, San Francisco,
505 Parnassus Avenue, M-917, San Francisco, CA 94143-0624, USA
[b]Alameda County Medical Center, Highland Hospital, 1411 East 31st Street,
Oakland, CA 94602-1018, USA
[c]Respiratory Care Service, University of California, San Francisco,
513 Parnassus Avenue, S-758, San Francisco, CA 94143-0206, USA

In many practice environments, the act of intubating a patient sets off a cascade of events that quickly take the patient out of the emergency department and into the intensive care unit (ICU) or operating room. Increasingly, hospital overcrowding leads to a delay in transfer and ventilator management falls upon the emergency medicine (EM) physician. In addition, during nights and weekends in some facilities, the EM physician may be called upon to troubleshoot or stabilize mechanically ventilated patients in the ICU. This article reviews the common modes of mechanical ventilation, new technologies, and specific ventilator strategies that have been shown to be beneficial. Indications for mechanical ventilation, ventilator associated pneumonia (VAP) and liberation from mechanical ventilation are beyond the scope of this article.

Perhaps one of the most confusing aspects of mechanical ventilation is the plethora of terms and acronyms that are used. However, this subject can be simplified by keeping in mind some key questions.

- Why is the patient on the ventilator?
- Is the patient breathing spontaneously?
- Who is doing the greater work of breathing: the patient or the machine?
- Is a volume-targeted strategy in place? Or is a pressure-targeted strategy being used?
- Is it a dual controlled mode?
- What is the set respiratory rate?

* Corresponding author. Division of Critical Care Medicine, University of California San Francisco, 505 Parnassus Avenue, M-917, San Francisco, CA 94143-0624.
E-mail address: jsantanilla@gmail.com (J.I. Santanilla).

0733-8627/08/$ - see front matter © 2008 Elsevier Inc. All rights reserved.
doi:10.1016/j.emc.2008.04.007                                    emed.theclinics.com

- What is the total respiratory rate?
- What is the set extrinsic/applied positive end-expiratory pressure (PEEP)?
- Is there intrinsic PEEP (auto-PEEP) present?
- What is the inspiratory/expiratory ratio, flow rate, and trigger mode?
- What do the ventilator graphics indicate?

By convention, many clinicians order a standard "AC/RR14/Vt600/PEEP 5/FiO$_2$ 100%," however, these orders ignore important facets of care that might prove to be beneficial to our patients. Most ventilators can be set to achieve goals of spontaneous breathing, volume-targeted ventilation, pressure-targeted ventilation, or some combination. In volume-targeted (also known as volume-cycled or volume assist/control) ventilation, the ventilator is set to reach a preset volume regardless of the pressure required to do so. Pressure-targeted modes are set to reach a preset pressure independent of volume generated. Dual modes combine the benefits of both strategies.

The respiratory rate and tidal volume determine a patient's minute-ventilation. Patients intubated for airway protection due to trauma or toxicology often do well with a normal minute-ventilation and as such, initially setting respiratory rates at 10–14 breaths/minute and the tidal volume at 7–8 mL/kg ideal body weight (IBW) is usually sufficient. Adjustments can be made based on arterial blood gas (ABG) analysis, end-tidal CO$_2$, or venous blood gas and pulse oximetry. Patients who are septic or have a severe acidosis often require a higher minute-ventilation. Respiratory rates can be increased, as can tidal volume; however, volumes above 10 mL/kg IBW should not be used due to the risk of inducing ventilator associated lung injury. In addition, in special scenarios such as acute lung injury (ALI) and acute respiratory distress syndrome (ARDS), initial tidal volumes should be set as low as 6 mL/kg IBW. Some of these specific scenarios are discussed later in this article.

Although the fraction of inspired oxygen (FiO$_2$) is usually initially set at 1.0, most agree that quickly titrating down is beneficial due to the theoretic risk of oxygen toxicity. Adjustments can be made based on ABG or pulse oximetry, with a goal of keeping an arterial PO$_2$ above 60 mmHg or a arterial oxygen saturation above 90%. Extrinsic PEEP is typically set at 5–8 cmH$_2$O. It is used to offset the gradual loss of functional residual volume (FRC) in the supine mechanically ventilated patient. Care should be exercised when PEEP levels >8 cmH$_2$O are used in the setting of elevated intracranial pressures [1], unilateral lung processes, hypotension, hypovolemia, or pulmonary embolism.

Flow rate and waveform should be considered in the discussion with the respiratory therapist. The flow waveform is usually set to decelerate in an effort to optimize recruitment due to different time constants in the lung. Trigger mode can be set to detect either pressure or flow gradient. This should be set such that the patient can trigger the ventilator without great effort. If the trigger is set too high (not sensitive enough), the work of breathing incurred by the patient can be substantial. By convention, many ventilators are set to a flow trigger with a sensitivity of 1–3 cmH$_2$O [2]. If, the sensitivity is set too low (too sensitive), the ventilator can "auto-trigger" because of oscillating water in the ventilator tubing, or by hyperdynamic heartbeats, or when the patient moves.

## Spontaneous breathing

Spontaneously breathing patients can be supported on the ventilator by pressure support ventilation (PSV). In this mode, the ventilator provides a supplemental inspiratory pressure to each of the patient generated breaths. The clinician sets the FiO$_2$ and PEEP. The patient sets the respiratory rate and generates their desired flow rate. The applied pressure is turned off once the flow decreases to a predetermined percentage. The tidal volume is dictated by the pressure support given, patient effort and the lung compliance. There is no minimal rate, although there is a back-up apnea rate in most modern ventilators.

## Volume-targeted (control) modes

Volume-targeted modes are the most commonly used and the most familiar mode of mechanical ventilation. As its name implies, "volume" (ie, tidal volume) is the ventilator's targeted parameter. The ventilator will generate the necessary driving pressure to reach this "target." In addition to tidal volume, the clinician sets a desired respiratory rate, FiO$_2$, and PEEP. It should be noted that other important aspects of the mechanical ventilator can be controlled in this setting, such as waveform (decelerating or square), inspiratory/expiratory ratio (I:E ratio), flow rate, and trigger mode. However, many clinicians fail to consider these factors in their ventilator management.

Both assist control (AC) and synchronized intermittent mechanical ventilation (SIMV) can be set as volume-targeted modes. In these modes, both will provide the desired tidal volume at a preset, minimum respiratory rate; however, if the patient triggers the ventilator at a rate greater than the set rate, these two strategies diverge. In AC, each breath above the set respiratory rate will result in a full mechanically supported breath at the set tidal volume. In SIMV, the ventilator will only give the set number of breaths at the clinician selected tidal volume and each additional breath will require the patient to generate a spontaneous tidal volume without mechanical assistance. Furthermore, a patient-generated breath must overcome any resistance caused by the artificial airway and/or ventilator circuitry. Pressure support can be added to SIMV for patient-generated breaths in efforts to alleviate or reduce any increase in work of breathing related to resistance imposed by the ventilator circuit and endotracheal tube (see below). Assist control and SIMV, set at rates greater than the patient's intrinsic respiratory rate, are virtually identical.

Caution should be exercised to avoid auto-PEEP (also known as breath-stacking) when using volume-targeted AC modes. Because each mechanically delivered breath is given at full tidal volume, patients with a high respiratory rate on AC may not have sufficient time to completely exhale between breaths. This results in progressive air trapping, leading to an increase in auto (intrinsic) PEEP.

## Pressure-targeted (control) modes

As its name implies, "pressure" is the ventilator's targeted parameter. The ventilator will generate an inspiratory pressure that has been set by the clinician. The resulting tidal volume will be a function of respiratory mechanics. In addition, the clinician sets the desired PEEP, respiratory rate, $FiO_2$, and inspiratory time or I:E ratio, and trigger mode. It should be noted that the clinician does not control waveform or peak inspiratory flow. As with volume-targeted ventilation, pressure-targeted ventilation can be set to either an AC or SIMV mode. Pressure-targeted modes might have better pressure distribution and improved dissemination of airway pressures [3] and their use has been growing in popularity. In this mode, the decelerating waveform optimizes distribution of ventilation.

The main drawback with this strategy is that any change in the system compliance and/or resistance will affect the generated tidal volume. For example, if the patient bites on the endotracheal tube or a mucus plug develops, the set pressures that were generating an adequate volume will no longer do so. In contrast, a sudden increase in system compliance might result in the generation of tidal volumes that may be considerably larger than desired. Thus, instead of the traditional pressure alarm limits, one must adjust and be cognizant of tidal volume and minute-ventilation alarm settings. Uncertainties like these have led many clinicians to favor volume targeted strategies or dual controlled strategies in the acute care setting.

## Alternative ventilator strategies

### Synchronized intermittent mechanical ventilation plus pressure support ventilation

Due to the increased work of breathing imposed by the ventilator circuit and endotracheal tube, SIMV plus pressure support ventilation (PSV) was developed. This strategy supplies inspiratory pressure during spontaneous breaths. In a way, this became the first use of a dual targeted mode. This mode was initially recommended by those who felt that as a patient's need for mechanical ventilatory support decreased, the set respiratory rate could be decreased and thus the patient "weaned" to pressure support ventilation alone and ensuing extubation. However, subsequent data has shown that this method of liberation actually increases the number of ventilator days (patient days on mechanical ventilation) [4].

## Dual control modes

These new modes use a closed-loop ventilator logic that combines the features of volume and pressure targeted ventilation. These modes automatically alter control variables, either breath-to-breath or within a breath, to ensure a minimum tidal volume or minute-ventilation [5].

### Breath-to-breath

Pressure-Regulated Volume Control (PRVC) (MAQUET, Servo 300 and Servo-i; VIASYS Healthcare, AVEA), AutoFlow (Drager Medical, Evita 4), Volume Ventilation Plus (VV+) (Covidien, Purtian Bennett 840), Adaptive Support Ventilation (ASV) (Hamilton Medical- Hamilton G5, Hamilton C2, Galileo, Raphael), and Variable Pressure Control (VPC) and Variable Pressure Support (VPS) (Cardiopulmonary Corporation, Venturi Ventilator) are all very similar proprietary modes. All use a pressure-targeted logic in which the ventilator determines after each breath if the pressure applied to the airway was sufficient to deliver the desired tidal volume. If, for example, the tidal volume did not meet the set target, the ventilator will adjust the pressure applied to the airway on the next breath. These modes can be thought of as pressure control on "autopilot." Some have described this as having a computerized respiratory therapist at the bedside at all times. Unfortunately, guidelines for the use of these modes have yet to be established. A concern with these modes is that they might spend an inordinate amount of time chasing the patient in an effort to deliver a desired tidal volume. In addition, if the patient begins to generate higher flows, as with pain or anxiety, the ventilator may misinterpret this effort and inappropriately decrease its output, thus increasing the patient's work of breathing.

### Within a breath

#### Volume Assured Pressure Support Ventilation and Pressure Augmentation

These modes, Volume Assured Pressure Support Ventilation (VAPSV) (VIASYS Healthcare, Bird 8400STi) and Pressure Augmentation (VIASYS Healthcare, BEAR 1000), alter the control parameter "within" the inspiratory cycle of a breath. The clinician sets a pressure-support level, peak flow and tidal volume. Thus, the ventilator provides an inspiratory support and inspiratory demand flow in the same manner as with PSV, but will adjust the inspiratory pressure to obtain assured tidal volume delivery if the set tidal volume is not achieved with initial settings.

## Other modes

### High frequency ventilation

High-frequency ventilation (HFV) attempts to achieve adequate gas exchange by using asymmetrical velocity profiles when combining very high respiratory rates with tidal volumes that are smaller than the volume of anatomic dead space. It is used more commonly in neonates and infants with neonatal respiratory failure. There has been a renewed interest in using HFV in adult patients with ALI/ARDS, with the rationale that the small tidal volumes may cause less ventilator associated lung injury. However, more trials are necessary to determine if HFV can improve mortality outcomes in these patients [6].

### Airway Pressure Release Ventilation and BiLevel Ventilation

Both of these modes, Airway Pressure Release Ventilation (APRV) (Drager Medical, Evita 4) and BiLevel Ventilation (Covidien, Puritan Bennett 840), are proprietary names, yet function essentially in the same manner. The clinician sets a pressure high, pressure low, and a time at each level (time high and time low). Ventilation occurs during the release from pressure high to pressure low. The time low is typically 0.2–0.8 seconds in restrictive lung disease and 0.8–1.5 seconds in obstructive lung disease. It is probably most prudent to start at 0.8 and titrate to meet individual patient requirements. The time low is also referred to as the release phase [7]. A common occurrence in this mode is setting the time low too long. This essentially mimics a pressure-targeted SIMV strategy. The patient typically spends 4–6 seconds in time high. In the paralyzed patient APRV/BiLevel is identical to pressure targeted inverse ratio ventilation. For these reasons, some have described this mode as inverse ratio ventilation (IRV). However, a major difference between APRV/BiLevel and IRV is that IRV typically requires chemical paralysis or heavy sedation. APRV/BiLevel allows for spontaneous breathing throughout both pressure levels, making it relatively more comfortable and typically does not require heavy sedation or paralysis. APRV/BiLevel has gained popularity in patients with hypoxemic respiratory failure because it improves oxygenation by optimizing alveolar recruitment and ventilation/perfusion (V/Q) matching [8].

### Proportional Assist Ventilation Plus and Proportional Pressure Support

Proportional Assist Ventilation Plus (PAV+) (Covidien, Puritan Bennett 840) and Proportional Pressure Support (PPS) (Drager Medical, Evita 4) are forms of synchronized ventilatory assistance, where the ventilator generates pressure in proportion to the patient's effort, ie, the greater the effort, the more pressure the ventilator generates. Therefore the clinician determines the level of resistive and elastic unloading, irrespective of patient volume or flow requirements.

## Specific scenarios

### Asthma and chronic obstructive pulmonary disease

Approximately 4% of patients that are hospitalized for asthma require mechanical ventilation [9]. Patients with obstructive pulmonary processes that require intubation can at times be very difficult to manage. Mortality rates for respiratory failure due to status asthmaticus before 1990 were reported to be as high as 38% [10]. However, there has been a dramatic drop to an estimated 7% in 2000 [9]. It is thought that the acceptance of permissive hypercapnia and improved understanding of the potential complications from mechanical ventilation, ie, auto-PEEP and ventilator induced lung injury (VILI), has lead to this decline [11].

The peri-intubation period can be quite dangerous and requires caution to prevent fatal events. These patients are often volume depleted and induction agents can precipitously drop blood pressures. Pre-induction crystalloid boluses of 500 mL to a liter are often prudent. In addition, care should be taken to prevent breath stacking and auto-PEEP. Patients typically have some level of hyperinflation and auto-PEEP at the time of intubation. Overzealous bag ventilation can lead to worsening of this auto-PEEP, potentiating hypoxia, hypotension, and VILI. In addition, auto-PEEP causes the patient's work of breathing to increase because the patient has to generate a larger drop in airway pressure to initiate a breath. For example, a patient with an auto-PEEP of 10 cmH$_2$O and a set pressure trigger of -2 cmH$_2$O (and no applied PEEP) has to generate an alveolar pressure of 12 cmH$_2$O to generate a breath. Assisted breaths should be limited to less than 8–10 breaths per minute and adequate time should be allowed for exhalation. The primary goal is to allow expiration of trapped air and minimize airway pressures. This is done by decreasing the inspiratory time and increasing the expiratory time. Strategies that can be implemented to achieve this goal include reducing the respiratory rate, reducing tidal volume (initially setting 6–7 mL/kg IBW), increasing the flow-rate (initially setting at 80–100 L/min) and using a square waveform. Several of these options will subsequently increase the peak inspiratory pressure; however, this is well tolerated below pressures of 50 cmH$_2$O [11,12] and is not a reliable marker of hyperinflation or the risk of VILI [13]. In addition, this strategy may worsen hypercapnia due to a decrease in minute-ventilation. This is termed "permissive hypercapnia".

As the treatment (β-agonists, steroids) takes affect, the peak pressures will begin to lower, the peak expiratory flow rate (PEFR) should increase and the expiration time (T$_E$) should become shorter (Fig. 1). These strategies to increase the expiratory time and shorten inspiratory time must be balanced with hypercapnia. Allowing patients to develop severe respiratory acidosis from permissive hypercapnia can result in cardiac arrhythmias and death. Sodium bicarbonate infusion or the administration of THAM (trishydroxymethyl aminomethane) may be required to keep the arterial pH at

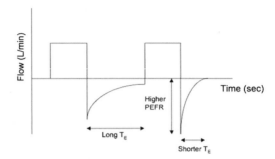

Fig. 1. Schematic of flow-time curve showing improvement in obstructive process. Note that peak expiratory flow rate (PEFR) increases and expiratory time ($T_E$) decreases with improvement.

a safe level above 7.15 to 7.20. Finally, it is necessary to adequately sedate these patients, as their hypercapnic state is a powerful stimulus to breath rapidly. Opiates such as fentanyl and sedatives such as propofol have gained increased roles in these patients. Occasionally, one will be required to chemically paralyze these patients to keep their respiratory rate and thus their expiratory time controlled. This should be a final option as steroids are part of the treatment in obstructive airway disease and the side effects of steroids and paralytics can be quite devastating [14,15]. However, paralysis cannot be avoided in certain cases.

Valuable information can be gained from flow-time curves and pressure-time curves. Improvement (see Fig. 1) or worsening of airway obstruction and air trapping (Fig. 2) can often be seen before becoming clinically apparent. In ideal situations, intrinsic PEEP (auto-PEEP) can be measured by using an end-expiratory hold (Fig. 3). This measurement is often inconsistent and difficult to obtain. Some authors have recommended that extrinsic PEEP be applied at 80% of the measured auto-PEEP [16]. However, due to the difficulties of accurately measuring auto-PEEP and the potential hazard of adding too much extrinsic PEEP [17], others have suggested that it should

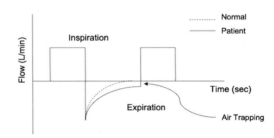

Fig. 2. Schematic of flow-time curve showing air trapping. Note that patient has not finished full exhalation prior to the initiation of the next breath. Square flow waveform is being used in this example.

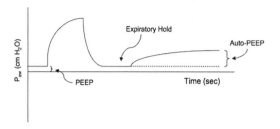

Fig. 3. Schematic of pressure-time curve showing an expiratory hold and subsequent auto-PEEP measurement.

be set at 50% of the measured intrinsic PEEP. If auto-PEEP becomes severe enough, it will begin to affect the end-inspiratory plateau pressures. Current recommendations for obstructive airway disease are to keep the plateau pressures below 35 cmH$_2$O [18,19]; however many clinicians follow the ALI/ARDS recommendations and keep the plateau pressures less than 30 cmH$_2$O. Extrinsic (applied) PEEP can be used to decrease some of the negative pressure that the patient has to generate to initiate a breath. Going back to the previous example, a patient with an auto-PEEP of 10 cmH$_2$O and a set pressure trigger of -2 cmH$_2$O (and no applied PEEP) has to generate an alveolar pressure of 12 cmH$_2$O to generate a breath. Adding an extrinsic PEEP of 5 cmH$_2$O means that the ventilator will trigger a breath when the alveolar pressure is 3 cmH$_2$O. Therefore, the patient now only has to generate a decrease of 7 cmH$_2$O (instead of 12 cmH$_2$O), thus reducing the required inspiratory effort.

Finally, if sudden hypotension occurs, a first step in troubleshooting is to remove the patient from the ventilator. Often times this is both diagnostic and therapeutic for air trapping. In addition, tension pneumothorax must be considered (see below).

## Acute lung injury and acute respiratory distress syndrome

The American–European Consensus Conference on Acute Respiratory Distress Syndrome (ARDS) defines this entity as a PaO$_2$/FiO$_2$ ratio <200 with bilateral pulmonary infiltrates on a chest radiograph consistent with pulmonary edema and no clinical evidence of left atrial hypertension or (if measured) a pulmonary capillary wedge pressure <18 mm Hg. Acute lung injury (ALI) has a similar definition with the exception being that it is a PaO$_2$/FiO$_2$ ratio <300 [20]. As recently as the 1990s, the mortality for patients with ARDS had been as high as 40%–50%. However, with the advent of lung-protective ventilation, mortality rates have decreased significantly. The ARDS Network showed that this strategy lead to a significant decrease in mortality [21]. Essentially, lung-protective ventilation attempts to prevent further damage to a patient's lung by avoiding overdistention of alveoli. Tidal volumes of 6 mL/kg IBW are used in conjunction with higher respiratory rates (initially set at 18–22 breaths/minute) to achieve an adequate minute-ventilation. Plateau pressures are limited to 30 cmH$_2$O [22], and tidal volumes can be further incrementally decreased down to 4 mL/kg IBW to achieve this goal. Permissive hypercapnia is allowed and tolerated as long as arterial pH is kept above 7.20. Sodium bicarbonate infusion or the administration of THAM may be required to keep the arterial pH at a safe level above 7.15 to 7.20. In addition, FiO$_2$ and PEEP are adjusted in a step-wise fashion to assure adequate oxygenation. It should be noted that although both volume-targeted and pressure-targeted modes can be used, the only firm data showing improved outcomes in ARDS to date involved volume-targeted ventilation. Finally, central venous pressure monitoring should be used to guide fluid management [23,24].

In the early phases of a resuscitation, it is often difficult to ascertain if pulmonary edema is cardiogenic or noncardiogenic. However, in light of the mortality benefit seen with a lung protective ventilation strategy, its relative simplicity, and minimal complications, one should consider implementing this strategy early in a patient's clinical course.

A common finding in lung protective ventilation is the occurrence of patient–ventilator dysynchrony. This dysynchrony is thought to be due to the patient wanting a higher flow rate than the ventilator is providing while on a volume-targeted strategy. This situation occasionally leads to double or triple cycling of the ventilator. It should be noted that in this situation, the patient is actually receiving higher tidal volumes and not benefiting from lung protective ventilation. Sedation needs to be optimized and, at times, different modes like pressure-targeted modes may be attempted. In addition, temporarily weakening the patient with paralytics may be considered.

To date there are several areas of uncertainty in the mechanical ventilation of patients with ALI/ARDS. Patients with traumatic brain injury, intracranial hemorrhage, fulminant hepatic failure, and elevated intracranial pressures (ICP) who develop ARDS must be managed carefully as lung protective ventilation may induce hypercapnia. Acutely hypercapnia may lead to cerebral vasodilation and an increase in ICP. In addition, there is little evidence to support the recommendation of any particular rescue therapy in patients with severe refractory hypoxia, such as recruitment maneuvers, high dose albuterol, inverse ratio ventilation, high frequency ventilation, prone ventilation and extracorporeal membrane oxygenation. In dire circumstances, these modalities may be used based on clinician preference and expertise.

## Troubleshooting

Respiratory distress in mechanically ventilated patients has a broad differential that includes anxiety, pain, inadequate ventilator settings, air-leak, endotracheal tube malfunction, pulmonary parenchymal process and extrapulmonary causes. Included in this list are: the acute life-threatening entities of tension pneumothorax and severe auto-PEEP. The troubleshooting process will be guided by the severity of the distress and the stability of the patient.

If the patient is hemodynamically stable a systematic approach can be taken. Obtain a focused history from the bedside nurse and respiratory therapist, perform a focused physical examination, check the ventilator, the circuit and respiratory mechanics (note current and past peak and plateau airway pressures), evaluate the chest x-ray and examine the pleural cavity with bedside ultrasound. This systematic approach will typically yield the cause of the distress.

Respiratory mechanics can be used to guide the troubleshooting process. Current peak pressures ($P_{peak}$) and plateau pressures ($P_{plat}$) should be compared with previous values when the patient was stable. This should be done in volume-targeted modes. Airway pressures are a function of volume and respiratory system compliance. A set volume and compliance results in a specific pressure. Peak pressures are obtained during inspiration and thus incorporate resistance to airflow. Plateau pressures are obtained during an inspiratory pause eliminating airflow and thus reflect pulmonary system compliance. An isolated increase in peak pressures (ie, an increase in $\Delta P_{peak}–P_{plat}$) points to a problem with airflow (Fig. 4). An increase in the plateau pressures leading to an unchanged or decreased $\Delta P_{peak}–P_{plat}$ points to a change in lung compliance (Fig. 5). Table 1 lists common causes of each.

Patients who are simply asynchronous with the ventilator should be evaluated for sufficient sedation, appropriate trigger mode and sensitivity, inspiratory time, tidal volume, and flow rate. Double-cycling (back-to-back ventilator delivered breaths) is typically seen in volume-targeted modes when the patient desires a higher flow rate than the set rate. Increasing

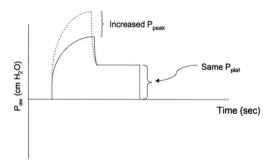

Fig. 4. Schematic of two superimposed pressure-time curves showing an isolated increase in peak inspiratory pressures ($P_{peak}$) with no change in plateau pressures ($P_{plat}$). This is characteristic of obstruction and increased airway resistance (see Table 1).

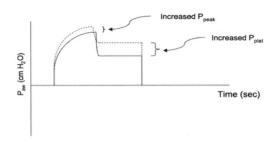

Fig. 5. Schematic of two superimposed pressure-time curves showing a small increase in peak inspiratory pressures (P_peak) with a greater increase in plateau pressures (P_plat). This is characteristic of decreased lung compliance (see Table 1).

the flow rate may alleviate this "air hunger." It is also commonly seen in patients on lung protective ventilation with low set tidal volumes. If increasing the flow rate does not improve synchrony and sedation is deemed to be adequate, one must decide between increasing the tidal volume or changing to a pressure-targeted mode. In addition, temporarily weakening the patient with paralytics may be considered.

Patients who become acutely hemodynamically unstable while on mechanical ventilation should immediately be removed from the ventilator and hand-ventilated with 100% oxygen. Special care should be taken with this maneuver in patients on high PEEP or on nitric oxide (NO). PEEP valves can be used to maintain recruitment if auto-PEEP has been ruled out and NO should not be acutely discontinued. Severe decompensation or continued deterioration requires quick action and empiric treatment of potentially life-threatening problems. Severe auto-PEEP should be considered and care should be taken not to worsen this process. Patients on volume-targeted modes, with an obstructive or reactive airways disease, receiving a high minute-ventilation, or on inverse ratio ventilation are at high risk for auto-PEEP. Patients should not be hyperventilated and special attention should be paid when the patient is initially disconnected from the ventilator. A prolonged expiration of trapped air with clinical improvement can be diagnostic of this process. Tension pneumothorax should also be considered and addressed by needle decompression, followed directly by tube thoracostomy. If time allows, a quick history and physical examination can potentially guide the decision of which side of the chest to needle decompress. Knowledge of a recent central line attempt, chest tube placed on water seal, or decreased breath sounds on one side may be helpful. Often times the history and physical examination is not be helpful and decompressing both sides may be necessary based on the condition of the patient.

If the patient quickly improves with manual ventilation (and auto-PEEP is excluded), then the likely culprit is the ventilator settings or circuit. Consider adjusting the settings and check the circuit for air leaks or condensation that has accumulated and is causing interference.

Table 1
Respiratory mechanics in mechanically ventilated patients

| Increase in $\Delta P_{peak}-P_{plat}$ | Unchanged or decreased $\Delta P_{peak}-P_{plat}$ |
| --- | --- |
| • Increased airway resistance caused by heat and moisture exchanger (HME) | • Pneumonia |
| • Patient biting endotracheal tube | • Atelectasis |
| • Kinked or twisted endotracheal tube | • Mucus plugging of one lung |
| • Obstruction of endotracheal tube by secretions, mucus, blood | • Unilateral intubation |
| • Bronchospasm | • Pneumothorax |
| • Obstruction of lower airways | • Pulmonary edema (noncardiogenic and cardiogenic) |
| | • Abdominal distention/pressure |

If the patient stabilizes with manual ventilation, note if any air is escaping through the mouth or nose and pay close attention to the resistance faced with each manual ventilation. Escaping air or an expiratory volume significantly smaller than the set tidal volume should lead to an inspection of the endotracheal tube positioning (ie, has it migrated out) and inspection of the pilot balloon. A deflated pilot balloon typically indicates a deflated cuff. Occasionally, adding more volume to the cuff may correct the problem. However, more commonly either the cuff has ruptured or the cuff apparatus has failed. At times the pilot balloon mechanism is the culprit and some respiratory therapists can easily replace the pilot balloon with commercially available kits. This may be a good starting point in a stable patient deemed difficult to reintubate, yet failure of the cuff apparatus typically requires replacement of the endotracheal tube. If there is a lot of resistance with manual ventilation—and auto-PEEP and pneumothorax have been ruled out—attempt to pass the suction catheter. Difficulty passing the suction catheter should prompt one to evaluate if the patient is biting on the endotracheal tube, or if the tube is kinked, twisted, obstructed, or out of position.

Finally, patients who are accidentally extubated (for example, during transport) or have an unplanned extubation (self-extubate) should promptly be reintubated if they are felt to be at high risk for respiratory failure or airway compromise. Of note, these patients should be treated as presumed difficult intubations, as accidental and unplanned extubations are notorious for causing trauma to the glottis leading to vocal cord edema. In a recent series, 22% of patients who failed unplanned extubation required multiple laryngoscopic attempts, 14% suffered hypoxemia, and 14% suffered esophageal intubations. One patient was unable to be ventilated and subsequently died [25]. Careful planning and preparation for difficult airway management can avert disasters and the need for emergent surgical airway.

## References

[1] Cooper KR, Boswell PA. Reduced functional residual capacity and abnormal oxygenation in patients with severe head injury. Chest 1983;84(1):29–35.

[2] Sassoon CS, Giron AE, Ely EA, et al. Inspiratory work of breathing on flow-by and demand-flow continuous positive airway pressure. Crit Care Med 1989;17(11):1108–14.

[3] Marini JJ, Crooke PS III, Truwit JD. Determinants and limits of pressure-preset ventilation: a mathematical model of pressure control. J Appl Physiol 1989;67(3):1081–92.

[4] Esteban A, Frutos F, Tobin MJ, et al. A comparison of four methods of weaning patients from mechanical ventilation. Spanish Lung Failure Collaborative Group. N Engl J Med 1995;332(6):345–50.

[5] Branson RD, Davis K Jr. Dual control modes: combining volume and pressure breaths. Respir Care Clin N Am 2001;7(3):397–408, viii.

[6] Krishnan JA, Brower RG. High-frequency ventilation for acute lung injury and ARDS. Chest 2000;118(3):795–807.

[7] Habashi NM. Other approaches to open-lung ventilation: airway pressure release ventilation. Crit Care Med 2005;33(3 Suppl):S228–40.

[8] Putensen C, Rasanen J, Lopez FA. Ventilation-perfusion distributions during mechanical ventilation with superimposed spontaneous breathing in canine lung injury. Am J Respir Crit Care Med 1994;150(1):101–8.

[9] Krishnan V, Diette GB, Rand CS, et al. Mortality in patients hospitalized for asthma exacerbations in the United States. Am J Respir Crit Care Med 2006;174(6):633–8.

[10] Mansel JK, Stogner SW, Petrini MF, et al. Mechanical ventilation in patients with acute severe asthma. Am J Med 1990;89(1):42–8.

[11] Darioli R, Perret C. Mechanical controlled hypoventilation in status asthmaticus. Am Rev Respir Dis 1984;129(3):385–7.

[12] Petersen GW, Baier H. Incidence of pulmonary barotrauma in a medical ICU. Crit Care Med 1983;11(2):67–9.

[13] Manning HL. Peak airway pressure: why the fuss? Chest 1994;105(1):242–7.

[14] Douglass JA, Tuxen DV, Horne M, et al. Myopathy in severe asthma. Am Rev Respir Dis 1992;146(2):517–9.

[15] Kupfer Y, Namba T, Kaldawi E, et al. Prolonged weakness after long-term infusion of vecuronium bromide. Ann Intern Med 1992;117(6):484–6.

[16] Gladwin MT, Pierson DJ. Mechanical ventilation of the patient with severe chronic obstructive pulmonary disease. Intensive Care Med 1998;24(9):898–910.

[17] Ranieri VM, Giuliani R, Cinnella G, et al. Physiologic effects of positive end-expiratory pressure in patients with chronic obstructive pulmonary disease during acute ventilatory failure and controlled mechanical ventilation. Am Rev Respir Dis 1993;147(1):5–13.

[18] Slutsky AS. Mechanical ventilation. American College of Chest Physicians' Consensus Conference. Chest 1993;104(6):1833–59.

[19] Papiris S, Kotanidou A, Malagari K, et al. Clinical review: severe asthma. Crit Care 2002; 6(1):30–44.

[20] Bernard GR, Artigas A, Brigham KL, et al. The American-European Consensus Conference on ARDS. Definitions, mechanisms, relevant outcomes, and clinical trial coordination. Am J Respir Crit Care Med 1994;149(3 Pt 1):818–24.

[21] Ventilation with lower tidal volumes as compared with traditional tidal volumes for acute lung injury and the acute respiratory distress syndrome. The acute respiratory distress syndrome network. N Engl J Med 2000;342(18):1301–8.

[22] Dellinger RP, Levy MM, Carlet JM, et al. Surviving sepsis campaign: international guidelines for management of severe sepsis and septic shock: 2008. Crit Care Med 2008;36(1): 296–327.

[23] Wheeler AP, Bernard GR, Thompson BT, et al. Pulmonary-artery versus central venous catheter to guide treatment of acute lung injury. N Engl J Med 2006;354(21):2213–24.

[24] Wiedemann HP, Wheeler AP, Bernard GR, et al. Comparison of two fluid-management strategies in acute lung injury. N Engl J Med 2006;354(24):2564–75.

[25] Epstein SK, Nevins ML, Chung J. Effect of unplanned extubation on outcome of mechanical ventilation. Am J Respir Crit Care Med 2000;161(6):1912–6.

**ELSEVIER
SAUNDERS**

Emerg Med Clin N Am
26 (2008) 863–868

EMERGENCY
MEDICINE
CLINICS OF
NORTH AMERICA

# Index

*Note:* Page numbers of article titles are in **boldface** type.